CLINICAL ASSESSMENTS IN PSYCHIATRY:
Mastering Skills and Passing Exams

EDITOR-IN-CHIEF

RAJESH R. TAMPI, MD, MS
Associate Clinical Professor of Psychiatry
Yale University School of Medicine
New Haven, Connecticut

ASSOCIATE EDITORS

SUNANDA MURALEE, MD
Assistant Clinical Professor of Psychiatry
Yale University School of Medicine
New Haven, Connecticut

NATALIE D. WEDER, MD
Clinical Instructor
New York University Child Study Center
New York, New York

KIRSTEN M. WILKINS, MD
Assistant Professor of Psychiatry
University of Oklahoma College of Medicine
Tulsa, Oklahoma

Wolters Kluwer | Lippincott Williams & Wilkins
Health

Philadelphia • Baltimore • New York • London
Buenos Aires • Hong Kong • Sydney • Tokyo

Acquisitions Editor: Lisa McAllister
Product Manager: Tom Gibbons
Vendor Manager: Alicia Jackson
Senior Manufacturing Manager: Benjamin Rivera
Marketing Manager: Brian Freiland
Design Coordinator: Teresa Mallon
Production Service: SPi Technologies

530 Walnut Street
Philadelphia, PA 19106 USA
LWW.com

Printed in China

Library of Congress Cataloging-in-Publication Data
Tampi, Rajesh R.
Clinical assessments in psychiatry : mastering skills and passing exams / Rajesh R. Tampi.
p. ; cm.
Includes bibliographical references and index.
ISBN 978-0-7817-9909-6 (alk. paper)
1. Psychiatry—Examinations—Study guides. I. Title.
[DNLM: 1. Psychotherapy—methods. 2. Clinical Competence. 3. Interview, Psychological—methods. 4. Mental Disorders—therapy. WM 420 T159c 2010]

RC457.T36 2010
616.890076—dc22

2009045869

---

10 9 8 7 6 5 4 3 2 1

RRS0911

CLINICAL ASSESSMENTS IN PSYCHIATRY:
Mastering Skills and Passing Exams

Drs. Tampi and Muralee would like to dedicate this book to their son Vaishnav, the greatest gift of their life, and to their parents who taught them the value of education.

Dr. Weder would like to dedicate this book to her mother and father, with love.

Dr. Wilkins would like to dedicate this book to all the psychiatry residents that she is privileged to teach. She would like to thank them for inspiring her to learn each and every day.

CONTRIBUTORS

Gustavo A. Angarita, MD
Resident in Psychiatry
Yale University School of Medicine
New Haven, Connecticut

Reji Attupurath, MD
Resident in Psychiatry
Richmond University Medical Center
Staten Island, New York

Margarita M. Cala, MD
Clinical Instructor
New York University Child Study Center
New York, New York

Nicole A. Foubister, MD
Assistant Professor of Psychiatry
New York University School of Medicine
New York, New York

Joshua Kantrowitz, MD
Research Assistant Professor
Nathan S. Kline Institute for Psychiatric Research
New York University
Orangeburg, New York

Gauri P. Khatkhate, MD
Staff Physician
Edward Hines Jr. VA Hospital
Hines, Illinois

Lekshminarayan R. Kurup, MD
Attending Physician
Mavelikara, Kerala, India

Robert T. Malison, MD
Associate Professor of Psychiatry
Yale University School of Medicine
New Haven, Connecticut

Vikrant Mittal, MD, MHS
Director of Psychiatry
Parkland Healthcare Center, BJC Healthcare System
Farmington, Missouri

Kalyani Subramanyam, MD
Resident in Psychiatry
Yale University School of Medicine
New Haven, Connecticut

Clarence Watson, JD, MD
Adjunct Assistant Professor of Psychiatry
New York Medical College
New York, New York
Clinical Associate in Psychiatry
University of Pennsylvania School of Medicine
Philadelphia, Pennsylvania

CONTENTS

PREFACE

Clinical assessments in psychiatry are usually taught during the training period. However, there is no standardized format on how these assessments are taught or how they are conducted in clinical practice. The organization and level of sophistication of these assessments also remain variable. It becomes a major problem when trainees are asked to perform such evaluations in an examination setting. The stress of time limitation, the complexity of the patient's presentation, and presenting this complex information leads to poor performance. The lack of standardized training for clinical examinations is clearly evident in the pass performances on such examinations throughout the world. Many examinees fail or do poorly on their first attempt. Failure in these examinations results in a mad scramble to find ways of learning to do a good clinical assessment. Examinees spend a lot of time and money to learn such assessments and the chances of success are not guaranteed.

A simple solution to prevent failures in clinical examinations is to practice standardized interviews on patients from the very beginning of one's training. This will help build confidence and the skill to do such interviews under the stress of the examination. It will also improve patient care by providing comprehensive and efficient assessments that aid in planning appropriate treatments and follow-up care. This way, examinees will not have to spend a lot of time and money on acquiring specialized training for the purpose of passing these examinations.

We have written this book to reach out to psychiatric trainees all over the United States and in the rest of the world, to help them learn how to conduct evaluations during examinations. It covers all the materials needed to pass oral examinations in psychiatry in an easy-to-use and step-by-step manner. The book starts with a chapter on preparing for clinical examinations in psychiatry. Chapter 2 describes the conduct of the psychiatric interview, case presentation and discussion. Chapter 3 focuses on various important case vignettes. This chapter also describes various important therapies and issues related to cross-cultural psychiatry. We have also added an appendix section that includes a brief outline of the psychiatric interview, important drug interactions, and a discussion on pertinent classes of drugs in psychiatry. To familiarize trainees with a standard psychiatric interview, we have included a web-accessed video.

Although geared towards trainees taking clinical examinations in psychiatry, this book will be helpful to anyone who wants to learn the skills needed to be a good clinician/diagnostician in psychiatry. Psychiatric trainees will not have to spend a lot of extra time and money to acquire the clinical interviewing skills that are important to their career. This book aims to be a 'one-stop-shop' in acquiring those skills.

Rajesh R. Tampi, MD, MS
Editor-in-Chief

CHAPTER 1

Preparing for Clinical Examinations in Psychiatry

Kirsten M. Wilkins, MD, Rajesh R. Tampi, MD, MS

INTRODUCTION

Whether you are preparing for the certification by the American Board of Psychiatry and Neurology (ABPN) or any other clinical skills examination, the prospect of a clinical examination in psychiatry can be anxiety provoking. Although we have all interviewed hundreds of patients and presented cases to multiple colleagues and supervisors throughout our careers, there is something distinctly different about interviewing a patient and presenting a case in an examination setting. The conditions may feel artificial and unfamiliar, and there is also a time limit with which to contend. Often there are serious-looking examiners who seem to be scrutinizing you all the while you are conducting the examination. Not to mention the amount of pressure behind the idea of a single pass/fail examination; there are no "do-overs" and no refunds on the money or time that you have expended on the process. It is enough to make anyone want to turn and embark on a second career. However, any clinical psychiatry examination can be mastered with the right quality and quantity of preparation! This book aims to help you do just that.

First, it is important to keep in mind the purpose of these kinds of examinations, or maybe better yet, to keep in mind what the purpose of these examinations is NOT. The purpose of any clinical examination in psychiatry is not to prove that you are an expert in psychodynamic formulations or psychopharmacology, or that you have the entire diagnostic systems memorized word for word. The purpose is not to prove that you are an exceptionally "warm and fuzzy" physician who knows just the right words to comfort any distressed patient. The purpose is also not to astound the examiners with your extensive research knowledge of the latest diagnostic or research tools in psychiatric patients. The only purpose of the examination is to show that you are a safe and competent physician who can conduct a psychiatric assessment, organize pertinent patient data into a logical presentation, and discuss a reasonable diagnostic formulation and treatment plan.

THE ABPN EXAMINATION

The exact conditions of your clinical examination will depend on whether you are taking the actual ABPN certification examination or (for the residents beginning their PGY-1 year on July 1, 2007 or after, or their PGY-2 year on July 1, 2008 or after) a clinical skills examination at your training program.

In general, however, oral psychiatry examinations include two sections: (1) a live patient interview and case discussion (lasting a total of 1 hour) and (2) clinical vignettes (usually four vignettes, lasting a total of 1 hour). In the live interview, the examinee has 30 minutes to interview a new patient in front of two (or more) examiners. Following the interview, the patient leaves the room. The examinee then has 30 minutes for the presentation and discussion of the case, which includes answering any questions posed by the examiners. (Any clinical topic is fair game during the case discussion portion, though typically, the questions are relevant to your proposed diagnosis and treatment plan.) In the clinical vignettes section, the examinee is presented with four separate vignettes (typically, three written, one video). The examinee has approximately 12 to 14 minutes to read (or view) the vignette and discuss the case with the examiner, before moving on to the next vignette.

When to Start Preparing for the Examination

By the time you reach the stage of taking the clinical skills examination, you have already taken and passed the clinical knowledge part of the examination process. Preparing for an oral examination, however, involves much more than just memorizing the diagnostic criteria. Preparation in the form of practice or "mock" examinations is essential. In our experience, beginning formal examination practices about 6 months prior to the actual examination is usually sufficient. However, you really begin preparing for oral psychiatry examinations from day 1 of your residency. Interviewing patients and presenting cases are the two things that psychiatry residents are given countless opportunities to do throughout residency. The key differences in the examination setting are that there is a time limit and that you are being observed. The best way to prepare for such conditions is to practice, practice, and practice more. This can be done formally, as in mock oral examinations, as well as informally in your daily clinical work. While it is certainly not advisable to begin worrying about the clinical examinations from day 1 of your training, making an early habit of organized patient interviews, concise presentations and formulations is something that will benefit you throughout your career and in your examinations.

WHAT TO STUDY FOR THE EXAMINATION

Preparing for an oral examination includes two major components: studying and practicing. Much of the studying you have already done for the clinical knowledge part of the examination will stand you in good stead for the clinical skills examination. Depending on the length of time since you last prepared for such an examination, you may want to review some of that material.

When it comes to the discussion portion of the patient interview or the clinical vignettes, anything is fair game—from the diagnostic criteria for schizo-affective disorder to the therapeutic range of lithium to the difference between cognitive behavioral therapy and psychodynamic therapy. However, it is not necessary (nor productive) to spend hours memorizing minutia. It is important to have working knowledge of the diagnosis and treatment, as well as basic epidemiology and etiologic theories, of the major psychiatric disorders. The subsequent chapters of this book will provide you with high-yield study material, including the DSM-IV-TR diagnostic criteria, for all the major psychiatric disorders that you might encounter in the examination setting.

HOW TO PREPARE FOR A CLINICAL EXAMINATION IN PSYCHIATRY

A. The Patient Interview

The best way to reduce anxiety about the clinical skills examination in psychiatry is to practice under similar conditions. Practice allows you to become more comfortable with the examination setting and raises your confidence in your ability to perform well under stress.

Preparation should include mock clinical examinations as well as informal practice in your daily clinical work. Many training programs hold annual mock clinical skills examinations, in which the trainee enacts the real examination conditions by conducting a 30-minute live patient interview in front of one or more supervisors. This is then followed by a presentation and a discussion, to simulate the actual examination. Following the actual examination, direct feedback and constructive criticism are provided to the trainee.

Some training programs hold review courses, in which the examinees are assigned to study groups led by a supervisor who serves as a mock examiner. Over the course of a few months, the examinees then rotate interviewing live patients and presenting cases to the mock examiner in front of the group. The examinee then receives feedback from the examiner and the group. Group members get the benefit of learning from each other's experiences as well as their own. Whether in a group setting or 1:1, the value of practice examinations cannot be overemphasized and is not limited to psychiatrists in training. Often, training programs welcome psychiatrists in the community who are preparing for the examination to join their annual practice sessions and board review courses.

In preparing for a clinical skills examination, the examinees should not limit themselves to practicing with one mock examiner exclusively. There is no way to predict who will be your examiner during the actual examination—you may have someone younger, older, university-based, community-based, research-oriented, psychotherapy-oriented, etc. Hence, it behooves the examinee to practice with a number of different examiners prior to the examination. Mock examiners can be supervisors, senior residents/fellows, or peers. Examinees will find it most helpful to practice with examiners who have taken and passed the clinical skills examinations themselves.

Equally as important as the variety of examiners with whom to practice is the variety of patients. In the examination setting, you may encounter outpatients or inpatients from any number of hospital settings and demographic backgrounds. Therefore, it is best to practice interviewing different types of patients if at all possible, including those in outpatient as well as inpatient settings. Keep in mind where your experience and inexperience lie. If, for example, you are an addiction psychiatry fellow, you may have had plenty of practice interviewing and presenting patients with substance use disorders. However, you may be a little rusty in interviewing geriatric patients and may benefit from some extra practice in that area.

Each examinee has his or her own strengths and weakness; therefore, there is no specific number of practice interviews that each examinee must complete in order to become proficient in these examinations. The number of practice examinations one needs to complete depends entirely on each individual's experience, confidence level, and skill set. In general, we have found that examinees do best with five to ten practice examinations. You may never feel 100% prepared; having some anxiety about the examination is only natural. However, you should practice enough that you feel comfortable with the examination conditions and become confident in your ability to pass.

Board preparation can also take place in your daily clinical work. Whether you are a trainee rotating in the psychiatric emergency room or a psychiatrist performing a consultation in a medical hospital, you can practice interviewing patients in a self-imposed 30 minute time segment. It takes practice to gather all the essential data in this time frame. It takes practice to politely interrupt and redirect a tangential patient appropriately. The more you do these interviews, the more comfortable you will become. Trainees can and should practice giving concise, organized presentations in 10 minutes or less to supervisors and peers in any clinical setting. As you are driving home for the day, mentally practicing formulations on any new patient that you saw that day is also immensely helpful.

B. The Clinical Vignettes (For ABPN Examination)

The clinical vignettes, while less anxiety provoking for most, still require some preparation. Typically, the examinee is presented with four different "stations" (i.e., an office or small room), each with its own examiner(s). Three of the vignettes are one-page written cases; one is a video vignette. You will be given approximately 12 to 14 minutes per station, as there will be a couple of minutes between stations. The examinee will be provided with the vignette and given a few minutes to read (or view) the case. The examiner(s) will then begin a discussion and ask questions about the case. The questions asked may take either a "diagnostic focus" or a "treatment focus." Typically, the video vignette will call on your mental status examination skills. (For sample written and video vignettes, as well as sample questions, visit the ABPN website.)

Clinical vignettes can be developed for practice purposes and may also be available from your local training program. The ABPN website has examples of the vignettes. We have found it helpful to practice vignettes in a group setting, in which several examinees can rotate asking and answering each other's questions. The case discussion portion of your live interview practice will help prepare you for the vignette section as well, as these are times you will be asked to "think on your feet."

THE DAY OF THE EXAMINATION

Whether your clinical skills examination is out of state or in your own psychiatry department, the same general rules will apply. As with any examination, you should get a good night's sleep before the examination day. Sleep is absolutely essential the night before to prevent exhaustion and or loss of concentration. Make sure that you eat a normal breakfast. Low blood sugar combined with anxiety almost guarantees that you will not perform your best. Too heavy a meal may make you sleepy during the actual examination.

Dress professionally in business attire; this is not the time for experimenting with new clothing or hairstyles. Allow plenty of time to get to wherever you need to be; consider traffic, weather, the possibility of getting lost, restroom breaks, etc. You do not need the added stress of running late on an examination day. Find a quiet place to wait until it is your turn and stay focused on yourself, not those around you. Remember how well prepared you are! Be confident and appear confident!! If you have practiced well, there is no reason why you should not do well in the examination.

We believe in the mantra of the great golfer Gary Player, "The harder you work, the luckier you get!"

CHAPTER 2

Conducting the Psychiatric Interview

Sunanda Muralee, MD, Kirsten M. Wilkins, MD, Rajesh R. Tampi, MD, MS

1. SETTING THE STAGE

To conduct an appropriate psychiatric interview, we must first set the stage from where this interview can be conducted in a safe and nonthreatening manner. The "safety first" rule should always be kept in mind before planning the interview.

Although most psychiatric interviews are voluntary, some patients who may initially agree to do the interview may later find themselves ill equipped to deal with such an interview. Often, these interviews can be very emotionally charged and may bring out strong emotions in the interviewees. In such a situation, adequate physical space must be provided so that these patients can leave the room to take "time-out" without any obstruction. This space is also needed for the interviewer to exit in case of a behavioral emergency.

It is best to be seated at each end of the limbs of a "V," with about 3 ft of space between the interviewer and the interviewee. The pointed end of the "V" should face the exit. Sitting in this position is less threatening than sitting right across from the interviewee. Ensure that the only furniture that is in the room is being used to seat people. If loose furniture is available in the room, keep it as far away as possible and secured to the floor. It is ideal not to have any loose objects lying around that can be used as a potential weapon.

It is also the interviewer's responsibility to ensure that the room is well lit and is quiet so that the interview can be conducted appropriately. Even in a professional examination setting, after taking permission from the examiners, the examinee must demonstrate that he or she is setting up the room for an appropriate psychiatric interview.

2. INTRODUCTIONS

After setting the stage for the interview, the interviewer must ensure that the interviewee (patient) is comfortably seated before starting the actual interview process.

The next stage in the interview process is to make the introductions. A simple way to start this process would be to greet the patient, give your title and name, and to ask for the patient's name. "Good_____ (morning/afternoon/evening) sir/madam, my name is Dr/Mr ____ and your name is ...?"

The next part of the conversation would be to ask the patient as to how he or she would like to be addressed; Sir/Madam/Mr____/Mrs_____/Ms_____ or by first names?

The next task is to introduce anyone else in the room. A simple statement including the names and the nature of work of those present would suffice. Following the introductions, spend a minute or two explaining the basic rules of the interview process. Points to include are

1. The purpose of the interview.
2. The interview is confidential and that it is voluntary.
3. The duration of the interview: 30/45/60 minutes.
4. Importance of redirection during the interview, i.e., examination with time limit; "I may need to interrupt you from time to time to get important information and it is not meant to be disrespectful in any way."
5. It is important to acknowledge language barriers, if there are any, and to say that it is okay to clarify issues before proceeding further.
6. Indicate that any notes taken during the interview will be destroyed at the end of the session and will not form part of any records.

3. CONDUCTING THE INTERVIEW

Then ask the patient's permission to start the official interview process.

It is always useful to start the interview by getting the basic/demographic information about the patient. You can introduce the following questions with a statement such as, "I'd like to start by getting some important background information."

1. Age: "How old are you?"
2. Place of abode: "Where do you live?"
3. Marital status: "What is your marital status?"
4. Employment: "How do you support yourself?"
5. Receipt of mental health treatment: "Where do you receive your mental health treatment?"

If inpatient, make sure to ask: "How long have you been on the inpatient unit?"
"How did you get admitted: voluntary vs. involuntary?"

1. History of the Present Illness

As with any psychiatric interview following the collection of demographic information, proceed to the history of present illness. In a 30-minute interview, this process should take about 7 to 8 minutes. An easy way to start this process would be to ask open-ended questions such as the following:

For inpatients: "What led you to being hospitalized?"

For outpatients: "What is the reason for your receiving psychiatric care as an outpatient?"

Give the patient a few minutes to answer your question. If the patient is organized and giving good/pertinent information, let the patient talk. If not, redirect by saying,

"Would it be appropriate then for me to say that this _____ is the reason for your being admitted/receiving treatment?"

or

"I am not sure that I understand, would you kindly clarify?"

When doing a psychiatric interview remember that it is not what you ask that is important, but how you ask that matters. The construct and the conduct of the interview supersede the content of the interview. It is more important to show that you can listen and gently guide the interview to the important areas than to engage in rapid fire "check-list" questioning.

Always remember to ask questions about the current symptoms and then inquire if these symptoms have been present in the past. It is also appropriate to use link questions like...

"In many instances, patients with depression also have symptoms of anxiety. Would you say that it was true in your case?"

Allow the patients to think and answer for about a minute.

If they say "yes," follow up with.... "Tell me more about it."

If they say "no," try once more to clarify the answer by saying.... "Would you say that you are an anxious or a restless person?"

If they say "yes," follow up with.... "Tell me more about it."

Ask about the following symptoms:

A. MOOD SYMPTOMS

1. Ask about depressive symptoms including the neurovegetative symptoms. Ask how long they have been present and what impairments these symptoms have caused in their life.

   Symptoms include depressed mood; markedly diminished interest or pleasure in all, or almost all, activities most of the day, nearly every day (as indicated by either subjective account or observation made by others); significant weight loss when not dieting or weight gain (e.g., a change of more than 5% of body weight in a month), or decrease or increase in appetite nearly every day; insomnia or hypersomnia nearly every day; psychomotor agitation or retardation nearly every day (observable by others, not merely subjective feelings of restlessness or being slowed down); fatigue or loss of energy nearly every day; feelings of worthlessness or excessive or inappropriate guilt (which may be delusional) nearly every day (not merely self-reproach or guilt about being sick); diminished ability to think or concentrate, or indecisiveness, nearly every day (either by subjective account or as observed by others); recurrent thoughts of death (not just fear of dying), recurrent suicidal ideation without a specific plan, or a suicide attempt or a specific plan for committing suicide.

   A way to ask about these symptoms is to link them to the depressed mood.

   "When people feel depressed they may also have the following symptoms. Have you had anyone of these symptoms...? If so, which of the following symptoms have you had and for how long have you had them?"

2. Ask about manic and hypomanic symptoms. Ask how long they have been present and what impairments these symptoms have caused in their life.
   If the impairments are severe enough for the patient to be admitted to a hospital and there are associated psychotic symptoms, the condition meets the criteria for mania irrespective of the duration of symptoms.
   Mania includes a distinct period of abnormally and persistently elevated, expansive, or irritable mood, lasting for at least 1 week or any duration if hospitalization is necessary. During the period of mood disturbance, three (or more) of the following symptoms have persisted (four if the mood is only irritable) and have been present to a significant degree: inflated self-esteem or grandiosity, decreased need for sleep (e.g., feels rested after only 3 hours of sleep), more talkative than usual or pressure to keep talking, flight of ideas or subjective experience that thoughts are racing, distractibility (i.e., attention too easily drawn to unimportant or irrelevant external stimuli), increase in goal-directed activity (either socially, at work or school, or sexually) or psychomotor agitation, excessive involvement in pleasurable activities that have a high potential for painful consequences (e.g., engaging in unrestrained buying sprees, sexual indiscretions, or foolish business investments).
   One way to ask about these symptoms is to link them to elevated mood.
   "When people feel abnormally elevated or irritable they may also have the following symptoms. Have you had anyone of these symptoms...? If so, which of the following symptoms have you had and for how long have you had them?"
   If you suspect hypomania, confirm that there was no social or occupational impairment, yet the change in mood was observable by others.

B. ANXIETY

Ask about anxiety symptoms and try to classify the type of anxiety the patient has currently.

A good start would be to ask... *"Would you describe yourself as an anxious person?"*

If the answer is yes... state, "Tell me more about it."

You can also ask pointed questions to further clarify the type of anxiety the patient suffers from.

Panic attack: *"Do you have periods of intense apprehension, fearfulness, or terror that occur out of the blue?"*

"Is it often associated with feelings of impending doom?"

"During these attacks, do you have shortness of breath, palpitations, chest pain or discomfort, choking or smothering sensation?"

"Do you fear that you are going crazy or losing control?"

Agoraphobia: *"Do you avoid places or situations from which escape might be difficult or embarrassing or in which help may not be available in the event of having a panic attack or panic-like symptoms?"*

Specific phobia: *"Do you feel anxious in any specific situation or with a specific object or person?" If the answer is yes... state, "Tell me more about it." Then ask... "Do you avoid such situations?"*

Social phobia: *"Do you feel anxious in certain types of social or performance situations?"*

If the answer is yes... state, "Tell me more about it." Then ask... "Do you avoid such situations?"

Obsessive-compulsive disorder:

Obsessions: *"Do you think certain thoughts or have images that go through your head over and over again?" If the answer is yes... state, "Tell me more about it."*

Then ask... "Do they bother you or cause any distress?" "Do they affect your life in any way?"

Compulsions: *"Do you have certain urges to do things over and over again?" If the answer is yes... state, "Tell me more about it."*

Then ask... "Do they bother you or cause any distress?" "Do they affect your life in any way?"

Posttraumatic stress disorder: *"Have you ever experienced a situation in which your life or the life of anyone close to you was threatened?" If the answer is yes... state, "Tell me more about it."*

Then ask about reexperiencing phenomenon, symptoms of increased arousal, and avoidance of stimuli associated with the trauma.

Generalized anxiety disorder: *"Do you worry all the time?"*

If the answer is yes... state, "Tell me more about it."

"Is this worry so bad that you find it difficult to relax?"

Ask about symptoms associated with generalized anxiety disorder: *being restless, easily fatigued, difficulty concentrating, irritable, feeling tense, and having difficulty sleeping.*

If the answer is yes... state, "Tell me more about it."

Depersonalization: *"Do you have times in your life where you think that you cannot feel experiences or emotions?" If the answer is yes... state, "Tell me more about it."*

Derealization: *"Do you have times in your life where you think that other people are lacking in feelings or emotions?" If the answer is yes... state, "Tell me more about it."*

C. PSYCHOSIS

Psychosis is a term used to define abnormalities of thought content (overvalued ideas, delusions), form of thought (flight of ideas, loosened associations), perception (illusions/hallucinations), or motor activity (catatonic symptoms).

Overvalued ideas: They are thoughts that are not abnormal, but held with subjective certainty despite evidence to the contrary.

Delusions: They are abnormal thoughts that are not in keeping with a patient's social, occupational, cultural, or religious belief systems and are held with subjective certainty despite evidence to the contrary.

Paranoia: It only means that it is self-referential. Paranoid thoughts can be grandiose or persecutory.

"Have you had any experience where you felt that for some reason people were trying to hurt you or harm you." If the answer is yes... state, "Tell me more about it."

"Have you had any experience where you felt that your thoughts were not your own and someone else was controlling them." If the answer is yes... state, "Tell me more about it."

"Do you feel other people can read your thoughts?" If the answer is yes... state, "Tell me more about it."

Hallucinations: These are false perceptions in the absence of any external stimuli.

"Have you had any experience where you were hearing, seeing, feeling, or smelling strange things." If the answer is yes... state, "Tell me more about it."

Clarify, "Do you have these experiences when you are alone?"

"Have you checked it out with other people if they too are having these experiences?"

D. SUBSTANCE USE

1. Ask about current use of alcohol.
   How much do they drink usually? When was their last drink? Have they been drunk recently? Have they had any serious withdrawal symptoms like seizures or delirium tremens?

CAGE Questions:

Tried to **cut down** the alcohol use?
Get **annoyed** when people talk about their drinking habit?
Feel **guilty** about their drinking habit?
Had alcohol as an **eye opener?**

If yes to more than 2 responses, 80% chance of abusing alcohol

Try to differentiate abuse from dependence.

Abuse: *A maladaptive pattern of substance use leading to clinically significant impairment or distress, as manifested by one (or more) of the following, occurring within a 12-month period:*

- recurrent substance use resulting in a failure to fulfill major role obligations at work, school, or home.
- recurrent substance use in situations in which it is physically hazardous (e.g., driving an automobile or operating a machine when impaired by substance use).
- recurrent substance-related legal problems (e.g., arrests for substance-related disorderly conduct).
- continued substance use despite having persistent or recurrent social or interpersonal problems caused or exacerbated by the effects of the substance.

Dependence: *A maladaptive pattern of substance use, leading to clinically significant impairment or distress, as manifested by three (or more) of the following, occurring at any time in the same 12-month period:*

- tolerance, as defined by either of the following: a need for markedly increased amounts of the substance to achieve intoxication or desired effect or markedly diminished effect with continued use of the same amount of the substance.
- withdrawal, as manifested by either of the following: the characteristic withdrawal syndrome for the substance (refer to Criteria A and B of the criteria sets for Withdrawal from the specific substances) or the same (or a closely related) substance is taken to relieve or avoid withdrawal symptoms.
- the substance is often taken in larger amounts or over a longer period than was intended.
- there is a persistent desire or unsuccessful efforts to cut down or control substance use.
- a great deal of time is spent in activities necessary to obtain the substance (e.g., visiting multiple doctors or driving long distances), use the

substance (e.g., chain smoking), or recover from its effects.

- important social, occupational, or recreational activities are given up or reduced because of substance use.
- the substance use is continued despite knowledge of having a persistent or recurrent physical or psychological problem that is likely to have been caused or exacerbated by the substance.

2. Ask about other drugs of abuse including tobacco, which is the most common substance of abuse. Ask about caffeine intake as well. With regard to drugs, ask about the pattern of use, any medical, social, occupational, or legal consequences, and withdrawal symptoms. Always ask about intravenous drug use. Try to differentiate between abuse and dependence based on the aforementioned criteria.

E. COGNITION

Ask about any recent changes in memory. Find out if the changes are related to short-term memory or long-term memory.

Short-term: Ask if they have trouble remembering names, are misplacing objects, losing common items, forgetting conversations, or having word-finding difficulties.

Long-term: Ask for changes in long-term memory, such as difficulty remembering important life events including births, deaths, anniversaries, birthdays, and important events in the world.

Assess for functional impairment (which is required for a diagnosis of dementia) by inquiring about activities of daily living (ADLs). There are two types of ADLs: basic and instrumental activities of daily living (IADLs).

Basic ADLs: D—dressing; **E**—eating; **A**—ambulation; **T**—toileting; **H**—hygiene

Instrumental ADLs (IADLs): S—shopping; **H**—house work; **A**—accounting; **F**—food preparation; **T**—transportation.

F. SUICIDES AND HOMICIDES

Ask for *recent and current* suicidal or homicidal thoughts or behaviors.

Assess seriousness of any attempt:

- Premeditation
- Effort to conceal the attempt
- Suicide or homicide notes
- Previous attempts
- Use of alcohol prior to the attempt
- Use of more violent means
- Treatments

Premeditation, concealment, leaving notes, previous attempts, use of alcohol, more violent means, and not seeking treatment after the attempt, are all poor prognostic factors and increase the seriousness of the attempt.

2. Past Psychiatric History

Ask the following questions to clarify the psychiatric history:

- When did you first realize that you had mental health issues?
- What were these issues/symptoms?
- If you sought treatment, who did you go to for treatment?
- Were you given any psychiatric diagnosis?
- What was recommended; therapy and/or medications?
- What types of therapy and medications have you tried in the past?
- Did you ever have Electroconvulsive Therapy (ECT) treatments?
- Have you ever had thoughts of hurting yourself or others? (If they have a history, get details of the attempt(s) and subsequent treatment.)
- Have you ever had treatment for substance abuse? (If they have a history, get details of use pattern and treatments.)
- Have you ever had any psychiatric hospitalizations? If so, how may times and for what reason?

3. Past Medical History

Ask the following questions to clarify the medical history:

- What types of medical problems have you had?
- What were the treatments prescribed?
- Any sequelae from these medical problems?
- Any recent medical issues?
- Check for endocrine problems, especially thyroid disease, diabetes mellitus, problems with adrenal gland, and the liver.
- Ask about the presence of cardiac disease such as coronary artery disease, hypertension, hyperlipidemia, and atrial fibrillation.
- Inquire about neuropsychiatric conditions such as Parkinson's disease, multiple sclerosis, and Huntington's disease.
- Review for a history of head injuries, seizures, and cerebrovascular disease.

4. Current Medications

Get a list of all the current medications and their doses, if the patient is able to remember the list, particularly psychiatric medications.

5. Allergies

Get a list of allergies for the patient, including drug allergies.

6. Family History

- Inquire about the family history of mental health problems, especially in first-degree relatives.
- Find out about the treatment history of the first-degree relatives with mental health problems.
- Ask about history of completed suicides and homicides in the family.

7. Personal/Social History

- Ask about issues during birth, infancy, childhood, and as a teenager (including any history of abuse or neglect).
- Inquire about a history of behavioral problems, attention deficits, hyperactivity, truancy, and other school issues.
- Ask about level of education, military history (especially important if interviewing a patient at the Veterans Affairs (VA), legal history, and occupational history.
- Sexual orientation: We can ask about patient's sexual orientation by saying something like "It is important for us to know about our clients/patients sexual orientation?" "Would you be able to tell us about your sexual orientation?"
- Spiritual/religious: "Would you be able to tell us about your spiritual/religious belief"
- Inquire about current personal relationships, marital history, presence of living or deceased children, religious or cultural affiliations, and current social support network.

8. Mental Status Examination

The mental status examination begins as soon as the patient walks in the door.

Observe the physical characteristics of the patient. Note race, build, hygiene, dressing, gait, mannerisms, and cooperation during the interview.

Carefully note any abnormal movements and physical/neurological deficits.

Observe the patient's speech pattern. It could be lacking in spontaneity. It may be slow or fast. It may be with an accent. It could be with paraphasic errors.

Once you have inquired about the present illness, you do not really need to ask about current symptoms again. However, you can clarify any issue that you felt you had not covered during the initial part of interview process.

The parts of the mental status examination that you have to cover during your assessment include all of the following. *However, if you had asked most of this information in the history of present illness, it does not need to be repeated in the mental status examination.*

1. Patient's appearance and behavior
2. Patient's relation to the examiner
3. Patients' speech, noting all of the following:
   - Clear/slurred speech
   - Normal/fast/slow speech
   - Accents
   - Word salad/neologisms/paraphasic errors
4. Patient's affect: It is the transient emotional state of the patient as observed by the examiner. It is noted by observing the facial expressions of the patient.

   The range of affect should be described either as flat, restricted or constricted, or full range.
5. Patient's mood: It is the sustained emotional state of the patient as observed by the examiner and reported by the patient.

   It has a subjective and an objective component. Note both for your presentation.

   Mood can be euthymic/depressed/anxious/angry/irritable/frustrated/euphoric/labile.

   Mood can be congruent or incongruent with the person's current situation.
6. Patient's thought content:

   It includes content of thought as described by the patient and can be normal (e.g., a patient who is preoccupied with the recent illness or death of a loved one) or abnormal.

   Abnormal thought content includes

   1. **Obsessions:** One's own thoughts that are recurrent thoughts, impulses, or images that are experienced as intrusive and that cause marked anxiety or distress.
   2. **Overvalued idea:** The overvalued idea refers to a solitary, abnormal belief that is neither delusional nor obsessional in nature, but which is preoccupying to the extent of dominating the sufferer's life.
   3. **Delusions:** A false personal belief that is not subject to reason or contradictory evidence and is not explained by a person's usual cultural and religious concepts (so that,

e.g., it is not an article of faith). A delusion may be firmly maintained in the face of incontrovertible evidence that it is false. The following are examples of delusions that may be observed when interviewing a patient:

- **Delusion of control:** *This is a false belief that another person, group of people, or external force controls one's thoughts, feelings, impulses, or behavior. Thought broadcasting (the false belief that the affected person's thoughts are heard aloud), thought insertion, and thought withdrawal (the belief that an outside force, person, or group of people is removing or extracting a person's thoughts) are also examples of delusions of control.*
- **Nihilistic delusion:** *A delusion whose theme centers on the nonexistence of self or parts of self, others, or the world. A person with this type of delusion may have the false belief that the world is ending.*
- **Delusional jealousy (or delusion of infidelity):** *A person with this delusion falsely believes that his or her spouse or lover is having an affair. This delusion stems from pathological jealousy and the person often gathers "evidence" and confronts the spouse about the nonexistent affair.*
- **Delusions of guilt or sin (or delusion of self-accusation):** *This is a falsely based feeling of remorse or guilt of delusional intensity.*
- **Delusion of mind being read:** *The false belief that other people can know one's thoughts. This is different from thought broadcasting in that the person does not believe that his or her thoughts are heard aloud.*
- **Delusion of reference:** *The person falsely believes that insignificant remarks, events, or objects in one's environment have personal meaning or significance.*
- **Erotomania:** *A delusion in which one believes that another person, usually someone of higher status, is in love with him or her.*
- **Grandiose delusion:** *An individual exaggerates his or her sense of self-importance and is convinced that he or she has special powers, talents, or abilities.*
- **Persecutory delusions:** *These are the most common type of delusions and involve the theme of being followed, harassed, cheated, poisoned or drugged, conspired against, spied on, attacked, or obstructed in the pursuit of goals. Sometimes the delusion is isolated and fragmented, but at other times they are well-organized belief systems involving a complex set of delusions ("systematized delusions").*
- **Religious delusion:** *Any delusion with a religious or spiritual content. These may be combined with other delusions, such as grandiose delusions (the belief that the affected person was chosen by God, e.g.), delusions of control, or delusions of guilt. Beliefs that would be considered normal for an individual's religious or cultural background are not delusions.*
- **Somatic delusion:** *A delusion whose content pertains to bodily functioning, bodily sensations, or physical appearance. Usually, the false belief is that the body is somehow diseased, abnormal, or changed.*

7. Patient's thought process:

   It could be either normal or abnormal. Normal thought process is usually linear and goal directed. Abnormal thought process could be any one of the following:

   1. **Retardation:** *Abnormally slowed thought process.*
   2. **Flight of ideas:** *Rapidly verbalized train of unrelated thoughts or of thoughts related only via relatively coherent associations.*
   3. **Perseveration:** *Persistent repetition of words or ideas.*
   4. **Tangentiality:** *Replying to questions in an oblique, tangential, or irrelevant manner.*
   5. **Derailment/loose association (Knight's move thinking):** *Ideas slip off the track on to another which is obliquely related or unrelated.*
   6. **Clanging:** *Sounds (often rhyming), rather than meaningful relationships, appear to govern words.*
   7. **Blocking:** *Interruption of train of thought before completion.*
   8. **Circumstantiality:** *Long winded thought process with delay in reaching its goal.*
   9. **Echolalia:** *Echoing of one's or other people's speech.*
   10. **Neologisms:** *New word formations.*

8. Patient's perceptions: Perceptions could be normal or abnormal. Abnormal perception could be either of the following:

   Illusions: They describe misinterpretations of a true sensation. They could be optical, auditory, tactile, or olfactory.

Hallucinations: They are defined as perceptions in a conscious and awake state in the absence of external stimuli which have the qualities of real perception.

- *They are vivid, substantial, and located in the external objective space.*
- *Hallucinations may occur in any sensory modality: visual, auditory, olfactory, gustatory, tactile, proprioceptive, equilibrioceptive, nociceptive, and thermoceptive.*
- *Hypnagogic hallucinations and hypnopompic hallucinations are considered normal phenomena. Hypnagogic hallucinations can occur as one is falling asleep, and hypnopompic hallucinations occur when one is waking up.*

9. Suicidal thoughts or plans: Ask about any thoughts or plans. If plans are present, ask if they are imminent. Evaluate risk by asking about:
   - *Premeditation*
   - *Thoughts to conceal the attempt*
   - *Thoughts of writing a suicide note*
   - *Previous attempts*
   - *Use of alcohol*
   - *Thought of using and access to more violent means (i.e., firearms)*
10. Homicidal thoughts or plans: Ask about any thoughts or plans. If plans are present, ask if they are imminent. Evaluate risk by asking about:
    - *Premeditation*
    - *Identified victim*
    - *Thoughts to conceal the attempt*
    - *Previous attempts*
    - *Use of alcohol*
    - *Thought of using and access to more violent means*
11. Cognition: Every mental status examination should include a cognitive assessment.

    Although Mini-Mental State Examination is the most commonly used tool for cognitive assessment, it may be too long to do in an examination setting and does not assess the frontal lobe functioning. Given the case, an abbreviated cognitive testing that assesses the major areas of the cognitive functioning should be carried out. We do not recommend any specific tool for this purpose, but feel that the list enumerated below will suffice.

1. Orientation: Time: Day, Date, Month, and Year
   Place: City, State, and Country
   Person: Their name and the name of the examiner along with his/her profession.
2. Attention: It is the ability to focus and can be tested by spelling word/numbers forward and backward.

   Examples: Spell CHAIR or WORLD forward and then backward. Counting five numbers forward or backward (DIGIT SPAN). Usually, people can do a five-letter word forward and backward. If they are unable to do so, start with a four-letter word; if unsuccessful, go to a three-letter word.

   The normal DIGIT SPAN is 7 ± 2.
3. Concentration: It is the ability to maintain focus.

   It can be tested by asking the patient to do serial subtractions. Subtract 7 from 100 or subtract 3 from 20.

   Go for about five subtractions and stop.
4. Memory:
   A. Immediate memory: It is also called online memory and lasts for about 5 minutes. It can be tested by asking the patient to recall three items after 5 minutes. The duration can be shortened to 2 to 3 minutes in older patients and if time is short.
   B. Short-term memory: It is for events that happened in the last few hours to days. It can be tested by asking about news and events that happened in the last day or two.
   C. Long-term memory: It lasts for months to years. It can be tested by asking about major events in history like the world wars and the names of the previous presidents.
5. Praxis: It is the ability to do learned motor movements. Apraxia is the inability to carry out these movements. There are many types of apraxias, but the three most important ones are
   A. Ideomotor: Inability to carry out a motor command. It is the most commonly encountered apraxia. It can be tested by asking the patients to act as if they were brushing their teeth; combing their hair; saluting.
   B. Ideational: It is the inability to create a plan for a specific movement. It can

be tested by asking the patient to pick up the pen and write down his or her name or to show how he or she will get an envelope ready for mailing.

C. Constructional: It is the inability to draw or construct simple configurations. It can be tested by asking the patient to copy interlocking pentagons.

6. Agnosia: It is the loss of ability to recognize objects, persons, sounds, shapes, or smells while the specific sense is not defective, nor is there any significant memory loss. Although there are many forms of agnosia, the most commonly tested one is visual agnosia. It can be tested by asking the patient to recognize objects like a pen or a watch.
7. Executive functions: It includes the complex functions of the brain that are mainly located in the dorsolateral prefrontal cortex. They include all of the following:
   A. Planning/organizing/sequencing: It can be tested by doing a three-step command like taking a sheet of paper with the left hand, folding it into half, and placing it on the table.
   B. Response inhibition: It can be tested by asking the patient to stop an activity on command. Ask the patient to open his or her mouth and say "Aah…" till you command them to stop.
   C. Abstraction: It can be tested by asking patients to interpret proverbs. When doing this test, make sure that the patient is aware of the meaning of a proverb. It is a popular saying expressing some general truths.
   Examples include
   "Actions speak louder than words."
   "Better late than never."
   "Charity begins at home."
8. Insight and judgment:

   Insight is defined not only in terms of a person's understanding of his or her illness, but also in terms of understanding how the illness affects the individual's interactions with the world. It encompasses a complex concept which should be seen as a continuum of thinking and feeling that is affected by numerous internal and external variables.

   Judgment can be defined as the person's ability to make informed decisions.

   Most commonly, insight and judgment are tested together on a continuum.

   Four questions that can help determine the patient's insight and judgment include
   1. Do you have any psychiatric illness?
   2. If yes, "What is the illness?"
      If no, "What do you think is going on?"
   3. "What do you think needs to be done to help your condition?"
   4. "What will happen if you do not accept the recommended treatments?"

If the patient is aware of his or her illness, the treatments available and is able to make an informed decision about the treatments, then the patient has good insight and judgment. If not, the patient has limited or poor insight and judgment.

9. Closing Out the Interview

Make sure that you take a minute or two at the end of the allotted time to close out the interview well. A closure is essential to wrap up the interview process and get a sense of completion of the activity for the patient, you, and the examiners.

Here are a few tips that should help with a good closing:

- Thank the patient for his or her cooperation.
- Reframe what you have understood from the interview in a paragraph and ask the patient if it is the essence of his or her presentation.
- You do not want to end the interview with time remaining. If there is any remaining time, ask the patient if there is anything else he or she thinks you should know about their history. You can also offer the patient support and encouragement during this time.

Here are a few things that you should *not* do in the closing stages of the interview:

- Ask the patient for a lot of new information.
- Ask if the patient has any questions for you. Chances are, you will not be able to answer specific questions pertaining to his or her current treatment plan and you do not want to be in the awkward position of being asked to pass judgment on his or her current diagnosis and treatment.
- Discuss major issues like suicidality or homicidality.
- Discuss issues that are upsetting to the patient.

If you have forgotten to ask some pertinent information during the interview, there is no need to panic. You can always make it up in your presentation. However, it is of utmost importance not to try and cram this information into the final stage of the interview, thereby losing any patient cooperation and/or the structure of the interview.

4. WHAT TO DO IF YOU FORGET TO ASK IMPORTANT INFORMATION DURING THE INTERVIEW

All examiners are aware of the stress of conducting interviews during examinations. Examinees often miss out on some important information inadvertently due to anxiety and time limitation. Not acknowledging this missed information is not a good policy as it shows lack of honesty/transparency in the assessment process.

A strategy that would be helpful to make up for omissions during the interview is to

- Keep your cool.
- Make a mental note of the information that you have forgotten to ask.
- Make up for omissions during the case presentation.
- During the presentation, at the appropriate sections make a statement such as "If I had more time I would have asked the following... because..."

  Present the information that you had omitted to ask and state to why it is important to know this information.

Example: If you missed symptoms of Post-traumatic stress disorder (PTSD) in someone with a reported history of abuse.

"Mr Y reported that he was physically abused by his biological parents as a child. He was moved by the local children's protective agency to his foster family at 11 years of age. He still has symptoms from his abuse as a child. If I had more time, I would have asked about the following symptoms including

A. Reexperiencing phenomenon ...
B. Avoidance phenomenon...
C. Increased arousal...

"I would like to know this information as a high percentage of children (5% to 90%) exposed to traumatic events develop PTSD. The percentage varies depending upon the nature of the event, but the rate of children developing PTSD following traumatic events is higher than those reported for adults."

By using this strategy you acknowledge omissions but make up for it during the presentation. It shows the examiners that you are an honest clinician who acknowledges his omissions but also has the presence of mind to make up for it.

5. CASE PRESENTATION

The case presentation is usually about 10 minutes long, and it starts with the presentation of the demographic information and ends with the summary of the case.

Each part of the case must be presented in sequence and in a clear manner.

Usually, the narrative starts with the present illness and goes through all the items you have gathered on the interview with the patient. If the current presentation of the patient is an extension of an ongoing episode, it can be presented that way; but the presenter must first alert the examiner to the sequence of this presentation.

If some information was not gathered during the interview, it is wiser to say that you would have asked about it if you had the time rather than say that you forgot about it.

All pertinent positives and negatives should be presented. For example, when talking about mood disorders, if the patient only has symptoms for a depressive episode, state the depressive symptoms and also state that the symptoms for hypomanic and manic episodes are absent.

Remember, the examiners have already listened to the interview. They do not need the entire interview regurgitated. Try to summarize the pertinent symptoms of the history of the present illness using Diagnostic and Statistical Manual of Mental Disorders (DSM) criteria as opposed to repeating what the patient said verbatim. For example, do not say,

"The patient reports she's been feeling really down in the dumps for about 3 weeks. She says she can't fall asleep and is up and down all night. She says she hasn't felt like eating her usual snacks and meals lately. She reports she doesn't have the energy to take care of her children and her household chores and that really bothers her. She doesn't enjoy her favorite tv shows or her karate class anymore."

Try this instead: "The patient endorses 3 weeks of depressed mood, with anhedonia, insomnia, poor appetite, fatigue, and poor concentration. This has caused distress and has impacted her overall functioning at home." This nicely summarizes the patient's symptoms and shows the examiners you know the DSM criteria for a major depressive episode.

Only facts should be presented and opinions/views should be reserved for the discussion section of the case.

The presenter must indicate very clearly the major headings during the presentation. For example,

"Now I am going to talk about the past psychiatric history."

"The past psychiatric history includes...."

"The patient's medical history is significant for ...."

The presentation should end with the summary of the case. The summary is a brief description of the patient's case. It differs from the formulation in that there is no diagnostic clarification provided nor there is a discussion on the etiology, therapy, or prognosis for the case. It is a summary of the facts.

A summary should be about a paragraph long and have the following elements:

1. Demographic information: age, sex, racial identification, marital status, and the employment status.
2. Present symptoms; Example: Depressive symptoms including...; Manic symptoms including...
3. Past medical and psychiatric history; Example: The history is significant for depression, anxiety, alcohol abuse, hypertension, and hyperlipidemia.
4. Prominent stressors; Example: The stressors include a recent exacerbation of the Chronic Obstructive Pulmonary Disease (COPD) and loss of his job.
5. Risk of suicide or homicide; Example: The patient's risk of suicide remains high given the prominent depressive symptoms and alcohol abuse coupled with her multiple losses.
6. Current treatment and the appropriateness/adequacy of the plan.
7. Cognitive functioning and insight and judgment; Example: The patient did not have any gross cognitive deficits and has a good understanding of his illness and is willing to comply with the treatment plan.

An example of a summary is given below.

Ms Grace is a 24 year old single White woman, an employee at the local grocery store who was evaluated today for ongoing symptoms of depression and anxiety for the last 4 months. Prominent symptoms include depressed mood, decrease in appetite, poor sleep with early morning awakening, and increased worry about her future. The patient stated that she is unable to relax because of her worries. She did not report any symptoms of hypomania or mania or psychosis. Her history is significant for an episode of depression and anxiety at the age of 19 years in the context of a breakup with her boyfriend. Her current symptoms started after she had a falling out with her current boyfriend. There are no prominent medical issues at the present time. Ms Grace does not report any active suicidal or homicidal thoughts. She has never been suicidal or homicidal, and feels that aggression to self and others is against her religious beliefs. She is currently being treated with sertraline at 100 mg daily and weekly supportive psychotherapy. Ms Grace feels that she is dong better on this treatment regimen. Her cognitive functioning is good and she is willing to continue her current antidepressant therapy and follow up with her therapist for ongoing supportive psychotherapy.

6. PRESENTING THE MULTIAXIAL DIAGNOSES/DIFFERENTIAL DIAGNOSIS

There are many ways to present the differential diagnosis, but the most logical one is to place them in categories and present the most probable one first and then go down through the list to the least probable.

Usually, the differential diagnosis should be presented in bullet points with no explanation being provided for choice or order of diagnosis. Clarification of the diagnosis should ideally be done in the formulation part of the presentation.

As DSM-IV-TR remains the standard diagnostic criteria for most of our readers, we will be using it as the diagnostic framework for our differential diagnosis.

In psychiatry, except for substance use disorders, the diagnoses are either a primary psychiatric disorder or secondary to a general medical condition or substance use.

The differential diagnosis is usually presented on Axis I and then the other axes are presented.

Axis I. This axis is for reporting all the various disorders or conditions in the classification except for the personality disorders and mental retardation which are reported on Axis II.

Primary psychiatric disorder: Mood disorder/ anxiety disorder/ psychotic disorder/cognitive disorder/ substance use disorder.

Rule out a secondary disorder: either due to a general medical condition (name the disorder) or a substance use.

Record as many differential diagnoses as you feel are appropriate. Do not include diagnostic categories for completion sake.

Axis II. This axis is for reporting personality disorders and mental retardation. It may also be used for noting prominent maladaptive personality features and defense mechanisms. The coding of personality disorders on Axis II should not be taken to imply that their pathogenesis or range of appropriate treatment is fundamentally different from that for the disorders coded on Axis I.

When an individual has more than one Axis II diagnosis, all of them should be reported. When an individual has both an Axis I and an Axis II diagnosis and the Axis II diagnosis is the principal diagnosis, it should be indicated by adding the qualifying phrase "principal diagnosis" or "reason for visit" after the Axis II diagnosis. If no Axis II disorder is present, this should be stated as such. If an Axis II diagnosis is deferred, it should be noted as such.

Example: Axis II Paranoid personality disorder, frequent use of projection.

Below is a table indicating severity of mental retardation.

Mild Mental Retardation	*IQ level 50–55 to approximately 70*
Moderate Retardation	*IQ level 35–40 to 50–55*
Severe Mental Retardation	*IQ level 20–25 to 35–40*
Profound Mental Retardation	*IQ level below 20 or 25*
Mental Retardation, Severity Unspecified	*It can be used when there is a strong presumption of mental retardation but the person's intelligence is untestable by standard tests.*

Axis III. This axis is used for reporting current general medical conditions that are potentially relevant to the understanding or management of the individual's mental disorder.

When an individual has more than one clinically relevant Axis III diagnosis, all should be reported. If no Axis III disorder is present, this should be indicated by the notation "Axis III: None." If an Axis III diagnosis is deferred, pending the gathering of additional information, this should be indicated by the notation "Axis III: Deferred." When it is clear that the general medical condition is directly etiological to the development or worsening of mental symptoms and that the mechanism for this is judged to be a direct physiological consequence of the general medical condition, a mental disorder due to a general medical condition should be diagnosed on Axis I and the general medical condition should be recorded on both Axis I and Axis III.

Example: Mood disorder due to hypercalcemia, with depressive features, and the hypercalcemia should be noted again in Axis III.

Axis IV. This is the axis used for reporting psychosocial and environmental problems that may affect the diagnosis, treatment, and prognosis of mental disorders (Axes I and II). These psychosocial or environmental problems may include a negative life event, an environmental difficulty or deficiency, a familial or other interpersonal stress, an inadequacy of social support or personal resources, or other problem relating to the context in which a person's difficulties have developed. If an individual has multiple psychosocial or environmental problems, then they should be noted. However, only those psychosocial and environmental problems that have been present during the year preceding the current evaluation should be noted. When a psychosocial or environmental problem is the primary focus of clinical attention, it should also be recorded on Axis I, with a code derived from the section "Other Conditions That May Be a Focus of Clinical Attention." These problems can be grouped into the following categories for convenience.

1. Problems with primary support group
2. Problems related to the social environment
3. Educational problems
4. Occupational problems
5. Housing problems
6. Economic problems
7. Problems with access to health care services
8. Problems related to interaction with the legal system/crime
9. Other psychosocial and environmental problems

Example: Job loss, poverty, and victim of sexual abuse

Axis V. This axis is used for reporting the clinician's judgment of the individual's overall level of functioning. This reporting of overall functioning on Axis V is done using the global assessment of functioning (GAF) scale. The GAF scale is rated with respect to psychological, social, and occupational functioning only. The impairments in functioning due to physical or environmental conditions are not rated. In most instances, ratings on the GAF scale should be for the current period. To account for day-to-day variability in functioning, the GAF rating for the "current period" can be operationalized as the lowest level of functioning for the past week. The GAF scale rating can be done at the time of admission and at time of discharge from a hospital. The GAF scale may also be rated for other time periods, for example, the highest level of functioning for at least a few months during the past year.

Global Assessment of Functioning Scale

91–100: No symptoms or superior psychosocial functioning.

81–90: Absent or minimal symptoms or good psychosocial functioning.

71–80: Mild but transient symptoms or slight impairment in social, occupational, or school functioning.

61–70: Mild symptoms or some difficulty in social, occupational, or school functioning.

51–60: Moderate symptoms or moderate difficulty in social, occupational, or school functioning.

41–50: Serious symptoms or serious impairment in social, occupational, or school functioning.

31–40: Some impairment in reality testing or communication or major impairment in several areas, such as work or school, family relations, judgment, thinking, or mood.

21–30: Behavior is considerably influenced by delusions or hallucinations or serious impairment in communication or judgment or inability to function in almost all areas.

20–11: Some danger of hurting self or others or occasionally failing to maintain minimal personal hygiene or gross impairment in communication.

10–1: Persistent danger of severely hurting self or others or persistent inability to maintain minimal personal hygiene or serious suicidal act with clear expectation of death.

0: Inadequate information.

7. CASE FORMULATION

Formulation is the theoretical framework on which we base the patient's presentation. It differs from the summary in the following ways:

- It clarifies reasons for choosing the diagnoses in Axes I and II.
- It explains the probable etiology for the patient's presentation.
- It summarizes the treatment framework for the patient.
- It comments on the patient's prognosis.

We believe that the formulation should be summarized under four separate subheadings. Whether the examinee wants to present these subheadings separately or present the entire narrative as one block of information is up to the individual. However, when presenting the formulation, these four subheadings should be kept in mind.

The four subheadings in the formulation are:

1. Diagnostic
2. Etiologic
3. Therapeutic
4. Prognostic

1. Diagnostic formulation: This section clarifies the diagnoses that we picked in Axes I and II. It prioritizes the diagnoses that were chosen and provides reasons for the priority. It also provides a link between the primary and secondary diagnoses. This section can also be used to highlight your knowledge of the DSM-IV-TR diagnostic criteria.

Example: Patient with borderline personality disorder (BPD).

Important mood disorders to rule out in this case include a major depressive disorder, bipolar disorder, cyclothymia, and dysthymia. The duration of her depressed mood does not meet criteria for either a major depressive disorder or dysthymia. In addition, she denied any neurovegetative signs of depression, such as fatigue, poor concentration, or changes in her appetite or sleep patterns. She also does not meet criteria for a manic or hypomanic episode. Ruling out cyclothymia in this case can be particularly difficult. This patient presents a long-standing history of frequent mood swings and impulsivity, which are common in cyclothymia. However, her mood swings are very short lived and seem to only appear in reaction to a particular stressor. She also does not present with grandiose mood, pressured speech, racing thoughts, or psychomotor agitation, which would point to a hypomanic episode. Her mood swings and impulsivity are better explained by her underlying personality disorder and her emotional dysregulation. One will also need to rule out mood disorder due to a medical condition and substance-induced mood disorders. This patient denies any history of substance abuse and is not taking any medications known to induce mood symptoms. This patient does not meet criteria for other Axis I disorders, including anxiety disorders or substance abuse disorders. She also does not meet criteria for a psychotic or cognitive disorder.

This patient meets six out of the nine DSM-IV-TR criteria for BPD. She has a history of unstable relationships which she ends abruptly after devaluating them, chronic feelings of loneliness, impulsivity in quitting her job and spending money (unable to pay rent), recurrent thoughts of self-harm, marked reactivity to mood, and an unstable sense of self.

The distinction between BPD and several mood disorders can be challenging, and these two disorders commonly coexist. Important Axis II disorders to rule out in patients with BPD include narcissistic personality disorder and dependent personality disorder. However, this patient is not showing any signs of needing others to make decisions for her, or to give her continuous reassurance and support. On the contrary, she seems to make frequent impulsive decisions without being able to think before acting or getting advice from important people in her life. She also does not present with an arrogant attitude, a grandiose sense of self-importance, and does not seem to be focusing on success or needing to feel "special," which is characteristic of people with narcissistic features. Some of her behaviors could raise the diagnostic suspicion of antisocial personality disorder (ASPD) (e.g., her impulsivity, irritability, and failure to save money for her rent). However, there is no evidence of a history of conduct disorder during her childhood, she does not show any disregard to others, and does not seem to lack response either. Therefore, this patient's primary diagnosis is BPD.

2. Etiologic formulation: This is the most complex part of the formulation and uses the biopsychosocial model to bring to light the probable etiology for the patient's presentation.

1. Biological: It mainly describes the genetic loading for the various Axes I and II diagnoses. It also hints on the various comorbidities (medical and psychiatric) that predispose the patient to develop psychiatric diagnoses. Emphasis is also laid on medication nonadherence as a reason for symptom development.
2. Psychological: It describes the various psychological themes that may lead to the development of psychiatric disorders. These include
   A. Trauma: Abuse/neglect/life-threatening events
   B. Significant personal losses: Loved ones/relationships/jobs
   C. Self-concept/self-esteem
   D. Defense mechanisms
   E. Cognitive distortions
   F. Developmental themes:
      Erikson's psychosocial development
      Freud's psychosexual development
      Kohlberg's moral development
      Piaget's cognitive development
   G. Conflict/relationship issues with parents/spouse/children/significant others/world
3. Social: It describes the various social issues that can lead to the development of psychiatric disorders. These include
   A. Financial status: Poverty/bankruptcy
   B. Employment: Unemployment/disability
   C. Martial status: Single/bad marriage/divorced/widowed
   D. Living environment: Lower socioeconomic status, poor living condition
   E. Educational opportunities: Low educational achievement/disabilities
   F. Access to medical/psychiatric/rehabilitative care: Limited access to care

The etiologic part of the formulation also uses four anchor points to further subcategorize the biopsychosocial aspect of the etiology for a patient's diagnosis. They are usually used in conjunction with the above mentioned biopsychosocial construct to synthesize a formulation. The four anchor points are

1. Predisposing factors: Conditions that prime the patient to develop psychiatric disorders.
2. Precipitating factors: Conditions that act as a catalyst for development of psychiatric disorders.
3. Perpetuating factors: Conditions that maintain the risk of relapse or recurrence of psychiatric disorders.

Factors	Predisposing	Precipitating	Perpetuating	Protective
Biological	Family history Comorbidities: Medical and/or psychiatric Substance abuse/dependence	New medical events Substance abuse/dependence Medication nonadherence	Ongoing medical events Psychiatric comorbidities Ongoing substance abuse/dependence Ongoing medication non adherence	Absence of family history No medical or psychiatric comorbidities No substance abuse or dependence
Psychological	Trauma Losses Neglect Self-esteem issues	Trauma Losses Neglect Self-esteem issues	Ongoing trauma Ongoing neglect Ongoing self-esteem issues	No loss/trauma/neglect Good and stable self-concept
Social	Socioeconomic: Poverty/unemployment Low educational attainment Family conflicts	Socioeconomic: Poverty/loss of job/unemployment Family conflicts	Ongoing socioeconomic issues: Poverty/loss of job/unemployment Ongoing family conflicts	Stable socioeconomic status Good educational attainment Good family life

4. Protective factors: Conditions that reduce the risk of development of psychiatric disorders.

Example: Patient with schizophrenia.

Mr P appears to have a predisposing genetic risk for psychotic illness, given his brother's diagnosis of schizophrenia. The history of complications at childbirth increases his likelihood of developing a psychotic disorder. Chaotic childhood was characterized by the parents' significant marital discord and marked physical abuse by his father who was abusing alcohol. School years were marked by poor academic performance and very low self-esteem. Parental divorce saw his mother working long hours and she was never available for any parental support. Teenage years were characterized by maternal absence, arguments over money, abuse of cannabis, and continued poor school performance. The patient started using defense mechanisms of projection, splitting, and acting out as ways of dealing with his chaotic life. He also started using cognitive distortions of All-or-Nothing-Thinking and Disqualifying-the-Positives to make sense of what was going on around him.

He has a classic course of illness and response to treatment, as his relapses are often associated with, and possibly precipitated by, nonadherence to his psychotropic medication regimen and/or abuse of cannabis. In the past, his decompensations also appear to have been at least partially precipitated by a high expressed emotion (EE) environment in his household. His most recent relapse was temporally associated with the sudden death of his father, toward whom he had ambivalent feelings. His use of projection, splitting, and acting out as defense mechanisms and cognitive distortions of all-or-nothing thinking and disqualifying the positives made him vulnerable, difficult and to deal with. It also caused high EEs with the family. He has at baseline narcissistic traits as evidenced by his constant claims of wanting to be in charge. These traits may perpetuate his tendency to have grandiose delusions.

He does have the protective strengths of longstanding employment, and a generally independent life, with at least a few friends. He is also physically healthy and other than the abuse of cannabis, he does not have any substance use issues. He has also developed a good working relationship with his psychiatrist and his therapist, and for the past year he has been attending his appointments regularly and taking his medications fairly consistently.

3. Therapeutic formulation: This section describes the basic framework of treatment for patients. It does not go into the details of treatment, but gives reasons for why these treatment modalities would be most effective in helping the patient.

Example: Patient with bipolar affective disorder.

The severity of the patient's mood lability and the persistence of suicidal ideation mandate a psychiatric hospitalization for this patient. Important goals for treatment are stabilization of her mood, reducing impulsivity and eliminating suicidal thoughts. Before initiating psychopharmacologic intervention with an anticonvulsant mood stabilizer with or without an antidepressant, we will need to explore the patient's past exposure and responses to psychiatric medications. Such exploration may be helpful in gauging the likelihood of compliance with medications, especially if the patient has experienced unpleasant side effects in the past. As this patient had a clear history of noncompliance with medications, determining whether her noncompliance was secondary to side effects or due to the lack of insight into her mental illness is an important step in selecting a treatment regimen. This initial step also serves as a foundation for establishing a therapeutic alliance with the patient. Such an alliance is essential for improving the patient's long-term prognosis by increasing the likelihood that the patient will remain engaged in treatment. Since maintenance therapy following the resolution of acute symptoms is crucial for the patient's long-term prognosis, communication with her outpatient psychiatrist regarding issues related to treatment compliance is ideal. Given the patient's history of physical abuse in the past, psychodynamic psychotherapy may help her deal with her past and keep her treatment focused. Patient education is also necessary in order to improve the patient's insight regarding her mental illness. Educating the patient's family about the nature of the mental illness can also be of great benefit. Knowledgeable family members may aid the patient in recognizing the recurrence of symptoms and seek intervention when the patient is unable to do so. As the patient is having difficulty keeping a job due to the recurrence of her mood episodes, referral to social services for possible application for disability may be warranted.

4. Prognostic formulation: This section describes the overall prognosis for the patient. It takes into account the diagnoses, treatment compliance, psychological stability, social issues, and the patient's motivation level.

Example: Patient with ASPD.

Mr C presents with a series of deviant behavior, such as robbing, lying, and stealing money from friends. He also has a current diagnosis of alcohol abuse. These are considered poor prognostic factors for patients with ASPD. He is now 41 years old. Reaching the fourth decade of life seems to be a good prognostic factor for ASPD, since symptoms and involvement with the legal system tend to decrease after this age in patients with ASPD. In terms of his suicidal behavior, he has important risk factors for another suicide attempt. He has had prior suicide attempts, which is the most important risk factor for future suicidality; he is a White male, he abuses alcohol and meets criteria for a major mood disorder, which are all risk factors for future suicide attempts.

8. PRESENTING TREATMENT OPTIONS

When presenting the treatment options for the patient under review, follow an organized format. Before you start treating the patient, there is a need to first evaluate the data gathered, clarify the data, make appropriate diagnoses, and only then decide on the treatment plan.

It is most prudent to start by saying something like, "Based on my evaluation today and the fact that I have picked the following as the most important diagnoses in this patient, my treatment plan is as follows...."

When dealing with psychiatric patients, the "safety first" rule should always be followed. We first need to ensure the patient's physical safety.

The first task at hand to ensure safety is to decide whether the patient needs inpatient or outpatient treatment.

1. Inpatient Versus Outpatient

Inpatient treatment is warranted if the patient is at imminent danger to self/others or is gravely disabled. Inpatient treatment may also be necessary for refractory psychiatry disorders.

- Imminent danger may be due to suicidality, homicidality, self-neglect, abuse, untreated illness, or nonadherence with prescribed treatments.
- Grave disability may be due to undiagnosed and/or untreated medical or psychiatric disorders.

Once a decision to admit has been made, we then need to decide on voluntary versus involuntary admission. Involuntary admission should ideally be reserved for patients who need inpatient psychiatric treatment and are unwilling to take this treatment or are unable to give consent for this treatment.

For those patients who are not at imminent danger to self or to others and are not gravely disabled, outpatient treatment should be proposed. Those in need of more intense outpatient treatment should be referred to intensive outpatient programs or day-hospital programs.

2. Review of Data

The next step in treatment is to clarify/corroborate the information given by the patient. For this clarification, the following steps should be taken:

- A review of records
- Discussion with the previous or current clinicians; medical-MD/PA/APRN and or psychiatric-MD/APRN/PhD/LCSWs*
- Discussion with family/significant other*

The above mentioned steps help us to

1. Clarify the diagnoses
2. Rule out other medical and psychiatric comorbidities
3. Understand important psychological and social issues
4. Ascertain adequacy of previous treatments
5. Evaluate legal issues

**Only after receiving a written permission from the patient; the exception being an emergency room evaluation.*

3. Physical Examination

Once the information has been clarified, the next step in treatment is to conduct a physical examination. Physical examination helps to rule out underlying medical conditions that may cause or worsen psychiatric symptoms. Important physical findings include

1. Vitals:
   - Hyperpyrexia—Infections
   - Tachy/bradycardia—Cardiac or Endocrine: thyroid disease
   - Hypo/hypertension—Cardiac or Endocrine: thyroid/adrenal
2. General examination:
   - Anemia
   - Lymphadenopathy—Infections/Malignancy
   - Thyromegaly—Hypo/hyperthyroidsm
   - Gynecomastia—Endocrine disorders
   - Venipuncture sites—Drug abuse
   - Gait and balance—Musculoskeletal/Neurological disorders
3. Systems:
   - Cardiac—Congestive heart failure/coronary artery disease
   - Respiratory—COPD/heart failure/malignancy
   - Gastrointestinal—Liver/pancreaticdisease/malignancies
   - Neurological—Parkinson's/Huntington's/cerebrovascular accidents

4. Laboratory Investigations

Following the physical examination, we must do the laboratory investigations to confirm/rule out underlying medical conditions. Not all patients will require all of the studies below. It is important to consider the reason for ordering a lab or imaging study; the examiner may ask you why you are recommending this test in this particular patient.

1. Blood/Urine Tests:
   - Complete blood count with differential: Anemia/infections/malignancy
   - Critical chemistry: Electrolyte imbalance
   - Thyroid function test: Hypo or hyperthyroidism.
   - Liver function test: Primary liver disease or liver disease secondary to malignancy/medications/alcohol/drug
   - Vitamin B_{12} and folic acid: Nutritional deficiencies
   - Urine examination: Infections/electrolyte imbalance/malignancy
   - Urine culture: Infections
   - Urine drug screen: Illicit drug use
   - Urine pregnancy test
2. Cardiac Function:
   - Electrocardiogram: Cardiac arrhythmia/QTc prolongation (especially when on antipsychotics)
   - Echocardiogram: Congestive heart failure/valvular abnormalities/chamber dysfunction
3. Cerebral/Cerbrovascular Function:
   - CAT scan: Head injuries/brain: Trauma/tumor/bleed/strokes
   - MRI scan: Trauma/tumor/bleed/strokes (better resolution than CAT scan)
   - EEG: Seizures/encephalopathy: Metabolic or infectious
4. Neuropsychological Testing: These tests should be recommended in patients in whom the presentation indicates complex psychopathology and in those patients who have personality issues and/or cognitive deficits.

   Some common tests are
   - Psychopathology: Millon Clinical Multiaxial Inventory
   - Personality testing: Minnesota Multiphasic Personality Inventory
   - Intelligent quotient (IQ): Wechsler Adult Intelligence Scale

- Wechsler Intelligence Scale for Children (WISC-IV)
- Halstead-Reitan Neuropsychological battery
- Luria-Nebraska Neuropsychological battery

5. Presenting the Treatment Options

Once the data is reviewed, the physical examination and laboratory tests are completed, and the diagnosis ascertained, we can decide on a specific treatment plan.

The question is then to choose between psychotherapy and pharmacotherapy or a combination of both treatments.

If the patient's symptoms are mild and are deemed to be due to personality issues or issues from the past, psychotherapy alone can be recommended.

In patients in whom the symptoms are mild and deemed not to have any relationship with their past and there are no major personality issues, pharmacotherapy alone can be recommended.

In most psychiatric disorders, a combination of psychotherapy and pharmacotherapy is the recommended treatment modality.

A. Choosing the type of psychotherapy: The following list serves as a rough guideline for choosing the appropriate therapy for the patient.
- Supportive psychotherapy: This form of therapy is best suited for people who are trying to cope with an acute crisis, or for those people where attempting to promote fundamental changes may be more disruptive than helpful.
- Psychodynamic psychotherapy: This form of therapy is best suited for patients who are not in a crisis and are willing to work on fundamental changes to their cognitive style and personality structure.
- Cognitive behavioral therapy: This form of therapy is most suited for patients with specific psychiatric disorders in whom faulty thinking patterns cause maladaptive behavior and "negative" emotions.
- Interpersonal therapy: This form of therapy is most suited for patients in whom the development of psychiatric symptoms are thought to be due to their interpersonal interactions.
- Family therapy: This form of therapy is most suited for patients in whom the development of psychiatric symptoms is thought to be due to systems of interaction between family members.

(*Please see the chapter on psychotherapy for specific treatment modalities.*)

B. Choosing the pharmacotherapeutic regimen: The following list serves as a rough guide to choosing the right pharmacotherapeutic regimen.
- Antidepressants: Selective Serotonin Reuptake Inhibitors (SSRIs) are usually the first line treatment. Serotonin-Norepinephrine Reuptake Inhibitors (SNRIs) can be used in lieu of SSRIs especially if the patient has chronic pain and/or atypical symptoms. Bupropion can be used in patients with anegric/apathetic depression and in those patients where weight gain is a concern. Mirtazapine is mostly used in the anxious-depressed and in those patients in whom sleep and appetite are poor. Tricyclic Antidepressants (TCAs) are useful in depressed patients with poor sleep and/or with chronic pain. Monoamine Oxidase Inhibitors (MAOIs) are reserved for patients who do not respond to the other agents and have atypical symptoms (mood reactivity, weight gain, hypersomnia, leaden paralysis, and rejection sensitivity).

  Augmentation (combining an antidepressant with another class of drug) and combination (combining an antidepressant with another class of antidepressant) is most useful in patients in whom there has been some but not adequate response to monotherapy and in whom taper of the first drug is not recommended. Lithium and triidothyronine (T3) have the best efficacy as augmenting agents for antidepressants.
- Anxiolytics: SSRIs and SNRIs have the best known efficacy for the long treatment of anxiety disorders. Mirtazapine is also helpful in the treatment especially of the anxious-depressed patient. Other drugs that have some efficacy in the treatment of anxiety disorders include anticonvulsants (divalproex sodium/gabapentin), hydroxyzine, and antipsychotic medications. They are frequently used as monotherapy or in combination with antidepressants for refractory anxiety disorders and in special populations like patients with substance dependence and comorbid anxiety.

Benzodiazepines are very helpful in the short-term treatment of anxiety disorders. The data for their use in long-term treatment of anxiety is limited. When used, they should be combined with antidepressants. Their use is limited by their addictive potential and their propensity to cause sedation, motor incoordination, and cognitive dysfunction. Short-acting benzodiazepines, such as alprazolam, have a higher propensity to be habit-forming than long-acting drugs, such as diazepam.

- Antipsychotics: Typical and atypical antipsychotics were traditionally separated based on their propensity to cause extrapyramidal symptoms. However, recently, they are also being divided as being typical or atypical based on their metabolic profile and also their ability to treat negative and/or cognitive symptoms of psychotic disorders. Although earlier data indicated that atypical drugs were better for the treatment of negative and cognitive symptoms of psychotic disorder, this data is currently being challenged by newer findings.

  Typical and atypical antipsychotics appear to have equal efficacy in the treatment of psychotic disorders. Choice of antipsychotics is based on the patient's symptoms, previous documented trials/failures and the risk of extrapyramidal signs/symptoms, and/or metabolic/cardiovascular profile of the patient. The Texas algorithm is probably the best evidence-based algorithm currently available for the treatment of patients with psychotic disorders.

  Combination of two or more antipsychotics for the treatment of psychotic disorders has very little evidence. Available evidence for the combination of antipsychotics is limited to clozapine with other antipsychotics mainly risperidone and aripiprazole. Combination of antipsychotics with mood stabilizers and/or antidepressants has better evidence than combination of two antipsychotics. Clozapine has the least propensity to cause tardive dyskinesia.
- Antidementia drugs: There are two classes of drugs available for the treatment of cognitive dysfunction associated with Alzheimer's disease (AD). These are the cholinesterase inhibitors and NMDA (*N*-methyl-D-aspartate) antagonist memantine. The three cholinesterase inhibitors donepezil, rivastigmine, and galantamine have equal efficacy and are approved for by the FDA for the treatment of mild to moderate AD. Donepezil has also been approved by the FDA for the treatment of severe AD, but the data for this indication is not convincing. These drugs do not improve memory, but reduce the rate of decline of cognition in patients with AD. The gastrointestinal side-effect profile of donepezil also appears to be a little better than the two other cholinesterase inhibitors.

  Memantine is an uncompetitive antagonist at the glutamatergic NMDA receptors. It is approved for the treatment of moderate to severe AD. Its effect on the milder forms of the disease is less robust. Common side effects are confusion, drowsiness, and headache. It has also has shown to reduce the progression of AD when combined with donepezil and this combination is reasonably well tolerated by patients.

  There are no FDA-approved treatments for behavioral disturbances in dementia. Limited data point to the efficacy for antipsychotics such as risperidone and olanzapine for these symptoms, but their use is limited by their increased risk of causing cerebrovascular events and death in elderly demented patients.
- Hypnotics: There are two main classes of hypnotics. They are the benzodiazepines and nonbenzodiazepines. They are all indicated for short-term use (<4 weeks).

  The benzodiazepine hypnotics commonly used in practice are temazepam and triazolam. Temazepam is the longer acting of the two medications with a half-life of 10 to 12 hours. Triazolam is ultra short acting with a half-life of 2 to 3 hours. It is good for initial insomnia and not for sleep maintenance. These drugs can cause dependence and hence should be used only for short periods.

  The most commonly used nonbenzodiazepine hypnotic agent is trazodone. Half-life is 5 to 9 hours. It is most helpful in treating SSRI-induced insomnia. Its use is limited by its potential to cause daytime sedation and orthostatic hypotension at higher doses.

Diphenhydramine is an antihistamine and anticholinergic drug that is often used as a hypnotic. Data, however, indicates that it is a weak sedative. It can exacerbate confusion in elderly, cause urinary retention in elderly patients with Benign Prostatic Hyperplasia (BPH) and worsen narrow angle glaucoma.

The other nonbenzodiazepine hypnotics that are available in the market include eszopiclone, zaleplon, and zolpidem. Eszopiclone has a rapid onset of action and a half-life of 6 hours. It has a longer duration of action than the other nonbenzodiazepine hypnotics. Zaleplon has a rapid onset of action and it is good for initiating sleep. It has a half-life of 1 hour and hence repeat dosing may be needed to maintain sleep. Zolpidem has a half-life of 3 hours, has a rapid onset of action, and is good for initiating sleep. A long-acting preparation of the drug is available for sleep maintenance. None of these drugs are thought to cause dependence or withdrawal. They are all hepatically metabolized.

Ramelteon is a melatonin agonist that is marketed as a sedative-hypnotic. It has a half-life of 2.5 hours and is good for initiating sleep. It is not known to cause dependence or withdrawal. It is hepatically metabolized.

- Mood stabilizers: There are three groups of drugs that are commonly used as mood stabilizers. These include lithium, anticonvulsants, and antipsychotics.

  Lithium is the classic mood stabilizer and is usually the first-line treatment for euphoric mania. Its efficacy is limited in dysphoric manics, rapid cyclers, patients with mixed states and in people with comorbid substance abuse/medical problems. Its use is limited by its narrow therapeutic window and lethality in overdoses. However, it is the only drug that has been shown to decrease suicidality in bipolar patients.

  Anticonvulsants commonly used to treat patients with bipolar disorder include divalproex sodium, carbamazepine, oxcarbazepine, lamotrigine, and topiramate. Divalproex sodium, carbamazepine, and oxcarbazepine are more useful in dysphoric manics, rapid cyclers, patients with mixed states, and in people with comorbid substance abuse/medical problems. As with lithium, divalproex sodium and carbamazepine need to have their levels checked. Oxcarbazepine does not induce the cytochrome P450 enzyme system, but has a similar side-effect profile as carbamazepine. The levels of these drugs are checked to monitor toxicity rather than evaluate clinical response. Lamotrigine is helpful in rapid-cycling bipolar type II patients and is thought to be a safer drug for use in pregnant patients. Although topiramate has limited efficacy as a mood stabilizer, it causes weight loss and may be added as an adjunctive treatment with other mood stabilizers to counter weight gain. Anticonvulsants can be combined with lithium or with each other in more refractory cases. When combining these drugs, be mindful of side effects and drug-drug interactions.

  Antipsychotics have efficacy in the treatment of acute manic episodes and maintenance treatment of bipolar disorder. Atypical antipsychotics are preferred as they cause less extrapyramidal symptoms. They can be used as monotherapy or in combination treatment with anticonvulsants and/or antidepressants.

  For bipolar depression, lithium and lamotrigine can be used as monotherapy or in combination with each other. Quetiapine has been FDA approved for the treatment of bipolar depression. Antidepressants should not be used alone without mood stabilizer coverage in bipolar patients given the risk of hypomanic or manic episodes.
- Medications for treating substance dependence:
  1. Alcohol dependence:
     A. Acamprosate: It is used for maintenance of alcohol abstinence. The exact action is not known, but it may interact with glutamate and GABA neurotransmitters. Half-life is about 20 to 33 hours. It should only be used once the patient has achieved abstinence.
     B. Disulfiram: It is an aldehyde hydrogenase inhibitor with a half-life of 60 to 120 hours. It leads to elevated

levels of acetaldehyde and toxic effects when the patient consumes alcohol.

C. Naltrexone: It is an opioid antagonist with a half-life of 13 hours. It is thought to reduce craving and decrease the number of relapses.

2. Nicotine dependence:
   A. Bupropion: It is thought to alter dopamine and noradrenergic neurotransmission and has a half-life of 4 to 21 hours.
   B. Varenicline: It is a partial agonist of the $\alpha 4\beta 2$ nicotinic receptors. It is thought to block activity of nicotine in activating these receptors and stimulate dopamine, thus reducing craving and withdrawal. It has a half-life of 17 to 24 hours. It should be started 1 week before the patient quits smoking. It should be taken for 12 weeks after quitting smoking.
3. Opioid dependence:
   A. Buprenorphine: It is a partial agonist at the mu-opioid receptor and an antagonist at the kappa-opioid receptor. Its half-life is 37 hours. It is also available as a combined medication with naloxone. It should be administered at least 4 hours after the use of opioids and when early withdrawal signs appear. It should be used cautiously in patients using other sedative-hypnotics because of coma and death.
   B. Methadone: It is an opioid-receptor agonist. It can be used for detoxification and maintenance treatment. It has a half-life of 24 to 36 hours.

These medications for treating substance dependence should always be combined with a behavioral modification program to increase the possibility of maintaining abstinence.

9. CONDUCTING THE RISK ASSESSMENT

Most clinicians associate the term "risk assessment" with completing a suicide or homicide assessment. Although suicide and homicide risk assessment is a major part of the risk assessment process, there are many other risks involved when treating a psychiatric patient. The risk assessment is also situation specific and time limited. It is a process and not an event.

The risk assessment for a psychiatric patient could be divided into the following subheadings:

- Worsening of primary illness
- Worsening of comorbid conditions: psychiatric/medical
- Worsening of substance abuse/dependence
- Suicide risk
- Homicide risk
- Medication nonadherence
- Worsening of social issues: education/occupation/relationships

These factors can be further assessed based on the following factors:

- Previous history
- Severity of symptoms/disorders
- Motivation for change
- Previous treatments
- Adherence to treatments

Severe illness, untreated or poorly treated conditions, and nonadherence to recommended treatments are all poor prognostic indicators. Comorbid substance abuse and poor social and occupational functioning also worsen prognosis.

The risks can be further subdivided into short term and long term. If the patient has good short-term prognostic indicators, then the chance of long-term prognosis is also good.

Suicide and homicide risks can be specifically assessed based on the following:

- Intent
- Severity of attempt
- Premeditation
- Concealment
- Substance use
- Psychiatric comorbidity
- Treatment
- Adherence to treatment

Attempts with intent to die or kill, premeditation, and an effort to conceal increases the seriousness of an attempt. Comorbid substance use, untreated psychiatric disorder, and/or poor compliance with recommended treatments add to the risk.

10. ANSWERING DIFFICULT QUESTIONS

Often when the examinee is asked a question, he or she tends to jump to the answer without thinking about the question in depth. When a question is asked, it is better to think about it for a few seconds before beginning the answer. If the question is not clear, always clarify what is being asked before beginning the answer. Do not assume anything.

For every answer, start with the basics and work your way up. It is prudent not to say things that you are not clear on and to avoid controversial answers.

Do not argue with examiners, as it shows poor etiquette. If you do not agree with the examiner, you can always state that your understanding of the issue is different. Do not be rigid; show some flexibility in your thinking.

If you are not sure of the answer, say so clearly. No one is expected to know everything. Honesty is the best option in such situations.

Knowledge of nationally accepted guidelines for the treatment of common psychiatric disorders (APA, Royal College of Psychiatrists) is always a plus. You are expected to have a knowledge of the national practice standards but not the latest research data.

Suggested Readings

Albers LJ, Hahn RK, Reist C. *Handbook of Psychiatric Drugs*. Laguna Hills: Current Clinical Strategies Publishing, 2008:8–115.

Hales RE, Yudofsky SC, Gabbard GO. The *American Psychiatric Publishing Textbook of Psychiatry*. 5th Ed. Arlington, VA: American Psychiatric Publishing, Inc., 2008, http://www.psychiatryonline.com/content.aspx?aID=290004, last accessed on January 26, 2009.

Kaplan HI, Sadock BJ. *Kaplan and Sadock's Synopsis of Psychiatry*. 8th Ed. Philadelphia, PA: Lippincott Williams & Wilkins, 1998:240–317.

Quick Reference to the Diagnostic Criteria From DSM-IV-TR™. American Psychiatric Association, Washington DC, 2000:37–319.

Moore TA, Buchanan RW, Buckley PF, et al. The Texas Medication Algorithm Project antipsychotic algorithm for schizophrenia: 2006 update. *J Clin Psychiatry* 2007 Nov;68(11):1751–1762.

CHAPTER 3

Case Vignettes and Discussions

A. Psychotic disorders

Joshua Kantrowitz, MD, Kalyani Subramanyam, MD

I. SCHIZOPHRENIA

CASE HISTORY

PRESENT ILLNESS

Mr S is a 34-year-old, single, white man, who is seen in weekly outpatient therapy at the local state mental health center and takes aripiprazole 15 mg and olanzapine 5 mg daily. He reports that he is doing OK at present. He was last hospitalized about 2 months ago, after his father's death from a long battle with congestive heart failure. He had been at his baseline until about 3 months before his father's death. At this time, his father's health began to deteriorate, and he was hospitalized on multiple occasions. Mr S repeatedly stated that he was fine but would with increasing frequency state that his father was faking the illness, because "he was afraid that I will take over the business." He continued to show up for appointments on time, but his psychiatrist began to get calls from his work supervisor about his erratic behavior, such as "distrusting stares." He was hospitalized 2 days after his father's death and was discharged 1 week later after the addition of olanzapine 5 mg to his aripiprazole 15 mg. He was evasive on whether he was taking his medication as prescribed prior to admission.

On the current interview, the patient continues to complain about his father "messing up" his inheritance. He is able to accurately describe various aspects of the large collection of old books his father had collected. He admits to feeling like he should be in charge at work but has kept this to himself more often. On direct questioning, he states that people have been talking about him when he is alone in his apartment and knows that they do not like him because they put scratches on his car, although he is unable to provide details or a clear rationale of who might be doing this. These incidents are rarely spontaneously brought up. Other than work, he has a few friends with whom he socializes with about once a week.

He denies any sustained mood changes, neurovegetative symptoms, or any history of elated mood or decreased need for sleep for several days in a row. He does not use any illicit drugs, nor does he admit to any memory problems. He is not currently having any thoughts of hurting himself or others.

PSYCHIATRIC HISTORY

The patient's first contact with mental health services was at age 21, after being hospitalized for a psychotic breakdown. He stopped going to college after 1 year, "because I didn't feel like going." He lived at home with his father, rarely leaving his room except to argue with his father that he should be in charge of the family bookstore. He was first hospitalized after verbally harassing customers at the store and was started on haloperidol. He was rehospitalized four times in the next 5 years, typically after stopping his haloperidol (usually 10 to 20 mg). He described that haloperidol made his "eyes go up," which was why he frequently stopped it. His arguments with his father grew more intense, and eventually he left home, and was briefly homeless. He was started on olanzapine, obtained Social Security Disability, and began regular treatment at the local mental health center. He took olanzapine 15 mg for the next several years and was only hospitalized once in 6 years. He gradually became more connected to his treatment center and began working part time there through a vocational rehabilitation center.

Approximately 2 years ago, he began complaining that he was gaining too much weight, and laboratory screening revealed elevated LDL and total cholesterol and elevated LFTs, along with a weight gain of 30 lb over the past 6 years. He was slowly changed to aripiprazole monotherapy. His LFTs and cholesterol remained elevated, but his weight decreased by 10 lb. He remained on aripiprazole monotherapy until his most recent hospitalization. There is no evidence of sexual or physical abuse, but Mr S admits to frequent verbal altercations with his father. He denied any history of alcohol or illicit drug use. He has no known arrests but was brought to the hospital several times by the police earlier in his illness.

FAMILY HISTORY

The patient's sister was diagnosed with schizophrenia. His father died of congestive heart failure at age 78.

SOCIAL HISTORY

Mr S was born in upstate New York. His parents were in their mid 40s when he was born and they divorced when he was 9. He is Episcopalian. He completed one semester of college, before getting several "incompletes" in his spring semester and dropping out. He moved back home and lived with his father for several years before the constant altercations with his father led him to become briefly homeless. After a subsequent hospitalization, and with the help of case management, he found his own studio apartment and gradually became reconnected with his father. He began working part-time at the family bookstore. He also works part-time in a vocational rehabilitation center job at his mental health center. He does not appear to have had any intimate relationships, now or in the past, but occasionally talks about wanting to go on dates with women. He has no children.

PERTINENT MEDICAL HISTORY

Mr S has a history of hyperlipidemia and mild transaminitis of unknown etiology.

MENTAL STATUS EXAMINATION

Mr S presented as a mildly obese, white man who looked his stated age. He was slightly disheveled but his general personal hygiene was good. He was cooperative, with good eye contact, punctuated by occasional blinking and grimacing. His speech was of appropriate rate, rhythm, volume, and spontaneity. His psychomotor activity was normal. His affect was of constricted range and diminished intensity. He seemed inappropriately nonplussed when discussing his father's death. His mood was described as "fine." His thought process was linear at first but became rapidly tangential under moderate pressure or with longer utterances. His thought content was notable for probable paranoid delusions that people were conspiring against him in his apartment, attenuated grandiose delusions that he should be in charge at work and home, and possible somatic delusions that he is healthy, despite clear medical evidence against this. He also admits to probable auditory hallucinations that people in his building are saying bad things about him. He denied any suicidal or homicidal ideations, intent, or plan as well as any obsessions. On the Folstein Mini-Mental State Examination, he scored 30/30 indicating that he had good cognitive functioning. His insight was fair; he could admit to having schizophrenia but was unable to elaborate further. His judgment was poor; he attends every scheduled appointment but is intermittently compliant with medications and extremely reluctant to make changes in his regimen, even if strongly encouraged by his psychiatrist.

PERTINENT PHYSICAL FINDINGS

Other than obesity and blood pressure of 142/89, the physical exam was essentially within normal limits.

LABORATORY DATA

ALT was 75, and AST was 73. Total cholesterol was 250, triglycerides were 278, LDL was 165, and HDL 34. Other liver function tests, CBC, general chemistry, and TSH were within normal limits.

TWO-MONTH OUTPATIENT COURSE

Mr S continued to come to his outpatient appointments and showed no further signs of decompensation. He remained on the same outpatient medications and continued to socialize occasionally and to decline to follow up with his medical provider.

DSM-IV-TR MULTIAXIAL DIAGNOSIS

Axis I. Schizophrenia, chronic paranoid type
Axis II. None
Axis III. Dyslipidemia, obesity, chronic mild transaminitis, borderline hypertension, mild tardive dyskinesia
Axis IV. Severity of psychosocial stressor: severe, death of father
Axis V. Global assessment of functioning: 40

FORMULATION

A. Diagnostic

This patient meets the DSM-IV-TR criteria for schizophrenia, chronic paranoid type. He has multiple fixed delusions and hallucinations, which have been present for years and cause significant dysfunction. These symptoms do not take place solely during an affective episode. His symptoms produce significant dysfunction in both his social and his occupational activities. In addition, he does not have prominent disorganized speech or behavior, or flat or inappropriate affect.

The distinction between schizophrenia and schizoaffective disorder can be challenging, especially without a thorough psychiatric history. Since Mr S does not always appear to be fully forthcoming and reliable, it remains possible that earlier in his illness his loud, irritable explosions were part of a manic episode, and bipolar disorder with psychotic features and schizoaffective disorder should be considered in the differential diagnosis. Moreover, substances do not appear to be a part of his illness, and given his classic course, a general medical illness is unlikely to play a significant role in his symptoms. However, further history, especially prior records that may elucidate his early course and any laboratory data, especially urine toxicology, would be helpful in clarifying the diagnosis. Mr S also has clear evidence (grimacing and blinking) of mild tardive dyskinesia.

This patient does not meet criteria for other Axis I disorders, including mood or substance abuse disorders, which are frequently seen in patients with schizophrenia. He also does not meet criteria for an anxiety or cognitive disorder.

Important Axis II disorders to rule out in patients with schizophrenia include schizotypal and paranoid personality disorders. While Mr S does have some notable personality traits, including narcissistic personality traits, one cannot diagnose a personality disorder in the context of an active Axis I disorder. In regard to the different subtypes of schizophrenia, Mr S meets criteria for the paranoid subtype, due to the presence of prominent delusions and hallucinations and in the absence of prominent disorganization or flat affect (ruling out the disorganized subtype) or prominent catatonic behavior (ruling out the catatonic subtype). Some consideration should be given to residual subtype, given the attenuation of some of his major symptoms.

B. Etiologic

Biologically, Mr S appears to have a predisposing genetic risk for psychotic illness, given his sister's diagnosis. He also has a classic course and response to treatment, as his relapses are often associated with, and possibly precipitated by, nonadherence to his psychotropics. There is no evidence of substance use, particularly cannabis, nor any head trauma, seizures, or obstetric complications, which are all purported to increase the likelihood of developing psychosis. Psychologically, parental divorce prior to age 11 can predispose to major mental illness, particularly depression. His latest relapse was clearly temporally associated in time with the rapid deterioration and death of his father, whom he had ambivalent feelings toward. He also has, even at baseline, narcissistic traits, as evidenced by his constant claims of wanting to be in charge. These may perpetuate his tendency to have grandiose delusions. Socially, he has lost a major, if conflicted, social support. He does have the protective strengths of long-standing employment, and a generally independent life, with at least a few friends. In the past, his decompensations appear to have been at least partially precipitated by a high expressed emotion (EE) environment in his household.

C. Therapeutic

Antipsychotics remain the first-line biological treatment for schizophrenia. Currently, Mr S is on a combination of two antipsychotics—olanzapine

5 mg and aripiprazole 15 mg. Most major treatment guidelines suggest that patients be optimized on one antipsychotic agent as monotherapy before polypharmacy is tried. Clearly, Mr S is not on the maximal dosages of either agent, which leaves plenty of room to increase one medication while stopping the other. There is evidence, from the Clinical Antipsychotic Trials of Intervention Effectiveness (CATIE) and other studies, that olanzapine is among the most effective first-line antipsychotics, and Mr S seemed to stabilize after the addition of it, although this stabilization was accompanied by major social changes in his life as well. Olanzapine, however, is also clearly associated with a preponderance of weight gain and dyslipidemia, as has been noted by the patient in the past.

Each of his antipsychotics has room for a dosage increase to reach the maximum doses typically used, but a past efficacy and Mr S's preferences should play a role in this decision. Other biological treatments should include an examination of his general health, as he has clear health issues that he is not addressing, possibly because of delusional reasons. An effort should be made to contact his primary care provider to coordinate care. In addition, his mild tardive dyskinesia should be monitored.

A critical intervention in Mr S's treatment should be to prevent and treat the development of metabolic syndrome. His significant weight gain and hyperlipidemia should be monitored regularly, and he should be encouraged to follow a low-fat, low-calorie diet and to exercise regularly. If these measures prove not to be helpful enough, pharmacotherapy should be considered.

Psychological treatment should include a consideration of grief therapy for the death of his father, with special care given not to explore further than the patient is comfortable, as he has stated that he does not wish to discuss his father's death. This inclination may change over time, and one should follow the patient's lead, as his relationship with his father has clearly been both a precipitating and a propagating risk factor over the years. Supportive therapy, however, is usually the treatment of choice for schizophrenia. There is also evidence that Cognitive Behavioral Therapy can be helpful for delusions. Socially, Mr S is clearly benefiting from his vocational treatment but might benefit from more organized vocational intervention, as working is clearly a protective strength for him. Group treatment might also be helpful, given that Mr S is relatively socially isolated.

D. Prognostic

Over the short term, Mr S has a guarded prognosis. On the one hand, he has, for a number of years, done quite well in the community. On the other, he has just lost one of the closest, if conflicted, relationships in his life. He also has had a recent relapse associated in time with his father's death and probable nonadherence to his medication regimen. Over the long term, Mr S has actually done quite well for a patient with schizophrenia, as evidenced by several years of employment and independent living with only a few hospitalizations. He also seems to have weathered his father's death without serious incidents. If he continues to follow up with treatment, there is a good chance of at least maintaining his current state of functioning for the foreseeable future. His long-term prognosis for general health issues, however, is more worrisome, given his near delusional avoidance of his primary care doctor and clear history of lipid abnormalities. Positive prognostic indicators include lack of any suicidal or homicidal ideation in his history and no clear history of any substance use.

SCHIZOPHRENIA

1. Introduction

Schizophrenia is a complex condition, increasingly recognized as a neurodevelopmental disorder. DSM-IV-TR criteria include having at least two of the following five symptoms for a one-month period: (a) delusions, (b) hallucinations, (c) disorganized speech, (d) grossly disorganized or catatonic behavior, and (e) negative symptoms. Having only bizarre delusions, or hallucinations that affect behavior or hallucinations of conversing voices, would also meet criteria. Additionally, symptoms must last at least 6 months, associated with marked impairment in functioning and not be better explained by another condition. This is a chronic, usually severe, condition that affects multiple aspects of patients' lives and is a significant cause of disability.

2. Epidemiology

The prevalence of schizophrenia is commonly reported as 1% of the adult population worldwide, although some report lower percentages. Typical onset is during adolescence, with peak ages of diagnosis being 20 to 28 years for men and 26 to 32 years for women. The disease is often subdivided into several phases: premorbid, prodromal (attenuated symptoms), psychotic (full presence of symptoms), and residual (between prodromal and active psychosis, with a lack of a return to baseline). Often patients shift between periods of active psychotic exacerbations and residual phases. There does not appear to be any clear racial difference as far as prevalence goes.

The economic burden of schizophrenia is large, including psychosocial disability costs (unemployment, disability payments), hospitalization costs, and outpatient clinical and social rehabilitation costs. The acquisition costs of the newer antipsychotic medications also play a role in this large economic burden. The cost-effectiveness of the second-generation antipsychotics has been questioned, with recent studies raising serious doubts. The cost-effectiveness component of CATIE found that average monthly health care costs were $US300 to $US500 greater with the newer second-generation medications than with perphenazine, with generally no significant advantage in symptom control or quality of life. Other studies and systematic reviews have come to similar conclusions.

3. Etiology

Clear cause-and-effect relationships for schizophrenia are unknown, but advances have been made recently. Since the 1960s, the dopamine hypothesis has been prominent (i.e., schizophrenia is caused by excess dopamine in the brain), and although this explains part of the process, the pathophysiology is substantially more complex. Although a full survey is beyond the scope of this review book, the ultimate etiology of schizophrenia may be related to disturbances in regulation of trophic genes such as neuregulin or dysbindin, neurochemical alterations, and adverse environmental events. However, disturbances of specific neurotransmitter systems, particularly dopamine, glutamate, and gamma-aminobutyric acid (GABA) may be the proximate cause of symptoms and neurocognitive deficits. Other, not mutually exclusive, theories include a deficit in myelin or white matter, aberrant synaptic pruning, and an association with adolescent cannabis. Genetic evidence is sometimes conflicting, but several putative susceptibility genes (including COMT, DISC1, RGS4, GRM3, and G72) have been identified.

Postmortem studies have identified localized alterations of specific neuronal, synaptic, and glial populations in the hippocampus, dorsolateral prefrontal cortex, and dorsal thalamus. Inhibitory interneurons are particularly affected, demonstrated by a decrease in their number, diminished expression of synthesizing enzyme, diminished expression of neuropeptides, and decreased migration of neurons into the cortex from the underlying white matter. The total number of neurons is diminished in certain areas of the brain, and moreover, magnetic resonance imaging (MRI) demonstrates corresponding enlarged ventricles and diminished volume in the hippocampus and the superior temporal cortex.

4. Diagnosis

The DSM-IV-TR criteria are shown in Table 3A.1.

While the most striking symptoms of schizophrenia are the positive symptoms (easy-to-spot behaviors not typically seen in healthy people that usually involve a loss of contact with reality, i.e., delusions or hallucinations), it is often the less obvious symptoms that are more associated with poor functioning. Although the presence of positive symptoms does not automatically denote schizophrenia, it is difficult to make this diagnosis without them, particularly in a short interview.

Delusions are typically defined as fixed false beliefs not accepted by other members of one's culture. While phenomenological descriptions of delusions are not a hot area of current research, one recent study found evidence for the distress associated with delusions as well as beliefs involving persecution and loss of control to be the most relevant aspects in distinguishing persons with schizophrenia from persons without schizophrenia. Note that the delusions seen in schizophrenia are typically bizarre, in contrast to the non-bizarre delusions of delusional disorder.

Hallucinations (perceptions in the absence of stimulus) are also common in schizophrenia. As with delusions, hallucinations are not pathognomonic of schizophrenia but lie on a continuum, being present in a not insignificant percentage of normative populations, at least in an attenuated form. Nonetheless, auditory hallucinations are common in schizophrenia, being present in greater than 60% of patients. Visual hallucinations are not uncommon, nor are tactile or olfactory. The presence of the latter two should at least raise the suspicion for substance withdrawal or CNS pathology.

TABLE 3A.1 Diagnostic Criteria for Schizophrenia

Criterion A: Having at least two of the following five characteristic symptoms: (a) delusions, (b) hallucinations, (c) grossly disorganized behavior, (d) catatonic behavior, and (e) negative symptoms. Only one of these symptoms is required if delusions are bizarre (see above) or hallucinations consist of a voice keeping up a running commentary on the person's behavior or thoughts or two or more voices conversing with each other.
Criterion B: Social/occupational dysfunction, e.g., having impaired functioning in one or more major areas such as work, interpersonal relations, and self-care.
Criterion C: Continuous symptoms persist for at least 6 months, including at least 1 month of active phase symptoms (or less, if successfully treated) that meet criterion A and may include periods of prodromal or residual symptoms (only negative symptoms or two or more attenuated symptoms, e.g., odd beliefs, unusual perceptual experiences).
Criterion D: Excludes schizoaffective disorder and mood disorder with psychotic features because either (a) no mood episodes have occurred with the active-phase symptoms, or (b) the total duration of mood symptoms has been brief relative to the duration of the active and residual periods.
Criterion E: Excludes that the disturbance is due to a drug of abuse or a medication, or a general medical condition.
Criterion F: States that if there is a history of a pervasive developmental disorder, schizophrenia is diagnosed only if prominent delusions or hallucinations are also present for at least a month (or less, if successfully treated).

Adapted from American Psychiatric Association. *Diagnostic and Statistical Manual of Mental Disorders*. 4th Ed. Text Revision. Washington, DC: American Psychiatric Association, 2000.

Disorganized speech (e.g., frequent derailment or incoherence) is often found in schizophrenia. Such a formal thought disorder can make communication difficult. Classic examples of disorganized speech/thought include circumstantiality (meandering path to the point), tangentiality (continued connection between sentences, but clearly moving off track), loose associations (minimal connection between words, classically described with mania), and word salad (virtually incoherent and uninterviewable for the most part). These distinctions are of unclear clinical significance.

Negative symptoms, or reductions in normal emotional and behavioral states, are often associated with disability. Negative symptoms often manifest as reduction of certain normal functions or behaviors—impairment of normal affect and emotion—of normal social interaction, purpose, and motivation. An example of negative symptoms is a patient who rarely smiles (affective flattening) or leaves the house (amotivation), has few social contacts other than family (asociality), rarely bathes, has little to no sexual interest, and tends to answer questions with one to two sentences (alogia or poverty of speech). Screening questions can include "How do you spend a usual day?" and "Do you have any close friends outside the family?"

Additionally, schizophrenia often occurs with significant impairment in cognition and a substantial decline in premorbid IQ. Impaired performance on measures of neurocognition is closely linked to community outcome. It can be difficult to screen for this in a short interview, but testing abstract thought by asking for proverbs and similarities can be done quickly.

Substance abuse is common in patients with schizophrenia, with some studies reporting up to 50% comorbidity, and it has been associated with more severe symptoms and a poorer outcome. Screening for substance abuse can be done in the same way that it is done in other disorders. Schizophrenia is also correlated with poor physical health, including higher rates of obesity, diabetes, hypertension, metabolic syndrome, and cardiovascular disease. This risk is multifactorial, involving shared vulnerability, genetic factors, unhealthy lifestyle, and the potential impact of antipsychotics. For any patient on atypical antipsychotics, one should ask about diabetes, cardiovascular disease, and lipid abnormalities and be prepared to discuss their relationship with these medications.

The differential diagnosis for psychotic symptoms is broad, and one should rarely definitively diagnose a patient with schizophrenia on an initial interview.

5. Treatments

A. NONPHARMACOLOGICAL TREATMENTS

While the classic psychotherapy of choice for schizophrenia is supportive therapy, the evidence for its effectiveness is weak, and a familiarity with several other evidence-based treatments (see Table 3A.2 for a review of these treatments) is key. These treatment modalities work best in combination.

B. PHARMACOLOGICAL TREATMENTS

Antipsychotics are the mainstay of treatment for schizophrenia, and although agents with novel mechanisms of action are on the horizon, at present, all marketed antipsychotics have in common a blockade of the dopamine type 2 (D_2) receptor, and primarily are only effective on positive symptoms. There is evidence that all available antipsychotics, with the exception of clozapine and possibly olanzapine, have approximately equivalent efficacy. Others have found advantages for clozapine, olanzapine, amisulpride, and risperidone in a systematic review. As reviewed here, olanzapine and risperidone may be the most effective first-line choices.

Conventional or first-generation antipsychotics are primarily D_2 blockers, and can be divided into three groups: high, medium, and low potencies. High potency is generally associated with a higher rate of extrapyramidal symptoms (EPS), namely, acute dystonia, parkinsonism, or akathisia; haloperidol is a representative example. Low potency is generally associated with higher sedation and anticholinergic side effects; chlorpromazine is a representative example. Medium potency is generally somewhere in between, with perphenazine being a representative example.

TABLE 3A.2 Evidence-Based Therapies for the Treatment of Schizophrenia

1. Cognitive behavior therapy (CBT) for schizophrenia addresses residual positive symptoms that remain after medication treatment. CBT helps develop alternative explanations for symptoms to reduce their impact on behavior.
2. Cognitive remediation (CR) seeks to improve cognitive symptoms using a variety of tests requiring cognitive skills such as attention, planning, problem solving, and/or memory. Many successful CR programs work in tandem with psychosocial groups or other treatment modalities.
3. Social skills training seeks to improve social interactions, e.g., negative symptoms. Examples include nonverbal behavior such as appropriate eye contact and voice volume, conversational skills such as introducing oneself to a new person and taking the perspective of another person, and problem-solving skills such as expressing dissatisfaction and generating solutions to interpersonal problems.
4. Although traditional 12-step programs such as AA may be helpful for some patients, integrated treatments for dual-diagnosis (substance disorder and schizophrenia) patients include intensive case management, motivational interviewing, specialized 12-step programs, CBT, social skills training, contingency management, and family psychoeducation.
5. Supported employment programs emphasize rapid placement and often work best with a place-then-train philosophy in which training takes place in the job setting.
6. Family psychoeducation offers information and support for family members who care for their relatives who have schizophrenia, as high levels of criticism and overinvolvement by family members can increase the risk of relapse.

Adapted from Velligan DI, Gonzalez JM. Rehabilitation and recovery in schizophrenia. *Psychiatr Clin N Am* 2007;30:535–548.

Atypical or second-generation antipsychotics bind primarily to different degrees to both the D_2 receptor and the serotonin 2A receptor ($5\text{-}HT_{2A}$). In addition, all demonstrate some antagonism at other dopamine and serotonin receptors. All are distinguished from the first-generation antipsychotics by a lower propensity for causing EPS. In addition to paliperidone and risperidone, the second-generation agents currently marketed in the United States are clozapine, olanzapine, quetiapine, ziprasidone, and aripiprazole.

Adverse effects are a significant issue for all antipsychotics and, to a certain extent, distinguish the various medications, particularly the second-generation antipsychotics, from each other. Although more commonly seen with the first-generation antipsychotics, all have the potential of causing EPS. Tardive dyskinesia is a disfiguring, potentially disabling, and potentially permanent movement disorder associated with antipsychotics, which may be more common with first-generation drugs, although this is debated. Second-generation antipsychotics also have a higher propensity for weight gain and dyslipidemia, with this effect being less for risperidone and quetiapine compared with clozapine and olanzapine and least frequent with aripiprazole and ziprasidone. Glucose abnormalities are likely more common with second-generation agents as well. Other potential side effects of both first- and second-generation antipsychotics include hyperprolactinemia, orthostatic hypotension, blood dyscrasias, gastrointestinal distress, and neuroleptic malignant syndrome. Often, an individual drug's side effect profile must be matched with the individual patient.

6. Prognosis

Classically, there are several good prognostic indicators for the long-term course of schizophrenia. These include female sex and a sudden onset of symptoms after a previously normal development. Patients having the opposite attributes (males and patients with an insidious onset) more typically have a grim outcome. Follow-up studies of 15 to 25 years suggest that approximately 50% of patients with schizophrenia have moderately good outcomes. A recent review reported that recent studies suggest that poor insight predicts poor outcome, potentially because of poor adherence to medications. A longer duration of untreated psychosis can predict a poorer long-term outcome. Conversely, early positive treatment response predicts a better long-term outcome. Some cognitive deficits can also predict long-term functioning.

7. General Formulation for Schizophrenia

A. DIAGNOSTIC

Schizophrenia is a psychotic disorder, and a patient must meet the criteria detailed above. It is important to rule out prominent mood symptoms, active substance use, and medical problems that can confuse the diagnosis. The most common mood disorder in the differential diagnosis is bipolar disorder with psychotic features. In addition, an important psychotic disorder to rule out is schizoaffective disorder. A key difference is the presence of psychotic features in the absence of mood symptomatology seen in schizoaffective disorder. The use of substances such as LSD, PCP, or hallucinogens can cause psychotic symptoms that resemble schizophrenia. It is important to screen for delusions, hallucinations, negative and cognitive symptoms, and disorganized thought.

B. ETIOLOGIC

The etiology of schizophrenia is broad, but current theories emphasize a neurodevelopmental hypothesis and genetic vulnerability (both individual genes and family history). The etiology of relapses is clearer, and it is important to consider the presence/absence of psychological and social stressors, medication adherence, and substance misuse.

C. THERAPEUTIC

Despite their limitations, antipsychotic medications are the best treatment for this condition. A good therapeutic relationship and consideration of individualized psychotherapies detailed above are also important. Stable housing, financial support, and physical health are obviously important as well. With the widespread use of atypical antipsychotics, prevention and adequate treatment of metabolic syndrome are of paramount importance in this patient population, since it has a direct impact on their morbidity and mortality.

D. PROGNOSTIC

Perpetuating factors and factors associated with relapse in schizophrenia include medication noncompliance, male gender, concomitant substance use, and limited cognitive function. On the other hand, protective and good prognostic factors include initial response to treatment, female gender, and lack of negative symptoms.

8. Risk Assessment

Beyond the general diagnostic interview, one should do a careful risk assessment with patients with schizophrenia. These factors all contribute significantly to the frequently tragic outcome for these patients. Important areas to cover, as reviewed by Kooyman et al., include the following:

a. Substance dependence/abuse/misuse: 40% to 60% of patients misuse substances, raising the risk for most of these other risk factors.
b. Suicidality: Risk of suicide is 5% to 13%, especially early in illness. Other risk factors include recent loss, with fear of mental disintegration; agitation or motor restlessness; poor adherence to treatment; drug misuse; and previous depressive disorders and suicide attempts.
c. Medication adherence: Medication nonadherence can lead to worse outcome in virtually all of these risk factors.
d. Physical health: Patients are at higher risk for metabolic syndrome and early death.
e. Command auditory hallucinations: These can lead to violence and suicide and must be asked about.
f. Housing: 20% to 30% of patients are homeless at least at some point in their lives.
g. Unemployment: 80% to 90% are unemployed.
h. Violence: Schizophrenia patients are somewhat more likely than the general population to be violent, especially patients who are medication nonadherent, use substances, or are actively psychotic.
i. Victimization: Patients are twice as likely to be victims of violence, irrespective of the patient's own violent tendencies.

KEY POINTS (ABPN Examination)

A. When interviewing a patient with schizophrenia

1. Psychosis has a broad differential, including primary medical, affective, and substance use problems. Attempt to screen for these other disorders before settling on schizophrenia.
2. Building rapport by listening is obviously important, but little is gained by letting a disorganized patient ramble.
3. Schizophrenia is more than just positive symptoms; be sure to ask about negative and cognitive symptoms also.
4. Do not forget physical health, medication adherence, and the other risk factors noted above.

B. When presenting a patient with schizophrenia

1. If diagnosis is unclear, state that you would use a structured diagnostic interview like SCID-DSM-IV for clarification.

Suggested Readings

Akbarian S, Kim J, Potkin S, et al. Maldistribution of interstitial neurons in prefrontal white matter of the brains of schizophrenic patients. *Arch Gen Psychiatry* 1996;53:425–436.

American Psychiatric Association. *Diagnostic and Statistical Manual of Mental Disorders*. 4th Ed. Text Revision. Washington, DC: American Psychiatric Association, 2000.

Benes F, Kwok E, Vincent S, et al. A reduction of nonpyramidal cells in sector CA2 of schizophrenics and manic depressives. *Biol Psychiatry* 1998;44:88–97.

Boks M, Rietkerk T, van de Beek M, et al. Reviewing the role of the genes G72 and DAAO in glutamate neurotransmission in schizophrenia. *Eur Neuropsychopharmacol* 2007;17:567–572.

Butler RW, Braff DL. Delusions: A Review and Integration. *Schizophr Bull* 1991;17:633–647.

Castle E, Wessely S, Der G, et al. The incidence of operationally defined schizophrenia in Camberwell 1965–84. *Br J Psychiatry* 1991;159: 790–794.

Choong C, Hunter MD, Woodruff PWR. Auditory hallucinations in those populations that do not suffer from schizophrenia. *Curr Psychiatry Rep* 2007;9:206–212.

Citrome L. The effectiveness criterion: Balancing efficacy against the risk of weight gain. *J Clin Psychiatry* 2007;68:12–17.

Citrome L, Kantrowitz J. Using antipsychotics for the treatment of schizophrenia: Likelihood to be helped or harmed, understanding proximal and distal benefits and risks. *Expert Rev Neurother* 2008;8:1079–1091.

Correll C, Leucht S, Kane JM. Lower risk for tardive dyskinesia associated with second-generation antipsychotics: A systematic review of 1-year studies. *Am J Psychiatry* 2004;161:414–425.

Davis J, Chen N, Glick I. A meta-analysis of the efficacy of second-generation antipsychotics. *Arch Gen Psychiatry* 2003;60:553–564.

Davis KL, Stewart DG, Friedman JI, et al. White matter changes in schizophrenia. *Arch Gen Psychiatry* 2003;60:443–456.

Di Forti M, Lappin JM, Murray RM. Risk factors for schizophrenia—All roads lead to dopamine. *Eur Neuropsychopharmacol* 2007;17:S101–S107.

Emsley R, Chiliza B, Schoeman R. Predictors of long-term outcome in schizophrenia. *Curr Opin Psychiatry* 2008;21:173–177.

Goldner EM, Hsu L, Waraich P, et al. Prevalence and incidence studies of schizophrenic disorders: A systematic review of the literature. *Can J Psychiatry* 2002;47:833–843.

Green AI, Drake RE, Brunette MF, et al. Schizophrenia and co-occurring substance use disorder. *Am J Psychiatry* 2007;164:402–408.

Green M, Kern R, Braff D, et al. Neurocognitive deficits and functional outcome in schizophrenia: are we measuring the "right stuff"? *Schizophr Bull* 2000;26:119–136.

Hafner H, an der Heiden H. The course of schizophrenia in the light of modern follow-up studies: The ABC and WHO studies. *Eur Arch Psychiatry Clin Neurosci* 1999;249:14–26.

Harrison G, Hopper K, Craig T, et al. Recovery from psychotic illness: A 15- and 25-year international follow-up study. *Br J Psychiatry* 2001;178:506–517.

Harrison P, Weinberger D. Schizophrenia genes, gene expression, and neuropathology: On the matter of their convergence. *Mol Psychiatry* 2005;10:40–68.

Heresco-Levy U, Javitt DC, Ebstein R, et al. D-serine efficacy as add-on pharmacotherapy to risperidone and olanzapine for treatment-refractory schizophrenia. *Biol Psychiatry* 2005;57:577–585.

Hoffman RE, McGlashan TH. Synaptic elimination, neurodevelopment, and the mechanism of hallucinated "voices" in schizophrenia. *Am J Psychiatry* 1997;154:1683–1689.

Javitt DC. Glutamate as a therapeutic target in psychiatric disorders. *Mol Psychiatry* 2004;9:984–997.

Jeste D, Lohr J. Hippocampal pathologic findings in schizophrenia: A morphometric study. *Arch Gen Psychiatry* 1989;46:1019–1024.

Jones P, Barnes T, Davies L, et al. Randomized controlled trial of the effect on quality of life of second- vs first-generation antipsychotic drugs in schizophrenia: Cost Utility of the Latest Antipsychotic Drugs in Schizophrenia Study (CUtLASS 1). *Arch Gen Psychiatry* 2006; 63:1079–1087.

Keefe R, Perkins D, Gu H, et al. A longitudinal study of neurocognitive function in individuals at-risk for psychosis. *Schizophr Res* 2006;88:26–35.

Kooyman I, Dean K, Harvey S, et al. Outcomes of public concern in schizophrenia. *Br J Psychiatry* 2007;191:s29–s36.

Kubicki M, Shenton M, Salisbury D, et al. Voxel-based morphometric analysis of gray matter in first episode schizophrenia. *Neuroimage* 2002;17:1711–1719.

Lieberman JA, Stroup TS, McEvoy JP, et al. Effectiveness of antipsychotic drugs in patients with chronic schizophrenia. *N Engl J Med* 2005;353:1209–1253.

Lincoln TM. Relevant dimensions of delusions: Continuing the continuum versus category debate. *Schizophr Res* 2007;93:211–220.

McEvoy JP, Lieberman JA, Stroup TS, et al. Effectiveness of clozapine versus olanzapine, quetiapine, and risperidone in patients with chronic schizophrenia who did not respond to prior atypical antipsychotic treatment. *Am J Psychiatry* 2006;163:600–610.

Mitchell AJ, Malone D. Physical health and schizophrenia. *Curr Opin Psychiatry* 2006;19:432–437.

Moore TH, Zammit S, Lingford-Hughes A, et al. Cannabis use and risk of psychotic or affective mental health outcomes: A systematic review. *Lancet* 2007;370:319–328.

Muller N, Schwarz M. Schizophrenia as an inflammation-mediated dysbalance of glutamatergic neurotransmission. *Neurotox Res* 2006; 10:131–148.

Norton N, Williams HJ, Owen MJ. An update on the genetics of schizophrenia. *Curr Opin Psychiatry* 2006;19:158–164.

Patil ST, Zhang L, Martenyi F, et al. Activation of mGlu2/3 receptors as a new approach to treat schizophrenia: A randomized Phase 2 clinical trial. *Nat Med* 2007;13:1102–1107.

Polsky D, Doshi J, Bauer M, et al. Clinical trial based cost-effectiveness analyses of antipsychotic use. *Am J Psychiatry* 2006;163:2047–2056.

Reichenberg A, Weiser M, Rapp M, et al. Self-reported mental health difficulties and subsequent risk for schizophrenia in females: A 5-year follow-up cohort study. *Schizophr Res* 2005;82:233–239.

Rosenheck RA. Evaluating the cost-effectiveness of reduced tardive dyskinesia with second-generation antipsychotics. *Br J Psychiatry* 2007;191:238–245.

Rosenheck RA, Leslie D, Sindelar J, et al. Cost-effectiveness of second-generation antipsychotics and perphenazine in a randomized trial of treatment for chronic schizophrenia. *Am J Psychiatry* 2006;163:2080–2089.

Siegel S, Irani F, Brensinger C, et al. Prognostic variables at intake and long-term level of function in schizophrenia. *Am J Psychiatry* 2006; 163:433–441.

Stahl S, Buckley P. Negative symptoms of schizophrenia: A problem that will not go away. *Acta Psychiatr Scand* 2007;115:4–11.

Vacher CM, Gassmann M, Desrayaud S, et al. Hyperdopaminergia and altered locomotor activity in $GABA_{B1}$-deficient mice. *J Neurochem* 2006;97: 979–991.

Velligan DI, Gonzalez JM. Rehabilitation and recovery in schizophrenia. *Psychiatr Clin N Am* 2007;30:535–548.

Woo T, Whitehead R, Melchitzky D, et al. A subclass of prefrontal gamma-aminobutyric acid axon terminals are selectively altered in schizophrenia. *Proc Natl Acad Sci* 1998;95:5341–5346.

II. SCHIZOAFFECTIVE DISORDER

CASE HISTORY

PRESENT ILLNESS

Mr S is a 44-year-old white male who was admitted to the inpatient unit due to his family's concern that the patient was acting strange and was noted to be increasingly pressured, disorganized, and paranoid for the past 2 weeks. He was also noted to be yelling and frequently losing his temper.

On interview, the patient's speech was noted to be pressured, and he said that he felt "extremely happy." He reported that he had stopped taking medications for the past 2 weeks and felt elated. He felt that he was god and had the power to predict what would happen in the future. He also reported about voices from god that told him about what he should be doing every day. According to him, he had knowledge from the trees and the leaves that the world was coming to an end and that the devil would come and harm him knowing that he had special powers. Mr S reported having a revelation a few days back that he was not ready to discuss, and he also reported that other patients and staff on the unit were aware about his powers. He knew this because he felt that people were talking about it and when he entered the room, they stopped talking and turned their heads to the other side. He reported having racing thoughts and having difficulty concentrating on anything. During the interview, he was noted to be pacing around trying to do different things at the same time but having difficulty completing any of the tasks. He was also noted to be labile, at times laughing and at other times tearful. The patient stated that he had a lot of energy and needed only 3 to 4 hours of sleep every day. He denied any changes in appetite. The patient denied any anxiety symptoms, mood symptoms, suicidal or homicidal ideation. He denied any current use of alcohol or other illicit substances.

PSYCHIATRIC HISTORY

The patient has had three inpatient psychiatric hospitalizations and has been in outpatient treatment since age 25. His first contact with a psychiatrist was at the age of 25 when he ran amok following LSD ingestion. During that presentation, he reported paranoid thoughts that included Christ's crucifixion and its connection to his age. He said that these thoughts were frightening and he reported being afraid that he might die. He also had said that children in the schoolyard, which adjoins his apartment, were talking about him in a derogatory manner. He presented as disorganized and gravely disabled, requiring an inpatient hospitalization. During the course of that hospitalization, he remained psychotic, without significant mood symptoms, and was diagnosed with schizophrenia, paranoid type. He was started on a low dose of perphenazine, and the dose was tapered up to 48 mg. Although there was significant improvement in his symptoms and he became better functioning, some paranoid thoughts persisted. He was managed in the community with twice-a-week outpatient therapy and was doing fairly well, until about a year later when he presented to the psychiatric emergency room reporting a depressed mood, with low energy, feeling hopeless, reduced sleep and appetite, and some suicidal thoughts with a plan of overdosing on his medication; however, he was able to contract for safety. He also continued to have paranoid thoughts that the devil was going to harm him and that people around him were talking about him. He was admitted to the inpatient unit and was started on fluoxetine, and perphenazine was continued. There was significant improvement in his mood symptoms but the delusions continued; however they did not interfere with his functioning. Within a month of his discharge, he required his third inpatient hospitalization as he presented with floridly manic symptoms with delusions such as thinking of himself to be Christ, pressured speech, increased psychomotor activity, losing a large amount of money in gambling, and reduced sleep. He was started on valproate, 1,000 mg everyday, and a trial of risperidone and olanzapine was initiated. Once he was stabilized on this medication regimen, he was discharged back to the outpatient clinic. He gained a lot of weight and refused to take risperidone or olanzapine, so these medications were discontinued and he was restarted on perphenazine. Subsequently, he became increasingly noncompliant with his treatment. When his symptoms improved, he would discontinue medications, resulting in frequent manic episodes with delusions and auditory hallucinations. He would insist on taking charge of his medications and would not show up for appointments with his clinician.

SUBSTANCE HISTORY

The patient has a history of alcohol use from the age of 16. He was drinking about two to three beers on weekends, usually with friends. He stopped drinking when he was 30 years old. He has also experimented a few times with mushrooms, LSD, marijuana, and cocaine in his 20s. He denies any current use of illicit substances.

FAMILY HISTORY

The patient has a brother with a history of alcohol dependence and a sister with bipolar disorder.

SOCIAL HISTORY

Mr S was born in Massachusetts. He is the oldest of four children, three brothers and one sister. He is still connected to his family and the family is very supportive. He is Catholic. He completed his GED and worked as a truck driver for a few years. He is currently on disability due to his psychiatric problems. He has his own studio apartment. Brothers and parents live close by. He had a girlfriend in his 20s and broke up with her. He is not in any intimate relationship currently. He has never married and has no children.

PERTINENT MEDICAL HISTORY

Medical history is significant for hypertension and appendectomy.

MENTAL STATUS EXAMINATION

Mr S presented as an obese white male who looked older than his stated age. He looked disheveled and was poorly groomed. He was cooperative, with fleeting eye contact throughout the interview. He displayed some psychomotor agitation. His speech was coherent, with slightly increased tone, tempo, and volume. His speech was also pressured and was difficult to interrupt. He stated his mood as "I feel happy" and displayed a labile affect, tearful at times and laughing at other times. The thought process was tangential; the thought content was significant for grandiose delusions that he is god and that he has the power to predict the future and for paranoid delusions that the devil would come and harm him as he had special powers. He also reported self-referential delusions and felt that people were talking about him. He denied any suicidal or homicidal ideation, intent, or plan as well as any obsessions. He reported experiencing auditory hallucinations of the voice of god telling him what to do every day. His insight and judgment were poor as displayed by his lack of awareness of having a problem and being noncompliant with medications and treatment.

Cognitive functions: The patient was oriented to person, place, and time. He had difficulty spelling "EARTH" backward, but could name objects, register and recall 3/3 items, follow commands, write a sentence, and draw intersecting pentagons.

PERTINENT PHYSICAL FINDINGS

Vitals: heart rate 95, blood pressure 162/81, temperature 98.2, respiratory rate 16.

He was obese. His pupils were equal and reactive to light and accommodation. No jaundice, pallor, or lymphadenopathy was noted. The first and second heart sounds were heard and there was no murmur. Lungs were clear. Abdomen was soft, nontender, and there was no organomegaly. Bowel sounds were heard normally. Extremities showed normal capillary perfusion. Neurological examination was normal.

LABORATORY DATA

CBC, general chemistry, TSH, urinalysis, and LFT were within normal limits, urine toxicology screen was negative, and valproate level was undetectable.

HOSPITAL COURSE

The patient was restarted on valproate and the dose was increased gradually to 1,000 mg. He was also restarted on perphenazine and the dose was increased up to 48 mg. After starting this medication, the patient's mood lability was reduced. He started to have some insight into his problems. He understood the need for taking medication and agreed to take it regularly. A family session was conducted and the family agreed to help remind him about his medication. They were also educated about the early signs of relapse so that he could be brought to the hospital immediately. The patient continued to have some delusions of devils trying to harm him but he reported that these thoughts were not bothering him too much. He agreed to follow up with his primary clinician.

DISCHARGE MEDICATIONS

Valproate 1,000 mg at bedtime
Perphenazine 48 mg daily

DSM-IV-TR MULTIAXIAL DIAGNOSIS

Axis I: Schizoaffective disorder, bipolar type
Axis II: Deferred
Axis III. Hypertension, obesity, appendectomy
Axis IV: Unemployed, financial difficulties
Axis V: Global assessment of functioning
At admission: 21 to 30
At discharge: 31 to 40

FORMULATION

A. Diagnostic

This patient meets the DSM-IV-TR criteria for schizoaffective disorder, bipolar type. He has multiple delusions and auditory hallucination with concurrent mood symptoms. He also has delusions which are present for a duration of more than 2 weeks in the absence of mood symptoms. He meets the criteria for a bipolar subtype of schizoaffective disorder due to the occurrence of both manic episodes and depressive episodes with delusions and hallucinations. The patient has a history of occasional alcohol use but stopped using about 14 years back. He continued to have symptoms even after stopping alcohol, so the disturbance does not appear to be a direct physiologic effect of substance, and given his classical course, a general medical illness is unlikely to play a significant role in his symptoms. This patient does not meet the criteria for other Axis I disorders such as substance use disorder, anxiety disorder, and cognitive disorder.

On Axis II, Mr S does have some personality traits including narcissistic personality traits in view of his sense of entitlement. However, one cannot diagnose a personality disorder in the context of an active Axis I disorder.

B. Etiologic

The patient has a genetic predisposition for mood disorders and substance dependence in view of the bipolar disorder in his sister and alcohol dependence in his brother. His relapse of symptoms is often associated with or precipitated by nonadherence to medications. His initial episode appears to be precipitated by substance use, which included alcohol, cannabis, LSD, and mushroom. He does not have a history of head trauma or seizures, which can increase the likelihood of developing psychosis. He also had a breakup of an intimate relationship, which can further affect his mood symptoms. At baseline, he has narcissistic traits with a sense of entitlement to favorable treatment from others; this predisposes him to grandiose delusions that he has special powers. He predominantly uses the defense mechanism of projection and omnipotence. The delusion about special powers is both comforting and terrifying as he feels that it would evoke an attack by the devil, feeding into the delusion of persecution. Socially, his strengths are a good support system, living independently, having some connection with health care, and having no legal problems. Barriers are unemployment, financial difficulties, having few friends, and, though having health care, not keeping appointments.

C. Therapeutic

Mood stabilizers are the mainstay of the treatment of the bipolar-type schizoaffective disorder, and antipsychotics are important to treat the psychotic symptoms. The patient was started on valproate as a mood stabilizer for his manic symptoms. A trial of olanzapine and risperidone was tried earlier but the patient did not like these medications due to side effects. In view of this, perphenazine was started and it helped his psychotic symptoms. There are also data from CATIE that show that there is no difference in efficacy between typical and atypical antipsychotics for psychotic symptoms. The typical antipsychotics are also less expensive and add less to the economic burden for the patient compared to atypical antipsychotics. Mr S stabilized with the combination of valproate and perphenazine. Valproate has propensity to cause weight gain and as Mr S is already obese, it is important to monitor his weight and metabolic profile.

Psychological treatment should include consideration of supportive therapy and social skills training. Involving the family in his treatment is also important. Mr S may also benefit from vocational intervention.

D. Prognostic

In the short term, good prognostic factors for this patient are living independently, predominant mood symptoms, abstinence from substance use, no suicidal or homicidal ideation, good response to medication, and having a supportive family. Poor prognostic factors are presence of schizophrenia symptoms, social isolation, and medication noncompliance. In the long term, the patient had frequent hospitalizations though he has lived independently. His episodes have become more frequent probably owing to his treatment noncompliance. He had suicidal ideation during depressive episodes. His family has been a great source of support for him.

SCHIZOAFFECTIVE DISORDER

1. Introduction

The concept of schizoaffective disorder attempts to define patients who have features of both schizophrenia and affective disorders. It is an inherently difficult construct because it is an intermediate category that straddles the boundaries of schizophrenia and mood disorders. Confusion surrounding the term has persisted despite operationalized diagnostic criteria. DSM-IV describes an uninterrupted illness in which characteristic symptoms of schizophrenia are present concurrently with a depressive episode, manic episode, or a mixed episode. During the illness, more than 2 weeks of delusions or hallucinations in the absence of prominent affective symptoms are required, helping to set the schizoaffective disorder apart from psychotic depression or mania. Affective symptoms need to be present for a substantial portion of the total duration of illness so as to differentiate it from schizophrenia.

2. Epidemiology

The lifetime prevalence of schizoaffective disorder is less than 1%, possibly in the range of 0.5% to 0.8%. These figures, however, are estimates; various studies of schizoaffective disorder have used varying diagnoses. Family studies have shown an increased risk for both schizophrenia and mood disorders among relatives of patients with schizoaffective disorder.

3. Etiology

The cause of schizoaffective disorder is unknown. The disorder may be a type of schizophrenia, a type of mood disorder, or the simultaneous expression of each.

Studies designed to explore the etiology have examined family histories, biological markers, short-term treatment responses, and long-term outcomes. It is considered that a balance of the dopamine system and serotonin is particularly affected in schizoaffective disorder, leading to chronic psychosis and intermittent, but sustained, mood symptoms.

Studies of relatives of patients with schizoaffective disorder have reported inconsistent results; however, according to DSM-IV-TR, an increased risk of schizophrenia exists among relatives of probands with schizoaffective disorder.

4. Diagnosis

DSM-IV-TR diagnostic criteria are shown in Table 3A.3. According to DSM-IV-TR, the first criterion in making a diagnosis of schizoaffective disorder is that the psychotic illness meets criterion A for schizophrenia, which includes delusions, hallucinations, bizarre behavior, and

TABLE 3A.3 Diagnostic Criteria for Schizoaffective Disorder

A. An uninterrupted period of illness during which, at some time, there is a major depressive episode, a manic episode, or a mixed episode concurrent with symptoms that meet criterion A for schizophrenia.
B. During the same period of illness, there have been delusions or hallucinations for at least 2 weeks in the absence of prominent mood symptoms.
C. Symptoms that meet criteria for a mood episode are present for a substantial portion of the total duration of the active and residual periods of the illness.
D. The disturbance is not due to the direct physiological effects of a substance (e.g., a drug of abuse, a medication) or a general medical condition.
Specify type:
Bipolar type: if the disturbance includes a manic or a mixed episode.
Depressive type: if the disturbance includes only major depressive episodes.

Adapted from American Psychiatric Association. *Diagnostic and Statistical Manual of Mental Disorders*. 4th Ed. Text Revision. Washington, DC: American Psychiatric Association, 2000.

negative symptoms. Concurrent with the psychotic symptoms, there needs to be a depressive or a manic episode that meets full criteria for such an episode. To distinguish depressive symptoms from negative symptoms of schizophrenia, criterion A1 for a major depressive episode must be fulfilled, i.e., presence of "depressed mood" and not simply anhedonia or loss of interest.

It is also important to take a detailed temporal history of onset and offset of mood and psychotic symptoms to fulfill criteria B and C of schizoaffective disorder. First, to meet criterion B (psychotic symptoms in the absence of mood syndrome), it is important to know when an affective episode and psychosis continue. Second, to meet criterion C, the length of all mood episodes must be combined and compared with the total length of illness to see if mood symptoms are present for substantial portion of illness. The term "substantial portion" typically requires that mood symptoms are present during 15% to 30% of the total illness duration. This requirement makes the diagnosis of schizoaffective disorder unstable because it requires the exercise of clinical judgment, and any fluctuations in mood can lead to a change of diagnosis. As with most psychiatric diagnoses, schizoaffective disorder should not be used if the symptoms are caused by substance abuse or a secondary medical condition.

DSM-IV diagnosis of schizoaffective disorder can be further classified as schizoaffective disorder, bipolar type or depressive type. For the bipolar type, the disorder should include a manic or mixed episode with or without a history of major depressive episodes. The depressive subtype meets the criteria for a major depressive episode with no history of having had mania or a mixed episode.

5. Treatments

A. NONPHARMACOLOGICAL TREATMENTS

Patients benefit from a combination of individual supportive therapy, family therapy, group therapy, cognitive behavioral therapy, and social skills training. As the field of psychiatry has had difficulty deciding on the exact diagnosis and prognosis of schizoaffective disorder, this uncertainty must be explained to the patient. Many patients would be suitable candidates for assertive community treatment (ACT). Depending on the level of recovery, some of the patients may need rehabilitation services to assist them either in developing skills for some form of employment or in maintaining a job. It can be very difficult for family members to keep up with the changing nature and needs of these patients. Medication regimens can be complicated with multiple medications from all classes of drugs. The family can benefit from psychoeducation and support groups.

B. PHARMACOLOGICAL TREATMENTS

Systematic pharmacological treatment studies of schizoaffective disorder represent a relatively neglected area of research. Patients with schizoaffective disorder often end up with complex pharmacological regimens as clinicians attempt to target both psychotic and affective symptoms. There is no clear evidence that any one pharmacological strategy is superior to others, whether during acute or maintenance treatment: antipsychotic monotherapy, mood stabilizer monotherapy, antidepressant monotherapy, or combination therapy (antipsychotic with a mood stabilizer or antipsychotic with an antidepressant). Acute treatment usually requires antipsychotics because most acutely ill patients have prominent psychotic symptoms. With little evidence from controlled studies, the choice of maintenance strategy is often guided by the subtype of schizoaffective disorder; for example, mood stabilizers may be used in patients for the bipolar subtype and antipsychotics in patients with persistent psychosis. There is some evidence that atypical antipsychotics with their mood-stabilizing properties may provide ideal monotherapy for patients with schizoaffective disorder. In patients with treatment-refractory illness, a trial of clozapine should be considered.

6. Prognosis

Due to the evolving nature of the diagnosis and limited studies done thus far, much remains unknown. However, it is considered that schizoaffective disorder has better prognosis than schizophrenia and a relatively poorer prognosis than bipolar disorder. The factors that represent poor prognosis are poor premorbid history, insidious onset, absence of precipitating factors, predominance of psychotic symptoms, especially negative ones, early age of onset, unremitting course, and a family history of schizophrenia. The opposite of each one of these would represent better prognosis.

7. General Formulation for Schizoaffective Disorder

A. DIAGNOSTIC

Schizoaffective disorder is a psychotic disorder and a patient must meet the criteria detailed above. The critical step in every differential diagnosis is determining whether a substance use disorder or a medical disorder could account for the patient's symptoms. A mood disorder or a psychotic disorder due to a general medical condition is diagnosed when evidence from the history, physical examination, or laboratory tests indicates that symptoms are a direct physiological consequence of a specific general medical condition. A history of substance use (with or without positive results on toxicology screening tests) may indicate a substance-induced disorder.

The psychiatric differential diagnosis includes mood disorders and schizophrenia. In distinguishing between schizoaffective disorder and mood disorder with psychotic features, it is important to assess the relative persistence of psychotic symptoms in the absence of prominent mood symptoms for at least 2 weeks. It is also important to note that the diagnosis of schizoaffective disorder sometimes becomes clear only with longitudinal follow-up.

B. ETIOLOGIC

The etiology of schizoaffective disorder is unclear. The disorder may be a type of schizophrenia, a type of mood disorder, or the simultaneous expression of each. The etiology of relapses such as other psychiatric illness may be due to nonadherence to medications, presence of psychological and social stressors, and substance abuse.

C. THERAPEUTIC

Pharmacological treatment requires a combination of mood stabilizers or antidepressants with antipsychotics. There is some evidence that atypical antipsychotics with their mood-stabilizing properties may provide the ideal monotherapy for patients with schizoaffective disorder. In patients with treatment-refractory illness, a trial of clozapine should be considered. Apart from medications, a good support system, stable housing, and financial support are important as well.

D. PROGNOSTIC

Perpetuating factors and factors associated with relapse include medication noncompliance, predominant psychotic symptoms, especially negative symptoms, and concomitant substance use. Good prognostic factors include response to treatment and absence of predominant psychotic symptoms, especially negative symptoms.

8. Risk Assessment

It is also important to assess suicidality, substance abuse/dependence, physical health, command auditory hallucination which can increase the risk of violence, medication compliance, and socioeconomic problems.

KEY POINTS (ABPN Examination)

A. When interviewing a patient with schizoaffective disorder

1. It is important to keep in mind medical and substance use problems in the differential.
2. Schizoaffective disorder has both mood and psychotic symptoms. Ask about positive, negative, and mood symptoms.
3. It is also important to take a longitudinal history to show the presence of psychotic symptoms in the absence of mood symptoms for at least a period of 2 weeks.
4. Do not forget physical health, medication adherence, and the other risk factors noted above.

B. When presenting a patient with schizoaffective disorder

1. If the diagnosis is unclear, state that you would use a structured diagnostic interview like the SCID-DSM-IV for clarification.

Suggested Readings

Erfurth A, Walden J, Grunze H. Lamotrigine in the treatment of schizoaffective disorder. *Neuropsychobiology* 1998;38:204–205.

Evans JD, Heaton RK, Paulsen JS, et al. Schizoaffective disorder: A form of schizophrenia or affective disorder? *J Clin Psychiatry* 1999;60: 874–882.

Grossman LS, Harrow M, Goldberg JF, et al. Outcome of schizoaffective disorder at two long term follow-ups: Comparisons with outcome of schizophrenia and affective disorders. *Am J Psychiatry* 1991;148:1359.

Janicak PG, Keck PE Jr, Davis JM, et al. A double blind, randomized, prospective evaluation of the efficacy and safety of risperidone versus haloperidol in the treatment of schizoaffective disorder. *J Clin Psychopharm* 2001;21:360–368.

Levinson DF, Umapathy C, Mushtaq M. Treatment of schizoaffective disorder and schizophrenia with mood symptoms. *Am J Psychiatry* 1999;156:1138–1148.

Malhi GS, Green M, Fagiolini A, et al. Schizoaffective disorder: Diagnostic issues and future recommendation. *Bipolar Disord* 2008;10:215–230.

Puzynski S, Klosiewicz L. Divalproex amide in the treatment of affective and schizoaffective disorders. *J Affect Disord* 1984;6:115–121.

Robinson D, Woerner MG, Alvir JMJ, et al. Predictors of relapse following response from a first episode of schizophrenia or schizoaffective disorder. *Arch Gen Psychiatry* 1999;56:241–247.

Strawkowski SM, Keck PE, Sax KW, et al. Twelve month outcome of patients with DSM III R schizoaffective disorder: Comparisons to matched patients with bipolar disorder. *Schizophr Res* 1999;35:167–174.

Tollefson GD, Beasley CM Jr, Tran PV, et al. Olanzapine versus haloperidol in the treatment of schizophrenia and schizoaffective and schizophreniform disorders: Results of an international collaborative trial. *Am J Psychiatry* 1997;154:457–465.

Williams PV, McGlashan TH. Schizoaffective psychosis, I: Comparative long term outcome. *Arch Gen Psychiatry* 1987;44:130–137.

B. Mood disorders

Clarence Watson, JD, MD, Nicole A. Foubister, MD

I. DEPRESSIVE DISORDERS

CASE HISTORY

PRESENT ILLNESS

Ms V is a 24-year-old single female graduate student pursuing a doctorate in philosophy who presents to the emergency department after being found on the 20th floor roof of her apartment building. Ms V is accompanied by a counselor from her university, who reports that prior to today Ms V has never been seen at the counseling center. Ms V reports that she has no past psychiatric history; however, for the past 3 weeks, she has been feeling extremely sad and has had frequent crying episodes. Ms V states that she has a poor appetite and has lost 5 lb over the last 2 weeks. Ms V reports that she spends most of her days in her room, as she no longer enjoys most activities. She reports that she has difficulty falling asleep, wakes up very early in the morning, and feels sluggish and fatigued during the day. Ms V reports that she has little energy, has stopped showering daily, and feels as if she is moving in slow motion. Ms V also reports that she is unable to concentrate on her schoolwork. She reports that when she was found on the rooftop, she had intended to jump after several days of recurring thoughts of committing suicide. Ms V denies symptoms consistent with hypomania or mania. Ms V denies current or past symptoms of anxiety, obsessions, or compulsions. In addition, Ms V denies past or current symptoms of psychosis.

Upon arrival to the emergency department, Ms V is seen by the psychiatry resident, who notes that her hair appears slightly unkempt, she is tearful, and she repeatedly states that she wants to go home. Further history reveals that 1 week ago, Ms V stopped attending classes and returning her friends' phone calls. In addition, Ms V recently wrote a detailed suicide note. Ms V reports that she had a breakup with her boyfriend 1 month ago and has been feeling increasingly isolated and lonely since the termination of their relationship.

PSYCHIATRIC HISTORY

Ms V reports that she has never been seen by a mental health clinician and denies a past psychiatric history.

FAMILY HISTORY

Ms V reports that her mother suffered from postpartum depression following her birth as well as the birth of her younger brother. Ms V reports that her father has also suffered from depression.

SOCIAL HISTORY

Ms V reports that she is in the first year of her doctoral program where she is studying philosophy. She reports that she has a few close friends with whom she normally spends time during the week. Ms V reports that she was born and raised in Nebraska. Her father worked as an attorney and her mother was a homemaker. Ms V reports that her childhood was relatively normal and denies a history of physical, sexual, or emotional abuse. Ms V reports regular contact with her parents as well as with her younger brother; however, she states that she does not feel that they are a source of emotional support. Ms V denies current or past history of alcohol or use of illicit substances.

PERTINENT MEDICAL HISTORY

Ms V reports a history of neonatal jaundice, which was successfully treated with phototherapy. She denies a history of seizures, head trauma, or current medical conditions. She takes no medications on a regular basis.

MENTAL STATUS EXAMINATION

Ms V is a 24-year-old Asian American female of thin build who appears to be her stated age. She was dressed in jeans and a T-shirt and although her hair was mildly unkempt, she was, overall, fairly groomed with good hygiene. Ms V sat in her chair with a stooped posture, crying, and with poor eye contact. Ms V had no noticeable gait disturbance upon entry and she had no evidence of tics, tremors, gestures, dyskinetic movements, or akathisia; however, she was noted to have psychomotor retardation with infrequent spontaneous movements. Ms V was cooperative and engaged with the examiner. Her speech was fluent, with decreased rate and tone. Ms V's thought processes were linear and goal directed. Her thought content was notable for ruminations of hopelessness; however, she denied auditory, visual, tactile, or olfactory hallucinations. In addition, she denied paranoid ideations, ideas of reference, thought insertion, thought broadcasting, or thought withdrawal. Ms V reported her mood as depressed and her affect was congruent. Ms V reported having suicidal ideation with thoughts of jumping off of her roof. Ms V denied any thoughts or intent to harm others. On Folstein Mini-Mental State Examination, Ms V scored 30 out of 30. Ms V's insight into her illness was fair, as she reported recognizing that she is depressed. However, her judgment was poor as evidenced by her plan to jump off of her roof.

PERTINENT PHYSICAL FINDINGS

Ms V's physical examination was unremarkable and her vital signs were stable.

LABORATORY DATA

Ms V's complete blood cell count, liver function tests, serum electrolytes, BUN, creatinine, glucose, RPR, B_{12}, folate, and TSH were all within normal limits. Her urinalysis, urine toxicology screen, and serum pregnancy test were all negative.

HOSPITAL COURSE

Ms V was voluntarily admitted to the inpatient psychiatric unit for treatment as well as safety monitoring. Ms V was started on fluoxetine, which was titrated up to 20 mg, and she was engaged in group, milieu, and individual supportive therapies. Ms V responded well to treatment interventions with notable improvement in her mood and affect. After 3 days in the hospital, she denied suicidal ideation, and on hospital day six, she was discharged home on fluoxetine 20 mg PO daily and follow-up treatment was arranged with a local psychiatrist and her university counseling center.

DSM-IV-TR MULTIAXIAL DIAGNOSIS

Axis I: Major depressive disorder, single episode, severe without psychotic features
Axis II: None
Axis III: None
Axis IV: Recent breakup with boyfriend
Axis V: Global assessment of functioning at the time of discharge: 55

FORMULATION

A. Diagnostic

Ms V meets the DSM-IV-TR criteria for major depressive disorder, severe without psychotic features. In order to meet the diagnostic criteria for a major depressive episode, a patient must have either depressed mood or loss of interest or pleasure accompanied by four additional symptoms, which must have been present during the same 2-week period and must represent a change from previous functioning. As noted above, Ms V had a depressed mood for 3 weeks accompanied by suicidal thoughts, a decreased appetite, and a disturbance in her sleep. Her symptoms have caused significant dysfunction, both academically and socially, as she is no longer attending classes, finds it difficult to leave her dorm room, and is no longer returning phone calls from her friends.

It is essential to rule out other Axis I diagnoses when diagnosing major depressive disorder and the differential diagnosis may include bipolar disorder, schizophrenia, schizoaffective disorder, borderline personality disorder, anxiety disorders, mood disorder secondary to a general medical condition, substance abuse, and dementia. Patients with depressive symptoms should be screened for all of the aforementioned disorders. Ms V denies a history of symptoms consistent with mania or hypomania, which currently rules out a diagnosis of bipolar disorder. Ms V denies taking any medications or current medical conditions and her review of systems, physical examination, and laboratory studies were all within normal limits, making a mood disorder secondary to a general medical condition a highly improbable diagnosis. A substance-induced mood disorder must also be considered; however, Ms V has no known history of substance abuse and her urine toxicology screen was negative. Her symptoms, therefore, do not appear to be due to the direct physiological effects of a substance or a general medical condition. In addition, as noted above, one must consider schizophrenia and schizoaffective rdisorder, anxiety disorders, and personality disorders. Ms V denies current or past symptoms of psychosis and has no evidence of a formal thought disorder on examination. Her history is not currently suggestive of a personality disorder; however, additional evidence of a personality disorder may emerge over time. If depressive symptoms meet the criteria for major depression, even if the symptoms are attributable to a stressor, major depression and not an adjustment disorder should be diagnosed. Ms V's symptoms appear to have been precipitated by her recent breakup; however, because her symptoms meet the diagnostic criteria for a major depressive episode, a diagnosis of an adjustment disorder with depressed mood is ruled out. Finally, grief is generally described as occurring after a major loss or trauma, such as the loss of a loved one. Although the symptoms of grief often overlap with the symptoms of major depression, the symptoms of grief are generally considered appropriate for the situation and patients with grief rarely experience global feelings of worthlessness. In contrast to patients with grief who may express a passive wish for death in order to join the deceased, patients with depression more commonly experience suicidal ideation.

B. Etiologic

Biologically, we know that Ms V has a family history of psychiatric illness as her mother suffered from postpartum depression and her father suffered from major depressive disorder. As a result, Ms V is at an increased genetic risk for developing a mood disorder. Ms V's depression appears to have been in part precipitated by the psychosocial stressor of the recent breakup with her boyfriend. The combination of her biological predisposition and recent social stressor, her breakup with her boyfriend, is likely to contribute to her current presentation.

C. Therapeutic

Ms V presented to the emergency department with active suicidal ideation with a plan to jump off of the roof; therefore, the first-line intervention is to ensure her safety through acute inpatient hospitalization. Major reasons for hospitalizing a depressed patient include poor social support, concomitant substance abuse, inability to care for self, and high suicide risk.

General medical conditions and substance use were ruled out before initiating treatment with antidepressant medication. In treating depression, antidepressants remain the first-line biological treatment. Currently, Ms V is on fluoxetine, an antidepressant belonging to the class of selective serotonin reuptake inhibitors (SSRIs). Treatment guidelines suggest that a patient with major depressive disorder be treated with a therapeutic dose of an antidepressant for 6 to 8 weeks. If a partial response is obtained, treatment guidelines recommend adding an adjunctive agent, such as bupropion or buspirone. If no clinical response is seen, guidelines suggest either switching to another medication in the same class or utilizing a medication from another class of antidepressants, such as a serotonin and norepinephrine reuptake inhibitor (SNRI).

Treatment on the inpatient unit should include group, milieu, and individual supportive psychotherapies. In addition, efforts should be made to engage Ms V's social support system, which may be facilitated by inviting family or friends in to meet with the treatment team. Psychoeducation is also essential and may assist in Ms V's coping as well as compliance with the treatment. As an outpatient, Ms V will likely benefit from individual psychotherapy such as cognitive behavioral therapy (CBT) as well as medication management by a psychiatrist.

An effort should be made to contact Ms V's primary care physician to obtain collateral information as well as coordinate care. Finally, with Ms V's permission, contact can be made and a discharge summary can be sent to her outpatient treatment providers.

D. Prognostic

Ms V has a fair prognosis. When untreated, an episode of depressions is usually self-limiting and lasts 6 months or more. Ms V's absence of psychotic symptoms and short hospital stay are positive prognostic indicators as are her history of supportive friendships, stable family functioning, and generally sound social functioning. The absence of a comorbid psychiatric or personality disorder is also a positive prognostic factor. Negative prognostic factors include the severity of Ms V's symptoms. In addition, having one or more episodes of major depressive disorder increases a patient's risk of subsequent episodes.

Patients with severe depression often do not have the energy to commit suicide and as energy returns in response to treatment, the risk of suicide increases. This should be discussed with Ms V and she should be instructed to call her outpatient psychiatrist or go to the nearest emergency department if she should have thoughts of self-harm.

DEPRESSIVE DISORDERS

1. Introduction

Variations in mood are a normal part of life and sadness will occur in every person's life in which the cause is obvious and the reaction understandable. However, when prolonged unhappiness affects one's functioning, affects the ability to care for oneself, presents a danger, or is associated with abnormalities of behavior or judgment, these symptoms require assessment and possibly treatment.

Mood disorders have been described for centuries and our current understanding of mood disorders has evolved to include major depression, bipolar disorders, dysthymia, and cyclothymia. Major depression may cause disturbances in multiple spheres including a patient's emotions, behaviors, and cognition. In addition, neurovegetative symptoms may be seen. In depression, a patient's mood is typically down or sad for most of the day nearly every day and patients may also experience anxiety or irritability. Additional emotional symptoms include anhedonia, diminished emotional bonds, social withdrawal, and thoughts of death. Patients may exhibit cognitive symptoms such as guilty ruminations, self-criticism, pessimism, distractibility, poor concentration, memory impairment, perceptual changes including delusions or hallucinations which are generally mood congruent, and feelings of worthlessness, helplessness, hopelessness, despair, and indecisiveness. Neurovegetative symptoms that may be seen include lack of energy, insomnia (particularly terminal insomnia) or hypersomnia, anorexia or hyperphagia, weight loss or gain, psychomotor retardation or activation, impaired libido, and frequent diurnal variation in the intensity of symptoms. Additional signs of depression may include stooped posture, tearfulness, sad affect, dry mouth, and dry skin. Somatic symptoms including constipation, leaden paralysis, and gastric distress may also be reported. Many patients will present with a masked depression in which they are unable to recognize their own symptoms and will complain of vague somatic symptoms such as back pain, headache, and abdominal pain which do not resolve with medical treatment.

2. Epidemiology

The World Health Organization ranks major depression among one of the most burdensome diseases in the world. With a current lifetime prevalence of 15%, it is estimated to become the second leading cause of disability worldwide by 2020. Major depression tends to occur in women with a frequency twice that of men. The peak age of onset of depression is in the fourth decade of life; however, episodes may occur at any point in the life cycle.

Major depression is a relapsing, remitting illness in most patients and recurrence is common. Following the first episode, there is a greater than 40% recurrence rate over a 2-year period; after two episodes, the risk of recurrence within 5 years is approximately 75%. In patients who have had three or more episodes, the risk of recurrence is 90%. The risk of major depressive disorder is increased twofold to threefold in those having a first-degree relative with major depressive disorder. Ten to thirty percent of patients treated for a major depressive episode will have an incomplete recovery, with persistent symptoms or dysthymia. There are no significant differences in the prevalence of depression across cultural, racial, or socioeconomic groups.

The treatment of depression begins with an accurate diagnosis and numerous studies have found that the diagnosis of depression is often missed by many health professionals. Depression can have a significant impact on morbidity and mortality and, in and of itself, can be a lethal illness. Approximately 50% of individuals who commit suicide have a diagnosis of depression, with suicide being the eighth leading cause of death in the United States. In terms of functioning (social, familial, occupational, and health), depression has been found to have a profound impact, accounting for more missed workdays and unscheduled visits to doctors' offices and emergency rooms than many other common diseases including diabetes, hypertension, and heart disease.

3. Etiology

The etiology of major depression is likely multifactorial. The biological causes of mood disorders may include altered neurotransmitter activity, primarily decreased availability of serotonin, norepinephrine, and dopamine, as well as abnormalities of the limbic-hypothalamic-pituitary-adrenal axis.

Biological theories have focused on both genetic and biochemical models. Twin studies support a genetic contribution to the occurrence of major depression, with a 54% concordance rate for monozygotic twins and a 24% concordance rate for dizygotic twins. Biochemical hypotheses have focused on monoamines (serotonin, norepinephrine, and dopamine) and the known mechanisms of actions of antidepressants support this theory. The neuroendocrine system has also been considered in the etiology depression. Abnormalities in the hypothalamic-pituitary-adrenal axis often occur in depression. It has been demonstrated that dexamethasone administration does not produce the expected suppression of cortisol release in patients with depression; however, the dexamethasone suppression test is neither specific nor sensitive and can be positive in psychiatric disorders other than depression. More recently, the role of corticotropin-releasing factor (CRF) has been investigated. CRF release is regulated by neurochemicals such as serotonin, norepinephrine, and gamma-aminobutyric acid. In depression, there appears to be an excessive release of cortisol. Thyroid function abnormalities have also been observed: many patients with depression have a blunted TSH and growth hormone response to the administration of exogenous thyrotropin-releasing hormone. As a result of these findings, thyroid hormone is occasionally utilized as an augmenting agent in refractory depression.

Finally, some researchers have looked at altered sleep architecture as an etiological cause of depression. Sleep studies have shown characteristic changes, including decreased REM latency and decreased slow-wave sleep. Sleep discontinuity, middle and terminal insomnia, increased REM density, and decreased non-REM sleep are also seen; however, it is difficult to determine whether these changes in sleep represent a symptom of depression or a cause.

In addition to biochemical models, there have been several psychological theories to explain the condition of depression. The psychodynamic model proposed by Freud focused on the role of early life losses. The psychoanalytic model posits that the primary disturbance is a fixation in the oral stage of development. This is precipitated by a real or perceived loss of an ambivalently loved object, which leads to a vulnerability in later life to managing acute real, imagined, or threatened interpersonal loss. According to the psychoanalytic theory, the disruption of reassurance and support in early life leads to a fall in self-esteem, self-doubt, and ultimately depression.

The cognitive-behavioral hypothesis proposed by Aaron Beck holds that depression results from a patient's biased thinking, also known as cognitive distortions, which produce negative interpretations of life events. According to this theory, patients with depression acquire a negative cognitive schema of the world in childhood and adolescence as a result of stressful life events. Subsequently, when a patient is presented with a situation that in some way resembles the conditions in which the original cognitive schema was learned, the negative schemata of the patient are activated. Depression schemata activated then lead to additional symptoms of depression.

In summary, it is likely that depression has biological and psychological causative factors which may play a greater or lesser role in triggering depression, varying with each individual patient.

4. Diagnosis

A. MAJOR DEPRESSIVE DISORDER

A diagnosis of major depression is made when symptoms have been present for at least 2 weeks and are not better accounted for by an organic process or grief. The DSM-IV-TR criteria are shown in Table 3B.1.

Major depressive disorder, recurrent episode is indicated by the presence of two or more major depressive episodes. In order to be considered two separate episodes, there must be an interval of at least two consecutive months in which criteria are not met for a major depressive disorder. Criteria

TABLE 3B.1 Diagnostic Criteria for Major Depressive Episode

Criterion A. Five (or more) of the following symptoms have been present during the same 2-week period and represent a change from previous functioning; at least one of the symptoms is either (1) depressed mood or (2) loss of interest or pleasure.

1. Depressed mood most of the day, nearly every day, as indicated by either subjective report (e.g., feeling sad or empty) or observation made by others (e.g., appears tearful)
2. Markedly diminished interest or pleasure in all, or almost all, activities most of the day, nearly every day
3. Significant weight loss when not dieting or weight gain (e.g., a change of more than 5% of body weight in a month), or decrease or increase in appetite, nearly every day
4. Insomnia or hypersomnia, nearly every day
5. Psychomotor agitation or retardation, nearly every day
6. Fatigue or loss of energy, nearly every day
7. Feelings of worthlessness or excessive or inappropriate guilt, nearly every day
8. Diminished ability to think or concentrate or indecisiveness, nearly every day
9. Recurrent thoughts of death (not just fear of dying), recurrent suicidal ideation without a specific plan, or a suicidal attempt or a specific plan for committing suicide

Criterion B. The symptoms do not meet the criteria for a mixed episode.

Criterion C. The symptoms cause clinically significant distress or impairment in social, occupational, or other important areas of functioning.

Criterion D. The symptoms are not due to the direct physiological affects of a substance (e.g., drug of abuse, medications) or a general medical condition (e.g., hypothyroidism).

Criterion E. The symptoms are not better accounted for by bereavement (i.e., after the loss of a loved one, the symptoms persist for longer than 2 months or are characterized by marked functional impairment, morbid preoccupation with worthlessness, suicidal ideation, psychotic symptoms, or psychomotor retardation).

Note: Do not include symptoms that are clearly due to a general medical condition or mood-incongruent delusions or hallucinations.
Adapted from American Psychiatric Association. *Diagnostic and Statistical Manual of Mental Disorders: Text Revision*. 4th Ed. Washington, DC: American Psychiatric Association, 1994.

A–E listed above continue to apply in cases of major depressive disorder, recurrent episode.

Aside from the variety of symptoms that can be manifested, there are a few subtypes of depression that have been identified. *Atypical depression* is characterized by reversed vegetative symptoms, namely, mood reactivity, increased sleep, increased appetite, leaden paralysis, and rejection sensitivity. *Major depressive disorder with psychotic features* is characterized by the presence of perceptual disturbances including delusions and/or hallucinations. The perceptual changes are generally mood congruent (belief that one is dying, derogatory and accusatory hallucinations, etc.). *Melancholic depression* is associated with a pervasive loss of pleasure, lack of reactivity and diurnal variation with more severe symptoms of depression in the morning, terminal insomnia, psychomotor changes (either retardation or agitation), significant anorexia, and excessive guilt. *Seasonal affective disorder* (SAD) is characterized by the development of a mood disorder in which there has been a regular temporal relationship between the onset of major depressive episodes and a particular time of the year, as well as full resolution of symptoms occurring at a characteristic time of the year. Although the diagnostic criteria focus on the seasonal pattern of depressive episodes, many patients with SAD also experience atypical vegetative symptoms such as hypersomnia, hyperphagia, carbohydrate cravings, and weight gain. *Postpartum depression* is defined as beginning within 4 weeks after childbirth according to the DSM-IV-TR. Postpartum "baby blues" are seen in a majority of women, typically in the first week after delivery, and are characterized by irritability and crying spells, which do not impair function and usually resolve spontaneously. By contrast, postpartum depression usually has an insidious onset and is characterized by the typical symptoms of depression. In addition, affected women are at an increased risk for future depressive episodes.

B. DYSTHYMIC DISORDER

Dysthymia is similar to major depressive disorder; however, it is more chronic and requires fewer depressive symptoms. Dysthymia is defined as a depressed mood that occurs for more days than not for at least 2 years with no symptom-free interval of 2 months or longer. In addition, two or more additional symptoms of depression are required and function must be impaired (see Table 3B.2 for diagnostic criteria).

Dysthymic disorder has a lifetime prevalence of 3% to 6%, with higher rates found in women as well as individuals with a family history of depression. Individuals with dysthymia frequently suffer comorbid psychiatric disorders, including major depression. Dysthymic disorder can also occur concurrently with anxiety disorders and substance use disorders. Dysthymia is a treatable condition and antidepressant medications have been shown to be effective. In general, antidepressants are used at doses recommended for depression.

C. DEPRESSION DUE TO A GENERAL MEDICAL CONDITION

Depression due to a general medical condition is diagnosed when the symptoms of a depressive syndrome are considered to be the direct physiological result of a medical illness. Various

TABLE 3B.2 Diagnostic Criteria for Dysthymic Disorder

A. Depressed mood for most of the day, for more days than not, as indicated either by subjective account or observation by others, for at least 2 years.
B. Presence, while depressed, of two (or more) of the following: 1. Poor appetite or overeating 2. Insomnia or hypersomnia 3. Low energy or fatigue 4. Low self-esteem 5. Poor concentration or difficulty making decisions 6. Feelings of hopelessness
C. During the same 2-year period (1 year for children and adolescents) of the disturbance, the person has never been without the symptoms in criteria A and B for >2 months at a time.
D. No major depressive episode has been present during the first 2 years of the disturbance, i.e., the disturbance is not better accounted for by chronic major depressive disorder or major depressive disorder in partial remission.
E. There has never been a manic episode, a mixed episode, or a hypomanic episode and criteria have never been met for cyclothymic disorder.
F. The disturbance does not occur exclusively during the course of a chronic psychotic disorder, such as schizophrenia or delusional disorder.
G. The symptoms are not due to the direct physiologic effects of a substance (e.g., a drug of abuse, a medication) or a general medical condition (e.g., hypothyroidism).
H. The symptoms cause clinically significant distress or impairment in social, occupational, or other important areas of functioning.

Adapted from American Psychiatric Association. *Diagnostic and Statistical Manual of Mental Disorders: Text Revision*. 4th Ed. Washington, DC: American Psychiatric Association, 1994.

TABLE 3B.3 General Medical Conditions and Substances Causing or Contributing to Depressed Mood

Metabolic/endocrine	Neoplasia
Hypothyroidism	Carcinomatosis
Severe anemia	CNS neoplasm
Hyperparathyroidism	Drugs and poisons
Hypokalemia	Alcohol
Hyponatremia	Steroids
Cushing's disease	Interferon-alpha
Addison's disease	Isotretinoin
Uremia	Methyldopa
Hypopituitarism	Opiates
Porphyria	Barbiturates
Wilson's disease	Beta-blockers
Wernicke-Korsakoff's syndrome	Cocaine withdrawal
Neurodegenerative and demyelinating diseases	Amphetamine withdrawal
	Heavy metal poisoning
Multiple sclerosis	Cholinesterase inhibitors
Alzheimer's disease	Cimetidine
Parkinson's disease	Chemotherapeutic agents
Huntington's disease	Infections
Neurological	Mononucleosis
Stroke (especially left frontal lobe)	Encephalitis
Traumatic brain injury	Hepatitis
Epilepsy	Others
Subdural hematoma	Systemic lupus erythematosus
Normal pressure hydrocephalus	Vitamin B_{12} deficiency
Cerebral tumors	Congestive heart failure

medical conditions can directly cause depression; however, strokes, pancreatic cancer, and hypothyroidism are among the most common.

The DSM-IV-TR indicates that patients with a mood disorder due to a general medical condition have a persistent disturbance in mood, which may be characterized by depressed mood and/or markedly diminished interest or pleasure. In addition, there must be evidence from history, physical examination, or laboratory findings that the disturbance is the direct physiological consequence of a general medical condition. Symptoms may not occur exclusively during the course of a delirium and must cause clinically significant distress or impairment in social, occupational, or other important areas of functioning.

Depression secondary to a general medical condition does *not* include depressive episodes that occur as a reaction to a psychosocial stress caused by the development of a medical illness. Rather, it is diagnosed when the medical condition is felt to be the direct physiological cause of the depression.

Table 3B.3 lists the selected general medical conditions that may be associated with depressive mood episodes.

D. SUBSTANCE-INDUCED MOOD DISORDER

Medications, toxins, and drugs of abuse can produce depression. Individuals suffering from a substance-induced mood disorder demonstrate a prominent and persistent disturbance in mood characterized by depressed mood, irritability, or anhedonia. Evidence obtained from the history, physical examination, or laboratory findings must support that symptoms developed during or within *1 month* of substance intoxication or withdrawal and that the substance is etiologically related to the disturbance. The symptoms must cause clinically significant distress, must be sufficient to warrant clinical attention, and must be in excess of those usually associated with the intoxication or withdrawal syndrome.

The likelihood of depressive syndromes resulting from intoxication with, chronic use of, or withdrawal from substances, both illicit and prescribed, varies with the substance, dose, and duration of use. This disorder is only diagnosed when depressed mood and associated symptoms are considered to be the direct result of substance use or withdrawal. Substance-induced mood disorder is most commonly caused by the chronic use of alcohol or benzodiazepines or by withdrawal from cocaine or amphetamines. In addition, medications prescribed for medical illnesses can result in depressive symptoms (Table 3B.3).

5. Treatment

A. NONPHARMACOLOGICAL TREATMENT OF DEPRESSION

Psychotherapy either alone or in combination with medications is a viable treatment option for patients with mild to moderate depression. The research literature has demonstrated clinical efficacy for CBT and interpersonal therapy (IPT).

IPT is a short-term supportive psychotherapy directed at improving interpersonal skills that may have contributed to the development of depression. Treatment with IPT is based on the premise that depression occurs in a social and interpersonal context, which must be understood in order for improvement to occur. IPT posits that three interacting components contribute to the formation of depression: (a) biological, genetic, and/or psychodynamic processes; (b) social and interpersonal experiences; and (c) enduring personality problems. Interpersonal therapists focus on the functional role of depression rather than on its etiology. Treatment occurs over 12 to 16 sessions.

IPT emphasizes the ways in which a person's current relationships and social context cause or maintain symptoms rather than exploring the deep-seated sources of the symptoms. Goals of treatment are the improvement in current interpersonal skills with subsequent symptom reduction and improved social adjustment. Studies have demonstrated that IPT is significantly superior to placebo.

CBT is a short-term, highly structured treatment. In CBT, depression is viewed as a result of negative cognitions of the self and the world. Cognitive techniques involve eliciting automatic thoughts, challenging the automatic thoughts, identifying the cognitive distortion, and testing the validity of the distortion. The goal of CBT is to recognize and eliminate cognitive distortions and to develop alternative cognitive schemata. CBT is the most well-studied therapeutic treatment of depression and appears to be as effective as medications for mild to moderate depression.

B. PHARMACOLOGICAL TREATMENT OF DEPRESSION

Antidepressants are the mainstay of treatment for depression and are a heterogeneous group of medications with diverse chemical structures and receptor activities. These agents are often grouped by chemical structure into SSRIs, tricyclic and heterocyclic compounds, monoamine oxidase inhibitors (MAOIs), and atypical agents.

Mild to moderate levels of depression may respond to either medications or psychotherapy. First-line treatment with antidepressant agents rather than psychotherapy alone is indicated for patients with prior medication-responsive depression, recurrent depression, severe depression, or an incomplete response to psychotherapy alone. All antidepressants appear to be equally efficacious with approximately 70% of patients having a positive clinical response (defined as a 50% reduction of symptoms) versus 35% for placebo. Selection of an antidepressant may be guided by history of a positive response of the patient or a family member to a given agent as well as by side effect profile, safety, tolerability, comorbid medical and psychiatric conditions, cost, and ease of dosing. In addition, an assessment of any drug-drug interactions due to induction or inhibition of liver enzymes should also be considered.

SSRIs, which selectively block the reuptake of serotonin, are generally considered the first-line agents for the treatment of depressive disorders. In general, SSRIs are well tolerated and safe and have the advantage of being much less dangerous in overdose than older agents such as tricyclic antidepressants (TCAs) or MAOIs. Common side effects of SSRIs include headache, nausea, increased or decreased appetite, diarrhea, anxiety, sexual dysfunction, fatigue, and insomnia. Side effects may diminish or disappear after several days; however, if they persist or prevent compliance, a change to an alternative agent may be necessary.

Other first-line treatments for depression are the newer generation antidepressants which include venlafaxine, bupropion, mirtazapine, and duloxetine. *Venlafaxine* is a dual SNRI, which may cause the side effects noted above as well as dry mouth, sedation, diaphoresis, and a potential dose-dependent increase in blood pressure. *Bupropion*, an antidepressant which affects both norepinephrine and dopamine, may be more activating. Potential side effects of bupropion include anxiety, insomnia, tremor, and headache; however, it is less likely to cause sexual dysfunction or weight gain. Bupropion is also marketed for smoking cessation. Bupropion should generally be avoided in patients with eating disorders or a history of head trauma or seizures, as the medication may lower the seizure threshold.

Mirtazapine exerts effects on both serotonin and norepinephrine. Mirtazapine can cause dry mouth, weight gain, and sedation (though less sedation at higher doses), making it useful in patients with weight loss and insomnia but less appealing to patients who wish to avoid these effects. *Duloxetine* is another SNRI which is also approved for the treatment of diabetic neuropathy and fibromyalgia. Side effects include nausea, dry mouth, constipation, insomnia, fatigue, dizziness, decreased libido, tremors, anxiety, orthostatic hypotension, elevated blood pressure, and elevated liver transaminases.

Older agents include the heterocyclic or *tricyclic antidepressants*. TCAs block the reuptake of serotonin and norepinephrine in the synapse. TCAs may be particularly dangerous in overdose as they can cause the development of cardiac conduction abnormalities. Plasma levels for TCAs can be measured; however, with the exception of nortriptyline, there is no target drug level. Blood levels may be obtained to monitor compliance. Side effects of the TCAs include anticholinergic effects such as dry mouth, constipation, blurred vision, and urinary retention. Other side effects can include sedation, orthostatic hypotension, diaphoresis, palpitations, sexual dysfunction, weight gain, and prolongation of the Q-T interval on EKG. TCAs should not be used in patients with narrow angle glaucoma or a history of cardiac disease. Use of TCAs in the elderly should also be carefully considered due to the anticholinergic side effect profile and risk of orthostasis.

MAOIs are agents that irreversibly limit the activity of MAO and increase the availability of serotonin, norepinephrine, and dopamine in the synapse. MAO also metabolizes tyramine, a pressor in the gastrointestinal tract. If MAO is inhibited, foods that are rich in tyramine (e.g., wine, aged cheese, beer) can increase an individual's blood level of tyramine and cause a hypertensive crisis, which can cause a stroke or death. Typical side effects of MAOIs include orthostatic hypotension, weight gain, edema, sexual dysfunction, and insomnia. MAOIs are occasionally used in the treatment of atypical depression; however, their use is limited by the need to maintain a tyramine-free diet while taking these medications. MAOIs also carry the risk of extensive and severe drug-drug interactions, with prescription as well as over-the-counter medications. Comprehensive psychoeducation is required for any patient prescribed an MAOI.

STAR*D is an NIMH-funded study which is the largest and longest trial ever conducted to evaluate the treatment of depression. STAR*D consisted of four levels of treatment, with patients progressing to each successive level if they had either an incomplete response to the treatment or intolerable side effects from medication. Each of the four levels of the study tested a different medication or medication combination. Approximately half of the participants in the STAR*D study became symptom free after two treatment levels. Over the course of all four treatment levels, almost 70% of patients who did not withdraw from the study became symptom free. An overall analysis of the STAR*D results indicates that patients with treatment-resistant depression can get well after trying several treatment strategies, but the odds of remission diminish with each additional treatment strategy needed. In addition, patients who become symptom free are more likely to remain in remission than those who only experience symptom improvement. Finally, patients who need to undergo several treatment trials before they become symptom free are more likely to experience a relapse of their depressive symptoms.

Table 3B.4 reviews antidepressant medications by class.

A clinical response to antidepressant medication is ordinarily seen in 4 to 6 weeks. It is generally accepted that a medication response is defined as at least 50% reduction in symptoms, while remission indicates a near total resolution of symptoms with a return to premorbid levels

TABLE 3B.4 Antidepressant Medications by Class

Drug/Class	Trade Name	Typical Therapeutic Dose (in mg)
SSRIs		
Fluoxetine	Prozac	20–60
Sertraline	Zoloft	50–200
Paroxetine	Paxil	20–60
Paroxetine CR	Paxil CR	25–62.5
Citalopram	Celexa	20–40
Escitalopram	Lexapro	10–20
Heterocyclic agents		
Amitriptyline	Elavil	150–300
Doxepin	Sinequan	150–300
Clomipramine	Anafranil	25–250
Imipramine	Tofranil	150–300
Desipramine	Norpramin	150–300
Nortriptyline	Pamelor	75–150
Protriptyline	Vivactil	15–30
Tetracyclics		
Amoxapine	Asendin	200–300
Maprotiline	Ludiomil	100–225
MAOIs		
Tranylcypromine	Parnate	20–60
Phenelzine	Nardil	30–90
Isocarboxazid	Marplan	10–50
Atypical		
Bupropion	Wellbutrin	300–450
Bupropion SR	Wellbutrin SR	300–400
Bupropion XL	Wellbutrin XL	150–450
Mirtazapine	Remeron	15–45
SNRIs		
Duloxetine	Cymbalta	60–120
Venlafaxine XR	Effexor XR	75–300
Desvenlafaxine	Pristiq	50–100

of functioning. An adequate length of treatment before considering a patient as nonresponsive to an agent is typically 6 to 8 weeks. Strategies for dealing with inadequate clinical response include maximizing the dose of the medication, switching to an alternative medication, or augmentation with an additional medication. The decision to switch antidepressant medication versus augmentation is somewhat arbitrary. Practitioners should consider changing treatments if, at the end of 6 weeks, there is little clinical response. However, if there is a modest response, maximizing the dose or the medication or treatment augmentation may be pursued. Augmentation can be accomplished with the addition of lithium, thyroid hormone, buspirone, psychostimulants, modafinil, dopaminergic medications, atypical antipsychotics, electroconvulsive therapy (ECT), and psychotherapy.

Atypical antipsychotics appear to have some degree of antidepressant activity; aripiprazole has recently obtained FDA approval as an adjunctive agent in the treatment of depression.

Individuals respond differently to different agents, even within the same class. It is often a process of trial and error to find a medication that is well tolerated and effective for a given patient. Treatment with a single antidepressant is preferable; however, certain patients may require more than one agent. Patient and family education is an important factor in improving medication compliance and should include education about the side effects as well as the nature, treatment, and the time course of recovery for depression. The recommended length of treatment after the first episode of major depression is 6 to 12 months on the full antidepressant dose which achieved remission. When discontinuing treatment, tapering off the medication is recommended to avoid discontinuation syndromes, especially for antidepressants with shorter half-lives, such as paroxetine.

Current data reveal a very high rate of relapse in individuals with two or more episodes of depression after discontinuation of medication. In contrast, continuation on the dose of antidepressant that achieved remission of symptoms can cut the rate of relapse in half. Long-term prophylactic/maintenance antidepressant therapy is indicated after the third episode of major depression, when the onset of depression is after the age of 60 years, when episodes of illness are long, severe, and/or disabling, when there are only short symptom-free intervals between episodes, and in patients with an underlying dysthymia (double depression).

ECT is indicated for the treatment of depression that is refractory to antidepressants, in patients with a history of prior positive response to ECT or in a depression that is so severe that it represents a life-threatening condition. During ECT, patients receive the induction of a generalized seizure by passing a current of electricity across the brain. The exact mechanism of action of ECT is unknown; however, the remission of symptoms requires a series of adequate seizures (at least 25 seconds in duration). The current standard of using a brief anesthetic agent and a neuromuscular blocking agent has significantly reduced side effects such as fractures. There are no absolute contraindications to ECT; however, certain high-risk medical conditions include hypertension, cardiac arrhythmias, pacemakers, myocardial infarction, intracardiac thrombi, anticoagulant therapy, pregnancy, dementia, vascular aneurysms, respiratory disorders (e.g., COPD, asthma), increased intracranial pressure from a brain tumor or mass, epilepsy, orthopedic problems, and a personal or family history of problems with anesthesia. In these patients, the use of ECT must be reviewed with an appropriate consultant.

ECT is efficacious in treating MDD with response rates of 70% to 90%. Patients generally receive treatment three times per week with an average of 8 to 12 treatments in total. ECT may be given bitemporally, bifrontally, or unilaterally, with unilateral ECT less likely to cause confusion and memory disturbances. The primary side effects associated with ECT are headache, nausea, and memory loss. The memory loss can have both a retrograde and an anterograde component. Memory loss is usually reversible, with recovery of memory occurring predominantly in 3 to 6 months after the discontinuation of ECT treatments.

Another somatic treatment for depression is phototherapy. Patients with SAD often show good response to phototherapy, which utilizes a bright, full-spectrum artificial light.

6. Prognosis

In patients with depression, the presence of one or more recurrent episodes predicts an increased risk of future episodes of depression. Additional risk factors for recurrence include comorbid psychiatric conditions including dysthymic disorder, substance abuse, and anxiety. Female gender, social isolation, a negative attitude toward one's occupation, subsyndromal symptoms, prior episodes, a longer lasting index episode, being single, and a higher severity of symptoms also increase the risk of recurrence of future episodes. Positive prognostic factors in major depression include a history of solid friendships during adolescence, stable family functioning, stable premorbid social functioning, the absence of psychotic symptoms, a short hospital stay, and the absence of a comorbid psychiatric or personality disorder.

7. General Formulation for Major Depressive Disorder

A. DIAGNOSTIC

Major depressive disorder is a mood disorder characterized by one or more episodes of persistently depressed mood or a loss of interest or pleasure for a minimum of 2 weeks, with four or more of the following symptoms: sleep disturbance, fatigue or loss of energy, feelings of guilt or worthlessness, impaired concentration, changes in appetite, psychomotor agitation or retardation, and suicidal thoughts or attempts. One should always screen for past manic or hypomanic episodes in any patient presenting with symptoms of depression in order to rule out bipolar disorder. It is important to rule out other Axis I and II disorders as well, including schizoaffective disorder, adjustment disorder, bereavement, histrionic personality disorder, borderline personality disorder, dementia, anxiety disorders, and depression due to a general medical condition or substance-induced mood disorder. Clinicians must also rule out dysthymic disorder and cyclothymic disorder. Depressed patients vary widely in their clinical presentation and may present with sadness, irritability, or somatic complaints.

B. ETIOLOGIC

The etiology of depression is likely multifactorial. Current theories posit biological causes such as altered neurotransmitter activity, genetics, sleep dysregulation, and disturbances in the limbic-hypothalamic-pituitary-adrenal axis. Psychological theories include Freud's psychoanalytic theory of a real or imagined loss of an ambivalently loved object which causes an unconscious rage which is turned against the self, thereby lowering self-esteem and causing depression. Alternatively, cognitive theory postulates that a cognitive triad of distorted perceptions occurs in which a person's negative interpretation of life experiences causes a devaluation of himself and subsequently causes depression. Social factors may also precipitate or exacerbate depression, including divorce, death of a loved one, loss of job, etc.

C. THERAPEUTIC

The first and most critical decision in treating a patient with depression is whether to pursue inpatient versus outpatient treatment. Indications for hospitalization are high risk of suicide or homicide, incapacitation by the disorder with an impaired ability to maintain activities of daily living such as obtaining food and shelter, and the need for diagnostic procedures to assess potential medical, neurological, or pharmacological etiologies for the depressive symptoms.

Once the decision is made to attempt outpatient versus inpatient treatment, the treating clinician must determine whether to pursue psychotherapeutic and/or pharmacological treatment. Cases of mild to moderate depression may be successfully treated with psychotherapy alone. CBT and interpersonal therapy are both short-term psychotherapies that have been found to be efficacious in the treatment of major depression. In cases of more severe depression, treatment with medication or a combination of medication and psychotherapy is indicated. SSRIs remain the first-line medication for depression, although many alternatives are available. ECT should be considered for any patient with depression refractory to medications, history of prior response to ECT, or with severe, life-threatening depression.

D. PROGNOSTIC

Major depression is increasingly viewed as a chronic condition. A very severe initial episode of depression, the presence of a coexisting dysthymic disorder, or the existence of a serious medical condition is associated with a poorer prognosis. Left untreated, a depressive episode may last 4 months or longer. Although the majority of patients have a full remission from a given depressive episode, recurrence is common. Long-term studies of people with MDD indicate that about 60% of patients who have one episode of depression will have a second episode and with each succeeding episode, the odds of a subsequent episode increase. Patients who do not achieve remission between episodes are at a higher risk of recurrence. As noted above, positive prognostic factors in major depression include a history of solid friendships during adolescence, stable family functioning, stable social functioning preceding the illness, the absence of psychotic symptoms, a short hospital stay, and the absence of a comorbid psychiatric or personality disorder.

8. Risk Assessment

All patients with depression must have a careful risk assessment and must be evaluated for suicidality and homicidality. Risk factors for suicide include male gender; white race; divorced, separated, or single status; bisexuality or homosexuality; substance abuse; age greater than 45; panic attacks; early loss or separation from parents; family history of suicide; hallucinations; hopelessness; insomnia; lack of future plans; previous suicide attempts; high lethality of previous attempt(s); living alone; low self-esteem; chronic physical illness; severe pain; recent loss; sexual abuse; and unemployment. Although women are more likely to attempt suicide, men successfully commit suicide four times more often than women. Suicide often occurs at the onset or the end of a depressive episode. It is essential to always inquire about suicidal thoughts or plan and perform a risk assessment, including questions regarding access to firearms or potentially lethal methods.

KEY POINTS (ABPN Examination)

A. When interviewing a patient with depression

1. Depression has a broad differential diagnosis, including primary medical illnesses, affective disorders, and substance use.
2. Always screen for other Axis I and Axis II disorders.
3. Build rapport, be empathic, and observe for verbal and nonverbal information.
4. Always ask about suicidality and homicidality.

B. When presenting a patient with depression

1. Present pertinent positives and pertinent negatives leading you to your differential diagnosis.
2. Do not regurgitate the patient's story verbatim; summarize the patient's symptoms using DSM terminology.
3. Do not jump immediately to treatment with medications. First discuss the additional studies you would like to obtain in order to rule out a mood disorder secondary to a general medical condition.
4. Always include in your risk assessment a proposed safety plan for any patient who verbalizes a history of suicidal or homicidal ideations or attempts.

Suggested Readings

Adler DA, McLaughlin TJ, Rogers WH, et al. Job performance deficits due to depression. *Am J Psychiatry* 2006;163:1569–1576.

American Psychiatric Association. *Diagnostic and Statistical Manual of Mental Disorders: Text Revision*. 4th Ed. Washington, DC: American Psychiatric Association, 2000.

American Psychiatric Association. Practice guideline for the treatment of patients with major depressive disorder (revision). *Am J Psychiatry* 2000; 157(suppl 4):1–20.

Barrett JE, Barrett HA, Oxman TE, et al. The prevalence of psychiatric disorders in a primary care practice. *Arch Gen Psychiatry* 1988;45:1100–1106.

Beck AT. The current state of cognitive therapy: A 40-year retrospective. *Arch Gen Psychiatry* 2005; 62:953–959.

Belmaker RH, Agam G. Major depressive disorder. *N Engl J Med* 2008;358:55–68.

Butler AC, Chapman JE, Forman EM, et al. The empirical status of cognitive-behavioral therapy: A review of meta-analyses. *Clin Psychol Rev* 2006; 26:17–31.

Coyne JC, Fechner-Bates S, Schwenk TL. Prevalence, nature, and comorbidity of depressive disorders in primary care. *Gen Hosp Psychiatry* 1994;16:267–276.

Ebmeier KP, Donaghey C, Steele JD. Recent developments and current controversies in depression. *Lancet* 2006;367:153–167.

Fancher T, Kravitz R. In the clinic. Depression. *Ann Intern Med* 2007;146:ITC5-1–ITC5-16.

Gillespie CF, Nemeroff CB. Hypercortisolemia and depression. *Psychosom Med* 2005;67(suppl 1): S26–S28.

Goldapple K, Segal Z, Arson C, et al. Modulation of cortical-limbic pathways in major depression: Treatment-specific effects of cognitive behavior therapy. *Arch Gen Psychiatry* 2004;61: 34–41.

Hansen RA, Garlehner G, Lohr KN, et al. Efficacy and safety of second-generation antidepressants in the treatment of major depressive disorder. *Ann Intern Med* 2005;143:415–426.

Kendler KS, Gatz M, Gardner CO, et al. A Swedish national twin study of lifetime major depression. *Am J Psychiatry* 2006;163:109–114.

Kessler RC, Berglund P, Demler O, et al. Lifetime prevalence and age-of-onset distributions of DSM-IV disorders in the National Comorbidity Survey Replication. *Arch Gen Psychiatry* 2005; 62:593–602.

Kessler RC, Chiu WT, Demler O, et al. Prevalence, severity and comorbidity of 12-month DSM-IV disorders in the National Comorbidity Survey Replication. *Arch Gen Psychiatry* 2005;62: 617–627.

Kessler RC, Zhao S, Blazer DG, et al. Prevalence, correlates and course of minor depression and major depression in the national comorbidity survey. *J Affect Disord* 1997;45:19–30.

Kroenke K, West SL, Swindle R, et al. Similar effectiveness of paroxetine, fluxetine, and sertraline in primary care. A randomized trial. *JAMA* 2001; 286:2947–2955.

Lustberg L, Reynolds CF. Depression and insomnia: Questions of cause and effect. *Sleep Med Rev* 2000; 4:253–262.

Mann JJ. The medical management of depression. *N Engl J Med* 2005;353:1819–1834.

Miller L, Warner V, Wickramaratne P, et al. Self-esteem and depression: Ten year follow-up of mothers and offspring. *J Affect Disord* 1999;52: 41–49.

Nutt DJ, Baldwin DS, Clayton AH, et al. Consensus statement and research needs: The role of dopamine and norepinephrine in depression and antidepressant treatment. *J Clin Psychiatry* 2006; 67(suppl 6):46–49.

Pampallona S, Bollini P, Tibaldi G, et al. Combined pharmacotherapy and psychological treatment for depression: A systematic review. *Arch Gen Psychiatry* 2004;61:714–719.

Papakostas GI, Thase ME, Fava M, et al. Are antidepressant drugs that combine serotonergic and noradrenergic mechanisms of actions more effective than the selective serotonin reuptake inhibitors in treating major depressive disorder? A meta-analysis of studies of newer agents. *Biol Psychiatry* 2007;62:1217–1227.

Pincus HA, Pettit AR. The societal costs of chronic majordepression. *J Clin Psychiatry* 2001;62(suppl6): 5–9.

Rihmer Z, Angst J. Mood disorders: Epidemiology. In: Sadock BJ, Sadock VA, eds. *Kaplan and Sadock's Comprehensive Textbook of Psychiatry*. 8th Ed. Philadelphia, PA: Lippincott Williams & Wilkins, 2004:1575.

Robinson LA, Berman JS, Neimeyer RA. Psychotherapy for the treatment of depression: A comprehensive review of controlled outcome research. *Psychol Bull* 1990;108:30–49.

Rush AJ. STAR*D: What have we learned? *Am J Psychiatry* 2007;164:201–204.

Rush AJ, Trivedi MH, Wisniewski SR, et al. Acute and longer-term outcomes in depressed outpatients requiring one or several treatment steps: A STAR*D report. *Am J Psychiatry* 2006;163: 1905–1917.

Schulberg HC, Mulsant B, Schulz R, et al. Characteristics and course of major depression in older primary care patients. *Int J Psychiatry Med* 1998; 28:421–436.

Snow V, Lascher S, Mottuer-Pilson C. Pharmacological treatment of acute major depression and dysthymia. *Ann Intern Med* 2000;132:738–742.

Solomon DA, Keller MB, Leon AC, et al. Multiple recurrences of major depressive disorder. *Am J Psychiatry* 2000;157:229–233.

Sullivan PF, Neale MC, Kendler KS. Genetic epidemiology of major depression: Review and meta-analysis. *Am J Psychiatry* 2000;157:1552–1562.

Thase ME. Depression and sleep: Pathophysiology and treatment. *Dialogues Clin Neurosci* 2006;8: 217–226.

Thase ME, Greenhouse JB, Frank E, et al. Treatment of major depression with psychotherapy or psychotherapy-pharmacotherapy combinations. *Arch Gen Psychiatry* 1997;54:1009–1015.

Thase ME. Molecules that mediate mood. *N Engl J Med* 2007;357:2400–2402.

Trivedi MH, Rush AJ, Wisniewski SR, et al. Evaluation of outcomes with citalopram for depression using measurement-based care in STAR*: Implications for clinical practice. *Am J Psychiatry* 2006;163:28–40.

Tsuang MT, Faraone SV. *The Genetics of Mood Disorders*. Baltimore, MD: Johns Hopkins University Press, 1990.

Vos T, Haby MM, Barendregt JJ, et al. The burden of major depression avoidable by longer-term treatment strategies. *Arch Gen Psychiatry* 2004; 61:1097–1103.

Weinmann S, Becker T, Koesters M. Re-evaluation of the efficacy and tolerability of venlafaxine vs SSRI: Meta-analysis. *Psychopharmacology (Berl)* 2008;196:511–520.

Weissman MM, Bland RC, Canino GJ, et al. Cross-national epidemiology of major depression and bipolar disorder. *JAMA* 1996;276:293–299.

Weissman MM, Markowitz JC, Klerman GL. *Comprehensive Guide to Interpersonal Psychotherapy*. New York, NY: Basic Books, 2000.

Zisook S, Lesser I, Steward JW, et al. Effect of age at onset on the course of major depressive disorder. *Am J Psychiatry* 2007;164:1539–1546.

II. BIPOLAR DISORDER

CASE HISTORY

PRESENT ILLNESS

Mr P is a 44-year-old divorced male who was brought to the emergency room for "erratic" behavior by police responding to a motor vehicle accident. Apparently, police had been called to the scene of the accident to find Mr P yelling at bystanders after he drove his car into a parked vehicle. Police noted that Mr P was not injured, but his speech was loud, rapid, and disjointed and that his explanation of the accident "did not make sense."

Upon arrival to the emergency department, Mr P appeared agitated and irritable and was intrusive in attempts to converse with hospital staff and patients. During his examination, Mr P explained that he was on a cross-country road trip and had not slept for several days. Days before the trip, he had been awake "day and night" working on various home remodeling projects that he had been postponing. Mr P explained that he suddenly decided to go on the trip and did not inform family, friends, or coworkers of his plans for travel.

Mr P denied feeling fatigued from his lack of sleep and stated that he felt "fantastic" except for having to tolerate "ridiculous questions" by the physician. He stated that he should not have been transported to the hospital since he had "lots of plans and ideas," and the police responding to the accident were "too dense" to understand. Mr P's speech was rapid and difficult to interrupt. Efforts to redirect Mr P during the examination resulted in an increased volume and disorganization of his speech. Mr P stated that he found it "tiresome" that jealous doctors continually interfered with his plans to "save the world from itself."

PSYCHIATRIC HISTORY

Mr P reported a history of multiple inpatient hospitalizations. Prior to his first hospitalization, Mr P experienced an episode of depression in his sophomore year of college which resolved without treatment. At that time, he took a short leave of absence but was able to successfully return to college and graduate. Mr P reported that the first of three inpatient psychiatric hospitalizations occurred immediately following college during a cross-country road trip. He recalled that the trip was the "best time of my life" and was angry that the hospitalization interrupted his trip. He stated that the other two hospitalizations occurred under similar circumstances. He also reported experiencing suicidal thoughts in the past but denied previous suicide attempts.

Following each hospitalization, Mr P was referred for outpatient psychiatric treatment in order to continue medications that he received in the hospital. However, Mr P stated that he did not believe that he suffered from mental illness and refused to follow up with those referrals and could not recall his prescribed medications.

Regarding his history of substance use, Mr P reported that he usually drinks two beers twice a month with friends. He denied a history of binge drinking, blackouts, and withdrawal symptoms. He also denied the use of illicit substances. He had no history of drug rehabilitation treatment.

FAMILY HISTORY

Mr P's mother suffered from major depressive disorder and had been hospitalized on several occasions. His maternal uncle also suffered from an unspecified mental illness and was a victim of suicide. He denied a family history of substance addictions.

SOCIAL HISTORY

Mr P was born and raised in Richmond, VA, and was the oldest of three children. His parents are married and in good health. His father worked in construction, and his mother was a school teacher. He graduated college and worked as an electrical engineer for several years; however, his employment history was sporadic. Apparently, he had difficulty holding job positions for extended periods due to unexplained absences and incomplete projects. He also reported financial difficulties due to gambling and credit card debts. His two marriages ended in divorce and he has no children. He denied a history of legal problems. He also denied having access to firearms.

MEDICAL HISTORY

Mr P was recently diagnosed with mild hypertension and is currently being treated with dietary modifications. Otherwise, he is in fair health.

MENTAL STATUS EXAMINATION

Mr P presented as an African American male who appeared his stated age of 44 years. He was slightly disheveled but casually dressed. His demeanor was superficially pleasant but irritable overall. He was generally cooperative and displayed good eye contact. He exhibited psychomotor agitation as he constantly shifted in his chair. His affect was labile, alternating between euphoria and irritability. He described his mood as "fantastic." His speech was loud and pressured. His thought processes included flight of ideas. His thought content was grandiose, but he denied experiencing hallucinations and did not exhibit other delusions. He denied suicidal and homicidal thoughts. He exhibited poor concentration and was distractible. His immediate and long-term memories were intact. His fund of knowledge was above average. He possessed poor insight and judgment.

PERTINENT PHYSICAL FINDINGS

Mr P's vital signs included a temperature of 98.2°F, heart rate 96 per minute, blood pressure 136/84 mm Hg, and respiration rate of 16 per minute. His oxygen saturation on room air was 99.0%. His pupils were equal and reactive to light and accommodation. No jaundice or lymphadenopathy was noted. His heart sounds were normal with no murmur present. His lungs were clear to auscultation. His abdomen was soft and nontender with no organomegaly and with normal bowel sounds. His extremities showed normal capillary perfusion. His neurological examination was unremarkable. He was 6′2″ tall and weighed 190 lb on admission.

LABORATORY DATA

The laboratory data obtained at intake revealed a BUN of 16 mg% and creatinine 1.0 mg%. HCO_3 was 24 mEq/L with a chloride level of 104 mEq/L. The sodium level was 140 mEq/L with a potassium level of 4.1 mEq/L. The white blood cell count was 5,300/ccm. Hemoglobin was 13.9 gm% with a hematocrit of 39%. The platelet count was 440,000/ccm. VDRL was nonreactive. The fasting blood glucose was 100 mg%.TSH level was 2.4 mIU/L. The blood alcohol level and urine drug screens were negative. Head CT was also negative.

HOSPITAL COURSE

Mr P was voluntarily hospitalized for psychiatric stabilization. He initially refused medications, reiterating that "nothing was wrong" with him; however, following encouragement and patient education by the treating psychiatrist, he agreed to treatment. He was then treated with lithium, which was further supported by records obtained from previous hospitalizations indicating a good response to this medication. His clinical picture gradually improved, as his affect became less labile and his thought processes were more goal oriented. He began to sleep throughout the night and his speech became nonpressured. He agreed to have his family contacted to make them aware of his location and a family meeting was arranged. His psychiatric symptoms continued to resolve and he demonstrated improved insight into his mental illness. He expressed his desire to return to his home and to continue with psychiatric treatment on an outpatient basis. He was discharged following a 14-day inpatient admission.

DISCHARGE MEDICATIONS

Lithium 600 mg PO twice daily.

DSM-IV-TR MULTIAXIAL DIAGNOSIS

Axis I. Bipolar I disorder, most recent episode manic, severe, without psychotic features
Axis II. None
Axis III. Mild hypertension
Axis IV. Financial, social environment, occupational
Axis V. At admission: 25
At discharge: 65

FORMULATION

A. Diagnostic

This patient meets all of the criteria for a manic episode required for a diagnosis of bipolar I disorder. His most recent mood disturbance included elevated mood, decreased need for sleep, pressured speech, and grandiosity. He also experienced flight of ideas, distractibility, increased goal-directed activity, and excessive involvement in pleasurable activities as evidenced by his cross-country travel. As a result of these symptoms, his social and occupational functioning have been impaired. The patient's diagnosis of bipolar I disorder, most recent manic episode, is supported by his current manic episode and a history of major mood disturbances in the past.

It is important to rule out other Axis I diagnoses when considering bipolar I disorder. While this patient presented during a manic episode, had he presented as depressed, eliciting the history of mania would be critical to avoid the misdiagnosis of major depressive disorder. It is also important to distinguish bipolar I disorder from other bipolar spectrum illnesses. The severity of this patient's manic symptoms rules out a diagnosis of bipolar II disorder. The patient's past psychiatric history does not include numerous mood disturbances with hypomanic episodes over a period of 2 years as seen in cyclothymic disorder. This patient did not exhibit psychotic symptoms that would require the distinction between the psychotic features of a mood disturbance and the symptoms of a primary psychotic disorder, such as schizoaffective disorder. Careful consideration must be given to the diagnoses of mood disorder due to a medical condition and substance-induced mood disorders. This patient does not have a history of significant substance use and his toxicology screens were negative. Additionally, he is not taking any medications known to induce mood symptoms. There is no indication that the patient suffers any medical conditions that could generate manic symptoms, such as endocrine, neurological, autoimmune, or infectious diseases. The patient does not meet the criteria for an anxiety disorder or cognitive disorder.

Axis II diagnoses must also be ruled out. In particular, borderline personality disorder and narcissistic personality disorder may be difficult to distinguish, especially since these personality disorders are predisposed to major mood disturbances. Common features such as impulsivity, irritability, mood swings, and suicidal thoughts may be seen in both borderline personality and bipolar disorders. Grandiosity and irritability are features of narcissistic personality disorder and may be confused with manic symptoms. However, this patient's mood symptoms are episodic and do not represent a persistent pattern of maladaptive symptoms as required to diagnose personality disorders.

B. Etiologic

Biologically, the patient has a family history of psychiatric illness. His mother suffered from major depressive disorder and his maternal uncle suffered an unspecified psychiatric illness and was a victim of suicide. Accordingly, the patient likely has a genetic predisposition for a major mood disorder. There are no obvious medical issues or substances that contributed to his recent decompensation. As with the occurrence of most episodes of mania in bipolar I disorder, there is no definite psychosocial trigger for the patient's current episode. However, the patient's noncompliance with psychiatric medications, despite his history of both manic and depressive episodes, has left him vulnerable to further mood disturbances.

C. Therapeutic

The first line of intervention in this case was to ensure the safety of the patient through acute inpatient hospitalization. As evidenced by his impulsivity and the occurrence of a motor vehicle accident, the severity of the patient's symptoms mandated hospitalization. Under these conditions, the patient may be further examined and observed for safety. Mr P had a positive therapeutic response to the mood stabilizer, lithium, which has been found effective for acute treatment of mania. Important goals for treatment were stabilization of mood, while monitoring for signs of evolving depression, reducing impulsivity, and eliminating agitated behaviors. Other medications that have been shown to be effective in the treatment of mania include anticonvulsants, such as valproate and carbamazepine, and atypical antipsychotics, such as olanzapine, risperidone, and others.

Before initiating psychopharmacological interventions, it is usually helpful to explore the patient's past exposure and responses to psychiatric medications. Such exploration may be helpful in gauging the likelihood of compliance with medications, especially if the patient has experienced unpleasant side effects in the past. This patient had a clear history of noncompliance with medications; therefore, determining whether his noncompliance was secondary to experience with side effects or due to the lack of insight into his mental illness is an important step in selecting a treatment regimen. This initial step also serves as a foundation for establishing a therapeutic alliance with the patient. Such an alliance is essential for improving the patient's long-term prognosis by increasing the likelihood that the patient will remain engaged in the treatment.

Since maintenance therapy following the resolution of acute symptoms is crucial for the patient's long-term prognosis, communication with his outpatient psychiatrist regarding issues related to treatment compliance is ideal. Patient education is also necessary in order to improve the patient's insight regarding his mental illness. Educating the patient's family about the nature of the mental illness can also be of great benefit. Knowledgeable family members may aid the patient in recognizing the recurrence of symptoms and seek intervention when the patient is unable to do so.

D. Prognostic

Mr P has important positive prognostic factors including the lack of psychotic symptoms, the absence of substance abuse disorders, no history of suicide attempts, and positive responses to prior psychiatric treatment. However, his poor compliance with psychiatric medications and psychiatric outpatient follow-up and lack of insight into his mental illness represent poor prognostic factors. Given his history of financial, marital, and occupational difficulties in addition to the nature of his mental illness, Mr P is at an increased risk for future mood episodes without maintenance treatment. These ongoing disturbances in mood also place him at increased risk for suicide in the future.

BIPOLAR DISORDERS

1. Introduction

Patients with bipolar disorder suffer from recurrent episodes of significant mood instability over a lifetime. These episodes include periods of mania, hypomania, or major depression. During manic episodes, an individual may experience euphoria, irritability, impulsivity, and grandiosity. Hypomania is less severe than mania, often involves euphoria, and does not generally impair an individual's daily functioning. Episodes of depression experienced in bipolar disorder are indistinguishable from those seen in major depressive disorder and may include depressed mood, anhedonia, and suicidal ideation. The spectrum of bipolar disorders has been categorized in terms of severity and pattern of mood symptoms and includes bipolar I, bipolar II, cyclothymic disorder, and bipolar disorder not otherwise specified (NOS).

Bipolar I disorder involves a history of at least one manic episode over a lifetime, regardless of the presence or absence of major depression. This disorder may present as manic, depressed, or mixed episodes. Each of these episodes may be complicated by psychotic features and, accordingly, must be distinguished from primary psychotic illnesses. Bipolar II disorder involves episodes of hypomania and major depression over a lifetime. There are no episodes of mania identified in bipolar II disorder. Cyclothymic disorder is characterized by a chronic pattern of less severe mood symptoms than seen in bipolar I and II disorders; however, individuals affected by cyclothymic disorder experience symptoms over a period lasting at least 2 years. Bipolar disorder NOS may involve manic or mixed states but does not meet the full criteria of the other subtypes of bipolar disorder.

2. Epidemiology

Bipolar I disorder affects approximately 1% of the adult population. It affects men and women equally and appears at consistent rates across cultural and ethnic groups. The average age of onset of bipolar I disorder is 20 years old, with a peak age range between 15 and 19. Initial appearance of manic symptoms after 60 years old is likely related to a general medical condition. Women are at risk of recurrence of mood symptoms during the postpartum period. Women are also more likely to suffer from rapid-cycling bipolar disorder. Studies have shown that 10% to 15% of individuals with bipolar I disorder will become victims of completed suicide and that suicide attempts more likely occur during depressive or mixed states. Many individuals with bipolar I disorder also suffer from substance use disorders. Studies have also shown that first degree relatives of individuals with bipolar I disorder suffer significantly increased rates of mood disorders.

Bipolar II disorder affects approximately 0.5% of population and appears to be more common in women. Individuals with this disorder have a 5% to 15% risk of subsequently developing bipolar I disorder. Women with this disorder are at an increased risk of postpartum mood disturbances. Completed suicide occurs in 10% to 15% of individuals with bipolar II disorder. Individuals with this disorder are at increased risk for comorbid substance use disorders and eating disorders. First degree relatives of individuals with bipolar II disorder are more commonly affected by major depressive disorder and bipolar I or II disorder.

Cyclothymic disorder carries a lifetime prevalence of 0.4% to 1%. It affects men and women equally, although women appear to be more likely to seek treatment than men. Onset of illness is usually in adolescence or early adulthood. Individuals with this disorder have a 15% to 50% risk of subsequently developing bipolar I or II disorder. First degree relatives of individuals with cyclothymic disorder are more commonly affected by major depressive disorder and bipolar I or II disorder.

3. Etiology

No single cause for bipolar disorder has been identified, but several hypotheses have been formulated. The combination of genetic, biological, and environmental factors appears to influence the nature of the disorder. Twin and adoption studies have shown that bipolar disorder is a heritable mental illness. Although a genetic link has been revealed through twin and adoption studies, no specific mode of inheritance has been identified. The risk of developing bipolar disorder is 75% for monozygotic twins of patients with bipolar disorder. First degree relatives of patients with bipolar disorder have a 20% risk of developing bipolar disorder as well.

Biological factors such as monoamine neurotransmitters, second messenger systems, and hormonal dysregulation have been implicated in the development of bipolar disorder. It is unclear to what extent the environment influences the disorder, despite studies showing that environmental factors, such as stressful life events, can impact the course of illness. Stressful events, sleep deprivation, and substance abuse have all been shown to adversely affect the course of illness.

4. Diagnosis

Patients with a bipolar spectrum disorder frequently present with disturbances in mood which may include depression, mania, hypomania, or mixed states. It is important to note that thorough history taking is essential in order to reach to a proper diagnosis. The initial clinical presentation of a depressed patient must be placed in the context of his past psychiatric history in order to avoid missing the diagnosis of bipolar disorder. In addition, these disorders are not diagnosed if the mood symptoms are better accounted for by schizoaffective disorder, schizophrenia, schizophreniform disorder, delusional disorder, or psychotic disorder NOS or if they are due to the direct physiological effects of a substance or a general medical condition.

TABLE 3B.5 Diagnostic Criteria for Manic Episode

A. At least 1 week of abnormally elevated or irritable mood (any duration if hospitalized)
B. During the episode, three (or more) of the following are present (four, if only irritable): 1. grandiosity 2. decreased need for sleep 3. pressured speech 4. flight of ideas or racing thoughts 5. distractibility 6. increased goal-directed activity or psychomotor agitation 7. excessive involvement in pleasurable activities
C. Symptoms do not meet the criteria for a mixed episode
D. There is marked impairment in occupational or social functioning, hospitalization is needed to prevent harm to self or others, or there are psychotic features
E. Symptoms are not due to the effects of a substance or general medical condition

Adapted from American Psychiatric Association. *Diagnostic and Statistical Manual of Mental Disorders: Text Revision.* 4th Ed. Washington, DC: American Psychiatric Association, 2000.

TABLE 3B.6 Diagnostic Criteria for Mixed Episode

A. Criteria for both manic and major depressive episode are present nearly every day for at least 1 week
B. There is marked impairment in occupational or social functioning, hospitalization is needed to prevent harm to self or others, or there are psychotic features
C. Symptoms are not due to the effects of a substance or general medical condition

Adapted from American Psychiatric Association. *Diagnostic and Statistical Manual of Mental Disorders: Text Revision*. 4th Ed. Washington, DC: American Psychiatric Association, 2000.

A. BIPOLAR I DISORDER

According to the DSM-IV-TR, individuals with bipolar I disorder have met the criteria for mania (Table 3B.5) at least once in their lifetime. Most of these individuals will also experience episodes of depressive illness; however, depression is not necessary to establish the diagnosis of bipolar I disorder. Typically, depressive episodes predominate and cycles between mania and depression are unpredictable. Many patients experience mixed episodes where criteria for both mania and depression are present (Table 3B.6). The mood episodes must adversely impact the patient's social or occupational functioning. Another important diagnostic feature of bipolar I disorder is that psychotic symptoms may be present during mood episodes and symptoms may be severe enough to require hospitalization.

While the course of bipolar I disorder can vary, a typical course averages 8 to 10 major mood episodes over a lifetime. In about 15% of bipolar I disorder individuals, the *rapid-cycling* variant of the disorder is experienced. In these cases, patients suffer alternating manic and depressive episodes at least four times a year.

B. BIPOLAR II DISORDER

According to the DSM-IV-TR, individuals with bipolar II disorder have had at least one episode of hypomania (Table 3B.7 for criteria) and at least one episode of major depression in their lifetime. Hypomanic episodes are similar to mania but

TABLE 3B.7 Diagnostic Criteria for Hypomanic Episode

A. At least 4 days of persistently elevated or irritable mood, different from the usual nondepressed mood
B. During the episode, three (or more) of the following are present (four, if only irritable): 1. grandiosity 2. decreased need for sleep 3. more talkative than usual or pressured speech 4. flight of ideas or racing thoughts 5. distractibility 6. increased goal-directed activity or psychomotor agitation 7. excessive involvement in pleasurable activities
C. It is an uncharacteristic change in functioning from when the person is not symptomatic
D. The mood disturbance and change in functioning are observable by others
E. There is no significant impairment in social or occupational functioning, hospitalization is not required, and there are no psychotic features
F. Symptoms are not due to the effects of a substance or a general medical condition

Adapted from American Psychiatric Association. *Diagnostic and Statistical Manual of Mental Disorders: Text Revision*. 4th Ed. Washington, DC: American Psychiatric Association, 2000.

less severe and shorter in duration. By definition, individuals with bipolar II disorder have not experienced episodes of mania or mixed states. Hypomanic episodes do not interfere significantly with social or occupational functioning but cause a change in behavior or functioning which is observable by others. Symptoms of hypomania are not severe enough to require hospitalization and do not include psychosis. It should be noted that while bipolar II disorder patients experience the less severe symptoms of hypomania, they tend to suffer more depressive episodes than individuals with bipolar I disorder.

C. CYCLOTHYMIC DISORDER

Cyclothymic disorder is a chronic pattern of mood instability lasting at least 2 years (1 year for children or adolescents) without relief from symptoms for more than 2 months. It involves fluctuating periods of hypomanic and depressive symptoms. These symptoms are not sufficient to meet the criteria for mania or major depression and therefore do not meet the threshold for either bipolar disorder I or II. Further, the hypomanic symptoms involved in cyclothymic disorder do not need to meet the duration requirement for a hypomanic episode (i.e., 4 days or more). While cyclothymia may continue as a chronic condition, it may also evolve into more severe forms of bipolar disorder.

D. BIPOLAR DISORDER NOT OTHERWISE SPECIFIED

Individuals suffering from bipolar disorder NOS experience symptoms with bipolar features that do not meet the full criteria for the other bipolar disorders. These individuals may experience symptoms such as recurrent hypomanic episodes without depressive episodes or chronic mood disturbances that are too infrequent to qualify as cyclothymic disorder.

E. DIFFERENTIAL DIAGNOSIS

Several Axis I diagnoses must be ruled out when making a diagnosis of bipolar disorder. When the presenting mood disturbance is depression, one must examine the patient's history for evidence of mania or hypomania. Failure to do so will create a possibility of a mistaken diagnosis of major depressive disorder. In the presence of psychotic symptoms, one must consider the possible diagnoses of schizoaffective disorder or schizophrenia. With such presentations, however, a distinction must be made from bipolar I disorder with psychotic features. Critical examination of the patient's history of psychotic episodes and the timing and duration of mood symptoms during those episodes will aid to differentiate primary psychotic disorders.

Special consideration must also be given to substance disorders as they may present with prominent mood symptoms. As such, substance-induced mood disorders must be ruled out. Intoxication and withdrawal syndromes may mimic the symptoms of mania or depression; therefore, screening for substance use is an essential step. However, it must be noted that the presence of substance abuse alone does not eliminate the diagnosis of bipolar disorder. This is especially the case since up to 60% of patients with bipolar disorder abuse substances at some point during their illness. Again, assessment of the timing of mood symptoms and substance intoxication and/or withdrawal may help clarify the diagnoses. Also, the effect of prescription medications on mood should not be overlooked. Mood disturbances due to medications such as steroids and amphetamines (often prescribed for the treatment of attention-deficit hyperactivity disorder) must be ruled out prior to a diagnosis of bipolar disorder. Furthermore, given that general medical conditions such as thyroid and adrenal disorders may produce significant mood disturbances, such conditions must also be ruled out.

Axis II disorders are also an important consideration prior to reaching a diagnosis of bipolar disorder. This becomes apparent when examining common symptoms shared by bipolar disorders and some Axis II disorders. In particular, individuals with borderline personality disorder suffer from labile mood and may report recurrent mood swings. Persons with narcissistic personality disorder exhibit grandiosity and are predisposed to depressed moods. Careful examination of the patient's psychiatric history and previous level of social and occupational functioning often provides important details to distinguish these disorders. A distinguishing feature of personality disorders is the pervasive and enduring pattern of dysfunctional interactions in interpersonal and occupational settings. Unlike personality disorders, the episodic mood disturbances suffered by patients with bipolar disorder customarily resolve with a return to normal baseline functioning.

5. Treatment

A. NONPHARMACOLOGICAL TREATMENTS

Psychotherapeutic modalities are not recommended as the primary treatment for bipolar disorder patients. However, psychotherapy that focuses on patient education regarding the disorder, its pharmacological treatment, and signs of impending mood episodes may assist in improving long-term prognosis. A major obstacle for some bipolar disorder patients is the lack of insight regarding their mental illness. Psychotherapeutic efforts addressing the impact of mental illness in patients' lives may improve compliance with pharmacological interventions. CBT may be useful in improving patients' insight and in promoting acceptance of mental illness. Combination therapy with CBT and mood stabilizing medications has been found to decrease the frequency and duration of mood episodes versus treatment with mood stabilizers alone.

Interpersonal therapy may reduce the stress related to difficult interpersonal relationships which may adversely impact illness. Further, family therapy focusing on education regarding the nature of the patient's illness, signs of illness exacerbation, and strategies to follow during the patient's mood episodes may improve family support and the patient's prognosis. Further, attention to lifestyle habits such as sleep hygiene and exercise may also contribute to the reduction of mood symptoms.

B. PHARMACOLOGICAL TREATMENTS

Regardless of the presenting mood episode, whether manic, depressed, or mixed, mood stabilization is the critical first step. Mood stabilizers such as lithium and valproate are standard drugs of first choice in the management of mood exacerbations in bipolar disorders. Atypical antipsychotics have also found a role in the treatment of bipolar disorder patients. During depressive states, antidepressant medications may also be used as adjunctive therapy to mood stabilizers. Antidepressants, however, are not recommended as monotherapy given the potential risk of inducing manic episodes. Benzodiazepines and typical antipsychotics are sometimes used to manage acute mania until mood stabilizers can take effect. Mood stabilizers are also the first-line treatment for cyclothymic disorder.

1. Lithium

Lithium is a mood stabilizer that has shown effectiveness in the treatment of acute mania and bipolar depression and as maintenance therapy in bipolar disorder. Lithium is also used as adjunctive treatment for major depressive disorder. Lithium's effects on mood are not fully understood but have been proposed to affect neurotransmitters, ion transport, and second messenger systems. Lithium has been shown to be effective in 60% to 80% of all hypomanic and manic episodes and is often regarded as the first choice for pure manic and depressive states. Studies have also found that lithium reduces the risk of suicide.

Lithium is excreted entirely by the kidneys. The clinician must be aware of potential drug-drug interactions with lithium. Medications such as ACE inhibitors, NSAIDs, and thiazide diuretics have the potential to increase lithium levels and cause lithium toxicity. Side effects of lithium include tremor, weight gain, gastrointestinal symptoms, polyuria, polydipsia, sedation, and cognitive dulling. It may also cause benign ECG changes, such as T-wave flattening or inversion. In addition, patients treated with lithium are at risk for developing hypothyroidism. Further, long-term therapy with lithium more than 10 years places patients at risk for kidney changes and, ultimately, renal failure. Prior to initiating lithium treatment, the clinician should obtain baseline labs, including BUN, creatinine, CBC, and thyroid stimulating hormone. ECG should also be considered, particularly for an older patient or a patient with cardiac disease. Pregnancy testing is critical since lithium treatment during the first trimester of pregnancy may result in fetal development of Ebstein's anomaly. Lithium is Category D in pregnancy.

Blood testing for lithium levels should occur about every 6 months in stable patients. Testing of renal and thyroid function should occur every 6 months. Serum lithium levels between 1.0 and 1.2 mEq/L for acute mania and between 0.6 and 0.8 mEq/L for maintenance therapy have been recommended; however, clinical response and not specific serum levels should direct medication management. Lithium levels above 1.5 mEq/L are likely to produce toxic effects (e.g., confusion, coarse tremor, increased deep tendon reflexes). Serious adverse events (e.g., vomiting, convulsions, stupor, coma) may occur at levels above 2.0 mEq/L and permanent neurological effects may occur above 2.5 mEq/L. Overdose of lithium may be fatal.

2. Valproate

Valproate, an anticonvulsant medication, is a mood stabilizer that is particularly effective in the treatment of rapid-cycling, depressive, and mixed states of bipolar disorder. It is also efficacious as maintenance therapy for bipolar disorder. It is metabolized by the liver and its use should be avoided in patients with liver disease. Valproate should be used with caution in patients taking lamotrigine, as valproate inhibits lamotrigine metabolism. This combination may cause a potentially significant increase in lamotrigine concentration and therefore increase the risk of severe rash.

Side effects include sedation, gastrointestinal symptoms, tremor, transient elevation in liver enzymes, weight gain, and hair loss. Dose-dependent, reversible thrombocytopenia may also occur with valproate treatment. Serious adverse reactions, such as hepatic failure and pancreatitis, have also been associated with valproate treatment. Polycystic ovarian syndrome has been seen in women treated with valproate. Prior to initiating treatment with valproate, the clinician should obtain labs, including CBC with platelets, hepatic function tests, and a pregnancy test. Pregnancy testing is critical since valproate treatment during pregnancy may result in fetal development of neural tube defects. Valproate is Category D in pregnancy.

Blood testing for valproate level, CBC including platelets, and liver function should occur at least every 6 months in stable patients. Serum valproate levels between 50 and 125 μg/mL have been found to be therapeutic for mood stabilization; however, clinical response and not specific serum levels should direct medication management. Overdoses with valproate are less likely than lithium to be fatal but do carry a risk of coma and death.

3. Carbamazepine

Carbamazepine, an anticonvulsant medication, is another mood stabilizing alternative for acute and maintenance treatment of bipolar I disorder. However, carbamazepine is not considered first-line treatment given its potential for serious adverse reactions. Common side effects include gastrointestinal symptoms, drowsiness, and ataxia. Skin rashes, hyponatremia, and mild thrombocytopenia and leukopenia may also be caused by this medication. Carbamazepine may also cause aplastic anemia, agranulocytosis, hepatitis, and Stevens-Johnson's syndrome, a potentially fatal side effect. Carbamazepine is metabolized by the liver and induces its own metabolism as well as the metabolism of many other medications.

Prior to initiating treatment with carbamazepine, the clinician should obtain CBC with platelets, serum electrolytes, hepatic function, and a pregnancy test. Pregnancy testing is critical since carbamazepine treatment during pregnancy may result in fetal development of neural tube defects. Carbamazepine is Category D in pregnancy. Monitoring of CBC with platelets, hepatic panel, and serum electrolytes should be performed every 2–4 weeks during the first 2 months of treatment. Monitoring can be decreased to every 3–6 months if testing remains stable.

As noted, carbamazepine is an autoinducer of its metabolism, as well as an inducer of the metabolism of other drugs. As a result, carbamazepine may lower the levels of other drugs, including antipsychotic, antidepressant, and oral contraceptive medications. The use of carbamazepine in patients on MAOIs is contraindicated. Carbamazepine may be fatal in overdose.

4. Lamotrigine

Lamotrigine, an anticonvulsant medication, is a mood stabilizing agent that is particularly effective in the treatment of bipolar depression. It is also useful in maintenance treatment of bipolar disorder. Common side effects include headache, dizziness, diplopia, and nausea. Another potential side effect of lamotrigine is a rash, which may herald the beginning of life-threatening reactions, Stevens-Johnson's syndrome, or toxic epidermal necrolysis. Approximately 8% to 10% of patients on lamotrigine will develop a benign rash within 4 months of drug initiation; however, given the serious risk of Stevens-Johnson's syndrome, lamotrigine should be immediately discontinued at the first sign of a medication-associated rash.

Gradual dose titration during drug initiation is recommended in order to decrease the risk of rash. Combination treatment with valproate should be done with extreme caution since valproate doubles the serum concentration of lamotrigine and increases the risk of rash. While development of rash is likely to occur early in treatment, it can occur at any time during treatment. Rash is more likely to occur in children.

5. Other Anticonvulsants

Gabapentin, topirimate, and tiagabine are anticonvulsant medications that have been used as alternatives for mood stabilization in bipolar disorder. The efficacy of these medications as primary mood stabilizers in bipolar disorder has yet to be established.

6. Atypical Antipsychotics

The atypical antipsychotics (olanzapine, risperidone, quetiapine, ziprasidone, and ariprazole) have been approved by the FDA for treatment of acute mania. Olanzapine and quetiapine have also been approved by the FDA for maintenance treatment of bipolar I disorder. Currently, clozapine does not have FDA approval for the treatment of bipolar disorder; however, it has shown efficacy in treatment-resistant mania. Treatment with atypical antipsychotics is particularly beneficial when psychotic symptoms are present; these medications may be used as adjunctive therapy to lithium or valproate. Of major concern is the development of side effects such as extrapyramidal symptoms, sedation, and metabolic side effects of weight gain, dyslipidemia, and diabetes. Of the atypicals, olanzapine and clozapine are the most likely to cause metabolic side effects. All patients on atypical antipsychotics should have routine monitoring of weight, fasting glucose, and lipid profile. Patients treated with clozapine are also at risk for developing agranulocytosis and require frequent monitoring of CBC.

7. Antidepressants

Use of antidepressants for bipolar patients is controversial and antidepressant monotherapy for the treatment of bipolar depression is not recommended. Treatment with antidepressant medications alone may induce rapid-cycling, hypomanic, or manic episodes in bipolar disorder patients. Antidepressants are sometimes initiated as adjunctive therapy to mood stabilizers once therapeutic levels have been attained. A combination drug, Symbyax (olanzapine and fluoxetine), has been approved for the treatment of bipolar depression. Signs of mania or hypomania should result in discontinuation of antidepressants.

8. Electroconvulsive Therapy

ECT is an effective alternative for treatment of acute mania and bipolar depression. It is useful in treatment refractory patients and patients who are unable to tolerate standard treatment with medication. ECT may also be used to treat women suffering exacerbation of bipolar illness during pregnancy. ECT appears to be equally as efficacious as treatment with lithium. Studies have shown that treatment of acute mania with ECT resulted in significant improvement of symptoms in 80% of patients. Studies have also shown that maintenance ECT reduces the hospitalization rate of bipolar patients. Side effects of ECT include delirium, memory loss, headache, nausea, and arrhythmias. While there are no absolute contraindications for ECT, relative contraindications include coronary artery disease, hypertension, cardiac arrhythmia, cerebral vascular aneurysms, recent stroke, and intracerebral masses.

6. Prognosis

The course of illness in bipolar disorders varies among patients. In patients with bipolar I disorder, approximately 7% will not experience recurrence of symptoms, 45% will have more than one episode, and 40% will suffer a chronic course. Typically, an average of 8 to 10 major mood episodes will be experienced by individuals with bipolar disorder. Approximately one third of patients with cyclothymic disorder progress to bipolar I or bipolar II disorder. Overall, bipolar I disorder carries a poorer prognosis than major depressive disorder.

Poor prognostic indicators for bipolar disorder include male gender, drug and alcohol dependence, psychotic features, recurrent depressive episodes, and poor premorbid occupational status. Up to 60% of bipolar disorder patients abuse substances during their lifetime. More favorable prognostic indicators include advanced age at onset of illness, brief manic episodes, and absence of comorbid psychiatric or medical illnesses. Bipolar disorder patients must often cope with the negative social consequences related to impulsive behaviors during manic episodes. Such consequences may involve enduring stressors on interpersonal relationships and occupational functioning.

As above, studies have shown that 10% to 15% of individuals with bipolar I disorder will become victims of completed suicide and that suicide attempts more likely occur during depressive or mixed state.

7. General Formulation for Bipolar Disorder

A. DIAGNOSTIC

Individuals with bipolar spectrum illnesses experience episodes of significant mood disturbance that range in severity. Diagnostic criteria for bipolar I, II, and cyclothymic disorders have been detailed above. It is critical to rule out disorders which share similar features to the bipolar disorders. Primary psychotic disorders with mood symptoms, such as schizoaffective disorder, are particularly difficult to distinguish from bipolar disorder patients who experience psychotic features during their mood episodes. In these cases, special attention must be given to the duration and resolution of psychotic symptoms in comparison to the duration and resolution of the mood episode. Other factors such as substance abuse, general medical illness, and prescribed medications may mimic many of the mood symptoms seen in bipolar disorders and must be ruled out.

B. ETIOLOGIC

The etiology of bipolar disorder remains unclear. Abnormalities in neurotransmitter regulation, hormonal regulation, and intracellular cascade systems have been proposed as potential causes. Adoption and twin studies have firmly established the heritability of bipolar disorder. Research efforts currently focus on identifying specific gene markers involved in the transmission of susceptibility for bipolar disorder. Regarding the etiology of a current mood episode, there may or may not be a clear precipitating factor. Clinicians should evaluate for the possibility of noncompliance with medications, substance abuse, new onset medical conditions or medications, and environmental and psychosocial stressors.

C. THERAPEUTIC

The foundation of successful treatment of bipolar disorder includes pharmacological management with mood stabilizing medications. These medications may include lithium, anticonvulsants, or atypical antipsychotics. In addition, many patients benefit from some combination of nonpharmacological and pharmacological approaches. Psychotherapeutic efforts that establish therapeutic alliance, improve insight into mental illness, and encourage patients to utilize family support may improve compliance with long-term therapy and ultimately improve overall prognosis.

D. PROGNOSTIC

Long-term prognosis in bipolar disorders often depends on compliance with treatment. Good prognostic indicators include older age of onset, female gender, and the absence of comorbid psychiatric disorders. Poor prognostic indicators include alcohol dependence, the presence of psychotic features, and frequent depressive episodes.

8. Risk Assessment

It is important to assess safety risk factors in bipolar disorder patients suffering acute mood symptoms. Suicide and potential violence are significant risks that may result from mood instability and impulsivity. Between 10% and 15% of bipolar disorder patients successfully complete suicide. The risk of suicide is highest during depressive and mixed states. Comorbidity with anxiety disorders or substance dependence increases the risk of suicide. As a result, it is important to inquire about suicidal thoughts and plans. Also, suicide risk factors, such as a history of suicide attempts and access to weapons, must be determined.

KEY POINTS (ABPN Examination)

A. When interviewing a patient with bipolar disorder

1. Always look for a history of mania in patients who present with depressive symptoms.
2. Assess for triggering events, including noncompliance with medications.
3. Always ask risk assessment questions for suicidal and homicidal thoughts and plans to engage in risky behaviors.

B. When presenting a patient with bipolar disorder

1. Highlight the presence or absence of manic or hypomanic episodes.
2. Do not overlook common comorbid conditions such as substance abuse.
3. Discuss safety concerns such as access to weapons and impulsive behaviors.

Suggested Readings

American Diabetes Association, American Psychiatry Association, American Association of Clinical Endocrinologists. Consensus development conference on antipsychotic drugs and obesity and diabetes. *J Clin Psychiatry* 2004;65:267–272.

American Psychiatric Association. *Diagnostic and Statistical Manual of Mental Disorders: Text Revision*. 4th Ed. Washington, DC: American Psychiatric Association, 2000.

Bader CD, Dunner DL. Antidepressant-induced hypomania in treatment-resistant depression. *J Psychiatr Pract* 2007 July;13(4):233–237.

Calabrese JR, Kimmel SE, Woyshville MJ, et al. Clozapine for treatment-refractory mania. *Am J Psychiatry* 1996;153:759–764.

Gijsman HJ, Geddes JR, Rendell JM, et al. Antidepressants for bipolar depression: A systematic review of randomized, controlled trials. *Am J Psychiatry* 2004;161(9):1537–1547.

Hilty DM, Brady KT, Hales RE. A review of bipolar disorder among adults. *Psychiatr Serv* 1999;50:201–213.

Khanna S, Vieta E, Lyons B, et al. Risperidone in the treatment of acute bipolar mania: Double-blind, placebo-controlled study. *Br J Psychiatry* 2005; 187:229–234.

Kieseppä T, Partonen T, Haukka J, et al. High concordance of bipolar I disorder in a nationwide sample of twins. *Am J Psychiatry* 2004 Oct; 161:1814–1821.

Lam DH, Watkins ER, Hayward P, et al. A randomized controlled study of cognitive therapy for relapse prevention for bipolar affective disorder: Outcome of the first year. *Arch Gen Psychiatry* 2003; 60:145–152.

Lester D. Suicidal behavior in bipolar and unipolar affective disorders: A meta-analysis. *J Affect Disord* 1993;27:117–121.

MacQueen GM, Young LT. Bipolar II disorder: Symptoms, course, and response to treatment *Psychiatr Serv* 2001 Mar;52:358–361.

Mukherjee S, Sackeim HA, Schnur DB. Electroconvulsive therapy of acute manic episodes: A review of 50 years' experience. *Am J Psychiatry* 1994;151: 169–176.

Sonne SC, Brady KT. Substance abuse and bipolar comorbidity. *Psychiatr Clin North Am* 1999; 22:609–627.

Wong ICK, Mawer GE, Sander JW. Factors influencing the incidence of lamotrigine-related skin rash. *Ann Pharmacother* 1999;33:1037–1042.

C. Anxiety disorders

Margarita M. Cala, MD

I. OBSESSIVE-COMPULSIVE DISORDER

CASE HISTORY

PRESENT ILLNESS

Mrs D is a 30-year-old married woman and mother of one child, referred by her primary care physician for a psychiatric evaluation. She reports a 10-year history of recurrent obsessions about cleanliness, mostly related to food items and concerns with germs. She reports having to wash a food item three or four times before eating it out of fear of contracting an illness. She puts all the dishes and utensils through a 2-hour cleaning regimen before each meal. She also stopped dining in restaurants or anywhere she could not wash her own food. Her obsession with food cleanliness became so extreme that she only ate very few foods and had to be admitted to the medical unit for malnutrition at age 22. While in the hospital, she reports being placed on sertraline, which she took for the next 9 years, with moderate resolutions of symptoms. Although she had to deal with residual symptoms, she was able to overcome her fears of contamination and maintain an appropriate food intake.

Six months ago, Mrs D gave birth to her first child. She noticed that during her third trimester, her concerns with dirt, germs, and environmental toxins markedly worsened. She had intrusive thoughts of the fetus being contaminated and proceeded to take multiple showers a day that were progressively lasting longer, up to 2 hours each. She also washed her hands repeatedly during the day, especially after being in contact with metallic surfaces.

After delivery of her baby, Mrs D also noticed a dramatic increase in her checking behavior, which she initially attributed to increased responsibility as a new parent. Although at first she was satisfied with a quick glance at appliances, doors, and windows before leaving the house, her checking behavior became progressively more complicated and time consuming. Mrs D is terrified that a fire could start if something were left on accidentally. She does not want to be responsible for harming her family, and engages in ritualized and repeated checks of "dangerous items" that are time consuming. Before going to work every morning, she makes sure that the microwave, stove, toaster, and other appliances are off and unplugged. She must stare at each appliance's knob for exactly 15 seconds before telling herself "it's off." If she is interrupted she has to start all over again. She feels exhausted after she leaves the house every morning and the rituals have caused her to be late for work repeatedly. Mrs D has recently been asked to resign from her job.

At night she imagines her house being on fire and her child being caught in it, which gets her out of bed to engage in checking rituals. This is a source of severe marital discord, as her husband describes it as "unbearable to live with." Mrs D is aware of the irrationality of her symptoms and feels like she has no control over them. The patient admits to feeling sad occasionally, especially after the recent loss of her job and relationship difficulties with her husband. However, these episodes do not last longer than a few hours and are rapidly interrupted by her obsessional thoughts.

PSYCHIATRIC HISTORY

Mrs D had a brief course of weekly group psychotherapy at age 22, which she reported to have helped her deal with her fears of contamination with food and regain the weight she had progressively lost. However, her obsessions with germs and contamination never subsided completely. She has never had psychiatric hospitalizations, nor is there evidence of suicide attempts or self-injurious behaviors. She was placed on sertraline 200 mg daily, with some alleviation of symptoms. Unfortunately, she discontinued the medication almost 2 years ago when attempting to get pregnant out of fears that it may hurt the fetus.

She denies any history of childhood physical or sexual abuse, as well as any history of alcohol or illicit drug abuse. She also denies any prior arrests or involvement with the legal system.

FAMILY HISTORY

Mrs D's mother was diagnosed with obsessive-compulsive disorder (OCD) and depression at age 25, and a maternal uncle has Tourette syndrome (TS). There is no history of psychiatric illness in the paternal side of the family.

SOCIAL HISTORY

Mrs D was born and raised in Connecticut, and is the only child of whom she describes as "supportive and warm parents." She reports her childhood as "happy" and describes difficulties only during the last years of high school and college. Although she was excessively devoted to school work and careful with details, she had trouble finishing assignments, which affected her grades.

After finishing college, Mrs D was employed as a jewelry store manager. She lost her job recently after failing to submit her last four periodic reports on time and being repeatedly late to work.

Mrs D married 3 years ago, but has had marital difficulties secondary to being "rigid and stubborn", as described by her husband. However, she reports that she just likes to do things "properly" and "by the book." She acknowledges the irrationality of her compulsive behaviors, although states she "just wants to keep her family safe."

Mrs D has no close friends, and states she has no time to engage in hobbies or any other social activities.

PERTINENT MEDICAL HISTORY

The patient denies any history of serious medical problems.

MENTAL STATUS EXAMINATION

Mrs D presents as a thin woman who looks her stated age of 30 years. She is neatly dressed and her general hygiene is impeccable. She is mostly pleasant and cooperative but avoids eye contact and becomes tearful while talking about the exhaustion and strong sense of self-doubt she deals with. Her speech is soft, with appropriate rate and rhythm. She exhibits no psychomotor abnormalities. She has full range of affect and her mood is reported as depressed. Her thought process is goal-directed and appropriate. She admits to obsessions of doubt, contamination, germs, and fear that something terrible may happen to her family. She realizes these are her own thoughts but finds them repetitive, intrusive, and is unable to prevent their repetition. She denies any current suicidal or homicidal ideations, intent, or plan. She denies any delusions, auditory or visual hallucinations. On the Folstein Mini Mental State Examination she scores 27/30. Two points were subtracted during serial 7's and one during recall. She is future oriented and her insight and judgment are fair.

PERTINENT PHYSICAL FINDINGS

Her physical exam is unremarkable except for chapped hands with eczematoid appearance. Her height is 5′7 and her weight is 117 lb on admission.

LABORATORY DATA

The laboratory data reveals Blood Urea Nitrogen (BUN) of 14 mg%, creatinine 0.9 mg%. The HCO_3 is 23.5 mEq/L, with a chloride level of 106 mEq/L. The sodium level is 140 mEq/L with a level of potassium of 4.0 mEq/L. The white blood cells count is 7,000/cmm. The hemoglobin is 13.5 gm% with a hematocrit of 39%. The platelet count was 250,000/cmm. Venereal Disease Research Laboratory (VDRL) is nonreactive. The fasting blood glucose is 81 mg%. TSH level is normal at 3.0 mIU/L.

OUTPATIENT COURSE

Mrs D was treated as an outpatient and was offered a combination of pharmacological and psychotherapeutic interventions. Although she agreed to taking medication, she was reluctant to psychotherapy due to "lack of time." She attributed this to her markedly time-consuming symptoms preventing her from spending enough time with her daughter and "catching up with things at home." She was restarted on sertraline and the dose was slowly titrated up to 200 mg daily. After 3 months on this dose, she reported no significant alleviation of her symptoms, which was also reflected by the Yale-Brown Obsessive-Compulsive Scale (Y-BOCS) rating.

The patient was then switched to paroxetine and the dose was slowly titrated up to 80 mg daily. Three months later, she experienced clinically significant alleviation of her symptoms and agreed to psychotherapeutic intervention. She was referred to a cognitive behavioral therapist with time-limited weekly visits. Treatment involved exposure to obsessional cues with self-imposed prevention of compulsive responses. The patient was educated about the nature of OCD and the rationale for exposure and response prevention. She was asked to create a hierarchy of feared situations that trigger anxiety and rank them from provoking the least to the greatest distress. The exposure started with moderately challenging triggers, instead of the lowest. She gradually moved up the hierarchy list and confronted increasingly challenging distress-provoking situations, such as touching a dirty doorknob without washing her hands or leaving without checking if the stove was off.

Mrs D attended a total of 18 sessions of cognitive behavioral therapy (CBT) and continued to take paroxetine at the stated dose. At a 6-month follow-up session, Mrs D reported significant alleviation of her symptoms and was able to start a new job.

DSM-IV-TR MULTIAXIAL DIAGNOSIS

Axis I. Obsessive-Compulsive Disorder (OCD)
Axis II. Rule out Obsessive-Compulsive Personality Disorder (OCPD)
Axis III. None
Axis IV. Severity of psychosocial stressor: severe, unemployment, marital discord, social isolation
Axis V. Global assessment of functioning: 40

FORMULATION

A. Diagnostic

This patient meets DSM-IV-TR diagnostic criteria for OCD as manifested by the presence of obsessions and compulsions that cause marked distress and interfere with her normal life functioning. She exhibits obsessions of contamination as manifested by persistent thoughts and concerns about germs and dirt, and about becoming ill or making her baby ill when she was still pregnant. She also has obsessions of pathological doubt that are reflected by preoccupations about not having completed common tasks at home. The patient also has fears and mental images of hurting her family by leaving electric appliances switched on that could cause a fire at home. The patient's attempts to suppress or ignore these thoughts are unsuccessful. She is able to recognize them as a product of her own mind. This differentiates it from the thought insertion or delusional ideation commonly seen in patients with psychotic disorders such as schizophrenia.

Her compulsions involve excessive showering, ritualized hand washing, and repetitive checking of electric items around the house. They result from an attempt to neutralize her obsessions and alleviate the emotional distress. These rituals are time consuming and cause significant distress to the patient. Occupational and interpersonal functions have been severely affected as the symptoms have caused the patient to lose her job, to have constant marital discord, and to remain socially isolated.

This patient does not meet the criteria for other Axis I disorders, including other anxiety disorders or major depressive disorder, which are frequently seen in patients with OCD. She also does not meet the criteria for a psychotic or cognitive disorder.

An important Axis II disorder to rule out in patients with OCD is Obsessive-compulsive personality disorder (OCPD) and other cluster C personality disorders. This patient exhibits traits of OCDP manifested by a history of perfectionism interfering with task completion and some evidence of excessive devotion to school work in the past. She is described by her husband as rigid and stubborn, which are major character traits of persons with OCPD.

B. Etiologic

Results from twins and family studies suggest that OCD is genetically mediated. The patient's mother has been diagnosed with the disease, and her uncle suffers from an obsessive-compulsive spectrum disorder (OCSD), such as Tourette's syndrome (TS). Epidemiological studies have shown that 30% of OCD patients have a tic disorder and first-degree relatives of TS patients have higher rates of obsessive-compulsive symptoms and OCD. Therefore, this patient has a strong genetic vulnerability to OCD and OCPD.

Life events that have been associated with precipitation and exacerbation of symptoms of OCD include pregnancy and childbirth. Although this patient had been diagnosed with OCD in the past, her symptoms seemed to have responded to treatment with a selective serotonin reuptake inhibitor (SSRI). Discontinuation of the medication, pregnancy, and childbirth could have potentially contributed to exacerbation of preexisting symptoms and to the development of new ones.

This patient's absorption with rituals and obsessional thoughts has led her to a highly restricted personal experience and to social isolation. The effect of this on her normal development and poorly defined sense of self could contribute to relationship problems and a pose high risk for divorce or separation.

C. Therapeutic

This patient has had a meaningful response to treatment with sertraline in the past, which is a predictor of future response to this class of medications. If there is no clinical response after a trial of 3 months of the maximal-tolerated therapy, she should be switched to another serotonin reuptake inhibitor (SRIs) before considering pharmacological augmentations. Approximately one third of nonresponders to initial SRI monotherapy will respond when switching to a second SRI. Assessment of clinical response can be done by using the Y-BOCS. A decline in 25% to 35% in the score is considered a clinical response.

The patient should be offered CBT in addition to pharmacotherapy. CBT is an established treatment for OCD and it has shown to be equal or perhaps superior to pharmacotherapy. It is valuable for patients who are reluctant to take medications or who wish to discontinue pharmacological treatment. Evidence indicates that CBT may also be helpful in preventing relapses.

The patient should be told in advance about the delay in the onset of response to medication and the need for a rather prolonged trial (3 months). This helps with unrealistic expectations from the patient and the resultant pressure on the clinician to change the dose prematurely.

OBSESSIVE-COMPULSIVE DISORDER

1. Introduction

Obsessive Compulsive Disorder (OCD) is a neuropsychiatric disorder characterized by the presence of obsessions and/or compulsions, with remarkably diverse symptoms that may vary within patients over time.

OCD can cause substantial impairment in the patients' quality of life, by interfering with academic functioning, work performance, and interpersonal relationships. The World Health Organization ranked this illness in 2000 as one of the most debilitating disorders, and it was among the 20 top causes of illness-related disability for people aged 15 to 24.

It is estimated that 40% to 60% of patients do not respond adequately to currently available therapies, and a larger proportion fail to obtain full remission of symptoms. The Y-BOCS is the most widely used instrument to assess and evaluate clinical response. Patients with a greater than 25% to 35% decline in Y-BOCS score are considered clinical responders. However, most of them continue to exhibit considerable impairment from their residual symptoms.

2. Epidemiology

OCD is a debilitating disorder with an estimated lifetime prevalence of 2%. It is present in approximately 3% of the population. It affects men and women equally, and the onset of symptoms usually presents at 6 to 15 years of age for males and 20 to 29 years of age for females.

Many patients with OCD struggle with other comorbid conditions. It is estimated that 55% to 65% of patients with OCD have at least one other Axis I disorder, with major depressive disorder, social phobia, and generalized anxiety disorder among the most prevalent. Concomitantly, a recent study reported that 22% to 32% of individuals with OCD also meet the DSM-IV criteria for obsessive-compulsive personality disorder (OCDP). Twenty percent to thirty percent of OCD patients have a history of tics.

Single people are more frequently affected with OCD than married people. This data might reflect the difficulty that people affected with the disorder have in maintaining a relationship.

OCD is frequently underdiagnosed and undertreated. A recent study revealed that 59.5% of OCD patients worldwide receive no treatment for the disorder.

3. Etiology

OCD, as most psychiatric disorders, is believed to be polygenic. There is evidence that the symptom clusters seen in a wide variety of obsessions and compulsions may have separate genetic associations. This may explain why some symptoms are notoriously more difficult to treat than others.

Epigenetic modifications may also contribute to the biology of the disorder. There is limited data pointing to a variety of risk factors including prenatal and perinatal adversity, psychosocial stressors, and postinfectious immune-based factors.

Studies have shown that stress increases the likelihood of intrusive thoughts, which are the foundation for developing obsessions. The anxiety resulting from these unwanted and disturbing thoughts can be extreme and may lead to compulsive behaviors aimed at releasing the associated anxiety. Further research analyzing the roles of biological and psychological factors is ongoing.

There is evidence supporting neurobiological differences implicating the loops connecting the orbitofrontal cortex and anterior cingulate, the basal ganglia and the medial thalamus in OCD. Cortico-striatal-thalamic-cortical circuit volume and gray matter density are usually altered in patients with this disorder, with a beneficial response in the decreased volume after pharmacotherapy and behavioral therapy. Concurrently, neurosurgical interruption of this circuit can reduce symptoms and decrease striatal volume.

The latest magnetic resonance spectroscopy studies have revealed evidence of elevated glutamate levels in specific brain regions in patients suffering from OCD. This finding has led to new research evaluating the effectiveness of glutamate modulating agents in treatment-resistant OCD.

4. Diagnosis

OCD remains a clinical diagnosis. The disorder is characterized by the presence of obsessive thoughts and compulsive actions that cause significant distress to the patient and interfere with occupational and social functioning. While the obsessions and compulsions can be of various types, they tend to fall into four specific clusters. These include contamination fears with cleaning compulsions; aggressive, sexual, religious, and somatic thoughts with checking, ordering, arranging, and repetitive rituals; obsessions with symmetry with accompanying ordering behaviors; and obsessions of saving with accompanying hoarding. The majority of patients with OCD are aware of the irrationality of the obsessions and compulsions and view them as ego-dystonic. A few patients lack any insight and are convinced that their symptoms are reasonable.

Some studies have found that hoarding symptoms are related to higher levels of comorbidity compared to nonhoarding OCD. The comorbidity includes personality disorders especially from the anxious-fearful cluster, pathological grooming conditions (skin picking, nail biting, and trichotillomania), and social phobia.

OCD shares symptoms with what has been called by some authors as Obsessive Compulsive Spectrum Disorders (OCSD). These disorders are similar in terms of symptoms profile, biology, and response to treatment and include neurological disorders with repetitive behaviors such as tic disorders, impulse control disorders such as trichotillomania, somatoform disorders such as body dysmorphic disorder, and eating disorders such as bulimia and anorexia nervosa. The common factor among these disorders is the inability to inhibit repetitive behaviors regardless of the underlying motive. However, for a person to obtain the diagnosis of OCD, the content of the obsessions or compulsions should not be solely restricted to the OCSD, which is also present as an Axis I disorder. This is clearly indicated by the DSM-IV-TR diagnostic criteria (Table 3C.1).

OCD symptoms may coexist with other psychiatric disorders including mood disorders, anxiety disorders, and psychotic disorders. OCD can be differentiated from schizophrenia by the less bizarre quality of the clinical presentation and lack of other psychotic symptoms. OCD patients also have more insight into the disorder unlike most of the patients suffering from psychotic illnesses. Although OCD and OCPD have similarities in their symptoms and the two disorders frequently coexist, the latter does not have the degree of functional impairment seen in patients with OCD.

5. Treatments

A. NONPHARMACOLOGICAL TREATMENTS

CBT continues to be a first-line treatment for OCD. Effectiveness is proved to be equal or perhaps superior to pharmacotherapy. The main element of this treatment is the exposure to the source of anxiety and prevention of the response or ritual. In addition to CBT, some studies have shown that group therapy can be potentially effective for patients with OCD.

B. PHARMACOLOGICAL TREATMENTS

1. Antidepressants

OCD was considered to be a poorly treated disorder with a chronic and unremitting course until drugs that inhibit the reuptake of serotonin (SRIs) such as the SSRIs and clomipramine were introduced in the mid 1980s. Medications lacking these properties, such as standard tricyclic antidepressants and MAO-Is, have shown in randomized control trials overall to be ineffective. SRIs are currently the first-line pharmacological treatment for patients with OCD. However, only few patients show complete remission of their symptoms, and some patients show minimal improvement. No SRI has shown to be more effective than others, and individual patients can respond to one agent but not to another. It is impossible to predict which SRI will be more effective, therefore the selection is usually based on side effect profile, half-life, and cost. Most published consensus guidelines consider an adequate SRI trial in OCD to consist of 12 weeks of the maximum tolerated dose. FDA-approved SRIs for the treatment of OCD are fluoxetine, paroxetine, fluvoxamine, sertraline, and clomipramine. A better tolerability and acceptability over clomipramine make the SSRIs the treatment of choice, leaving clomipramine as a second agent.

There is some evidence suggesting that citalopram, venlafaxine, and mirtazapine could be

TABLE 3C.1 DSM-IV-TR Diagnostic Criteria for Obsessive-Compulsive Disorder

A. Either obsessions or compulsions:

Obsessions as defined by (1), (2), (3), *and* (4):

(1) recurrent and persistent thoughts, impulses, or images that are experienced, at some time during the disturbance, as intrusive and inappropriate and that cause marked anxiety or distress

(2) the thoughts, impulses, or images are not simply excessive worries about real-life problems

(3) the person attempts to ignore or suppress such thoughts, impulses, or images, or to neutralize them with some other thought or action

(4) the person recognizes that the obsessional thoughts, impulses, or images are a product of his or her own mind (not imposed from without as in thought insertion)

Compulsions as defined by (1) *and* (2):

(1) repetitive behaviors (e.g., hand washing, ordering, checking) or mental acts (e.g., praying, counting, repeating words silently) that the person feels driven to perform in response to an obsession, or according to rules that must be applied rigidly

(2) the behaviors or mental acts are aimed at preventing or reducing distress or preventing some dreaded event or situation; however, these behaviors or mental acts either are not connected in a realistic way with what they are designed to neutralize or prevent or are clearly excessive

B. At some point during the course of the disorder, the person has recognized that the obsessions or compulsions are excessive or unreasonable. **Note:** This does not apply to children.

C. The obsessions or compulsions cause marked distress, are time consuming (take more than one hour a day), or significantly interfere with the person's normal routine, occupational (or academic) functioning, or usual social activities or relationships.

D. If another Axis I disorder is present, the content of the obsessions or compulsions is not restricted to it (e.g., preoccupation with food in the presence of an eating disorder; hair pulling in the presence of trichotillomania; concern with appearance in the presence of body dysmorphic disorder; preoccupation with drugs in the presence of a substance use disorder; preoccupation with having a serious illness in the presence of hypochondriasis; preoccupation with sexual urges or fantasies in the presence of paraphilia; or guilty ruminations in the presence of major depressive disorder).

E. The disturbance is not due to the direct physiological effects of a substance (e.g., a drug of abuse, a medication) or a general medical condition.

Specify if:

With poor insight: if, most of the time during the current episode, the person does not recognize that the obsessions and compulsions are excessive or unreasonable.

Adapted from American Psychiatric Association. *Diagnostic and Statistical Manual of Mental Disorders: Text Revision*. 4th Ed. Washington, DC: American Psychiatric Association, 2000.

efficacious in treating OCD but additional data from controlled studies is necessary.

2. Mood Stabilizers

There is no convincing evidence to suggest that mood stabilizers are effective in the treatment of OCD.

3. Anxiolytics

Augmentation strategies with clonazepam and buspirone have been attempted to maximize treatment response, showing unsatisfactory results. Studies involving other benzodiazepines have overall given inconsistent results. Use of clonazepam might be beneficial in patients with comorbid panic disorder, insomnia, or high levels of agitation.

4. Antipsychotics

Antipsychotic augmentation in SRI-refractory OCD is indicated in patients who have been treated for at least 3 months with the maximal tolerated therapy of an SRI. However, studies have shown that only one third of these patients will have a significant treatment response. Studies using haloperidol and risperidone have demonstrated efficacy. The evidence for quetiapine and olanzapine is still inconclusive, and additional studies are needed to prove their efficacy as augmentation agents.

A particular beneficial response to augmentation with haloperidol and risperidone has been demonstrated in patients with OCD and comorbid tic disorders.

5. Other Treatments

Brain stimulation techniques should be considered for the more severe and refractory patients. They include repetitive transcranial magnetic stimulation (TMS) and deep brain stimulation (DBS). TMS allows stimulation of specific brain areas by using magnetic field induction in a noninvasive way, whereas DBS consist of a neurosurgical implant of electrodes in the anterior limbs of the internal capsule that is connected to a pulse generator located subcutaneously in the patient's anterior chest.

Electroconvulsive therapy (ECT) efficacy in the treatment of OCD is still unproven. Traditional neurosurgical interventions such as capsulotomy and cingulotomy have shown positive results in severe and refractory cases of OCD.

6. General Formulation for Obsessive-Compulsive Disorder

A. DIAGNOSTIC

The DSM-IV-TR requires the presence of recurrent obsessions or compulsions or both, severe enough to cause marked distress to the person, to make a diagnosis of OCD. Although the compulsive behavior may be carried out in an effort to release the resultant anxiety associated with the obsession, the completion of the resultant act may have no effect in the level of anxiety and may even increase it.

The major psychiatric considerations in the differential diagnosis of OCD are OCPD, phobias, depressive disorders, and schizophrenia.

B. ETIOLOGIC

OCD is a heterogeneous disorder with a wide variability in phenotypic expression. Neurobiological, genetic, and environmental factors contribute to the expression of symptoms, and attempts to identify susceptible genes are still ongoing. Epigenetic factors are etiologically important, as OCD is most likely the result of interactions between genes and environment during brain development.

OCD has long been identified as a "stress-sensitive" condition—symptoms wax and wane according to the presence or absence of stress in the patient's life. Onset or exacerbation of symptoms have been noted to be related to pregnancy, childbirth, and parental care for their children.

OCD is often complicated by serious impairment in occupational and social functioning, significantly affecting coworkers and family members, which contributes to worsening interpersonal functioning.

C. THERAPEUTIC

SRIs and CBT are the first-line treatment for OCD. Remission is not common and refractory cases may benefit from different treatment strategies including pharmacological augmentations, brain stimulation approaches, and neurosurgical interventions for severe refractory cases. Double-blind placebo-controlled trials have demonstrated that antipsychotic augmentation with risperidone or haloperidol is an effective intervention in treatment-refractory OCD. Research in new pharmacological strategies targeting the glutamate system, such as the use of riluzole, holds promise for alleviating symptoms of this disabling and difficult-to-treat disease.

D. PROGNOSTIC

A majority of patients with OCD do not recover; they only remit. Early onset of symptoms has a higher frequency of compulsions not preceded by obsessions, higher comorbidity with tics and TS, and worse response to monotherapy with SRIs or clomipramine. Patients with predominant hoarding and symmetry obsessions are less likely to respond to SRIs alone and more often require augmentation with dopamine blockers. The presence of a personality disorder, delusional beliefs, coexisting major depression, and need for hospitalization indicate poor prognosis. A good prognosis is indicated by good social support and occupational adjustment.

7. Risk Assessment

Suicide risk in OCD patients has been considered to be low compared to the general U.S. population. However, recent research suggests that the risk may be underestimated. About one third of patients with OCD have major depressive disorder, and this may pose a significantly increased suicide risk.

KEY POINTS (ABPN Examination)

A. When interviewing a patient with obsessive-compulsive disorder

1. The genetic transmission of OCD is indisputable. A detailed family history and assessment for other OCSDs is important to make a diagnosis and include or rule out comorbidites.
2. Look for symptoms of depressive disorders, other anxiety disorders, and character traits suggesting obsessive-compulsive personality disorder, which have a high prevalence among this population.
3. Do not forget to make a thorough assessment of safety, including suicidal ideations, intent, or plans.
4. Look for evidence of interpersonal difficulties or family discord resulting from relatives' participation in rituals and alteration of their daily routines in an effort to reduce the patient's anxiety, or to control the patient's expressions of anger.

B. When presenting a patient with obsessive-compulsive disorder

1. Acknowledge that symptoms of other OCSDs conditions may overlap with OCD or be the result of shared risk factors for vulnerability.
2. If diagnosis is unclear, state that you would use a structured diagnostic interview like SCID-DSM-IV for clarification.

Suggested Readings

American Psychiatric Association. *Diagnostic and Statistical Manual of Mental Disorders: Text Revision*. 4th Ed. Washington, DC: American Psychiatric Association, 2000.

Bjorgvinsson T, Hart J, Heffelfinger S. Obsessive-compulsive disorder: Update on assessment and treatment. *J Psychiatr Pract* 2007;13:362–372.

Bloch MH, Landeros-Weisenberger A, Kelmendi B, et al. A systematic review: Antipsychotic augmentation with treatment refractory obsessive-compulsive disorder. *Mol Psychiatry* 2006;11:622–632.

Bram T, Bjorgvinsson T. A Psychodynamic clinician's foray into cognitive-behavioral therapy utilizing exposure and ritual prevention for OCD. *Am J Psychother* 2004;58:304–320.

Dell'Osso B, Altamura AC, Mundo E, et al. Diagnosis and treatment of obsessive-compulsive disorder and related disorders. *Int J Clin Practice* 2007;61:98–104.

Erzegovesi S, Cavellini MC, Cavedini P, et al. Clinical predictors of drug response in obsessive compulsive disorder. *J Clin Psychopharmacol* 2001;21:272–275.

Foa EB, Liebowitz MR, Kozak MJ et al. Randomized, placebo controlled trail of exposure and ritual prevention, clomipramine and their combination in the treatment of obsessive-compulsive disorder. *Am J Psychiatry* 2005;162: 151–161.

Fontenelle LF, Mendlowicz MV, Versiani M. The descriptive epidemiology of obsessive-compulsive disorder. *Prog Neuropsychopharmacol Biol Psych* 2006:30:327–337.

Gabbard GO. *Psychodynamic Psychiatry in Clinical Practice*. 4th Ed. Washington, DC: American Psychiatric Publishing, 2005.

Goodman WK, Price LH, Rasmussen SA, et al. Efficacy of fluvoxamine in obsessive-compulsive disorder: A double blind comparison with placebo. *Arch Gen Psychiatry* 1989:46:36–43.

Goodman WK, Price LH, Rasmussen SA, et al. The Yale-Brown obsessive-compulsive scale. I. Development, use, and reliability. *Arch Gen Psychiatry* 1989;46:1106–1111.
Graybiel, AM, Rauch SL. Toward a neurobiology of obsessive-compulsive disorder. *Neuron* 2000; 28:343–347.
Hollander E, Friedberg JP, Wasserman S, et al. The case for the OCD spectrum. In: Abramowitz JS, Houts AC, eds. *Concepts and Controversies in Obsessive-Compulsive Disorder*. New York, NY: Springer, 2005:95–113.
Jenike MA. Clinical Practice: Obsessive-Compulsive Disorder. *N Engl J Med* 2004;350:259–265.
Khan A, Leventhal RM, Khan S, et al. Suicide risk in patients with anxiety disorders: A meta-analysis of the FDA database. *J Affect Disord* 2002;68:183–190.
Mataix-Cols D, Rosario-Campos MC, Leckman JF. A multidimensional model of obsessive-compulsive disorders. *Am J Psychiatry* 2005;162:228–238.
Mataix-Cols D, Wooderson S, Lawrence N, et al. Distinct neural correlates of washing, checking, and hoarding symptom dimensions in obsessive-compulsive disorder. *Arch Gen Psychiatry* 2004;61:565–576.
Math SB, Janardhan Reddy YC. Issues in the pharmacological treatment of obsessive-compulsive disorder. *Int J Clin Pract* 2007;61:1188–1197.
McDonough M, Kennedy N. Pharmacological Management of obsessive-compulsive disorder: A review for clinicians. *Harvard Rev Psychiatry* 2002;10:127–137.
Miguel EC, Coffey BJ, Baer L, et al. Phenomenology of intentional repetitive behaviors in obsessive-compulsive disorder and Tourette's Syndrome. *J Clin Psychiatry* 1995;56:246–255.
Miguel EC, Leckman JF, Rauch S, et al. Obsessive-compulsive disorder phenotypes: Implications for genetic studies. *Mol Psychiatry* 2005;10:258–275.
Pallanti S, Hollander E, Goodman W. A qualitative analysis of non response: Management of treatment-refractory obsessive-compulsive disorder. *J Clin Psychiatry* 2004;65:6–10.
Pauls DL, Towbin KE, Leckman JF, et al. Gilles de la Tourette's syndrome and obsessive-compulsive disorder: Evidence supporting a genetic relationship. *Arch Gen Psychiatry* 1986;43:1180–1182.
Stein DJ. Obsessive compulsive disorder. *Lancet* 2002;360:397–405.
The Clomipramine Collaborative study Group. Clomipramine in the treatment of obsessive-compulsive disorder. *Arch Gen Psychiatry* 1991;48:730–738.
World Health Organization. The World Health Report 2001-Mental Health: New Understanding, New Hope. Geneva, Switzerland: World Health Organization, 2001.

II. POSTTRAUMATIC STRESS DISORDER

CASE HISTORY

PRESENT ILLNESS

Mr W is a 35-year-old married white lawyer, referred for psychiatric evaluation by his primary care doctor for symptoms he developed 6 months ago after a motor vehicle accident. He lost control of his car during a snow storm, causing the collision of three other vehicles. He was trapped in his car for several hours until the rescue team was able to extract him. Although Mr W did not suffer any major physical injury, one of the passengers in another vehicle was thrown out of the car during the impact and died.

The patient reports intrusive thoughts about the accident and "vivid memories" of being trapped in the car. He also stated that he can still remember "the smell of smoked air." He reports having nightmares about the passenger who died, in which Mr W stares at him lying dead on the pavement. Mr W also finds himself tearful at times, thinking, "If I had stayed home that night, no one would have died." During these tearful episodes, he wishes he were dead. However, these thoughts are always transitory and do not present in other contexts.

Ever since the accident, Mr W has taken an alternative road when driving home. Driving to places now takes him much longer than previously, due to increased focusing on his environment, including other cars and transit signs. He refused to drive during the remainder of the winter season following the accident. He presently experiences extreme fear when driving while raining, to the point of having to pull over and wait until the rain ceases. These behaviors cause to miss important meetings with clients and work. He has "not been able to keep up with work" in the office, which is causing him significant concern.

Mr W reports occasionally experiencing brief episodes of palpitations and mild chest discomfort, particularly when starting his car in the morning. He denied other associated symptoms. He finds himself easily startled when hearing other cars' horns or even by minor sounds at work. His wife has noted that he changes the channel whenever a commercial for snow tires appears. He also stopped working out at the gym, going to happy hours after work and playing golf with friends on the weekends. He currently spends most of his free time reading books at home. His medical workup is negative.

When asked about symptoms of depression, he denies periods of consistent depressed or irritable mood lasting more than a few hours and denies neurovegetative symptoms. He finds himself reluctant to talk about the day of the accident, and states he "just can't remember how it happened." When answers are prompted during the interview, he becomes tearful. Prolonged pauses are noted before he starts narrating parts of the story. He denies any suicidal or homicidal ideations, intent, or plan at the time of evaluation as well as any presence of psychotic symptoms.

PSYCHIATRIC HISTORY

Mr W had a course of brief psychotherapy at age 26 for "feeling overwhelmed with anxiety" while studying for the bar exam right after law school. Otherwise, he has never had any other contact with mental health treatment providers until now. He has never been exposed to psychotropic medication.

He denies any history of childhood physical or sexual abuse, as well as any history of alcohol or illicit drug abuse. He also denies any prior arrests or involvement with the legal system.

FAMILY HISTORY

The patient's mother was diagnosed with major depressive disorder in her early 40s.

SOCIAL HISTORY

Mr W was born and raised in Massachusetts and has one older brother. He reports his childhood as "happy" until his father's death of cancer when Mr W was 11 years old. At that time, he remembered feeling sad, having difficulty with grades at school and having a difficult time falling asleep, which resolved spontaneously a few months later. His mother remarried 2 years later, and Mr W indicates feeling loved and supported by his stepfather and having a good relationship with him to this date. He finished college and attended law school subsequently. He currently works as an associate in a law firm. He has been married for the last 3 years and has no children. He is an avid reader. He also used to enjoy playing golf with friends on the weekends and traveling with his wife.

PERTINENT MEDICAL HISTORY

The patient denies any history of any serious medical problems.

MENTAL STATUS EXAMINATION

Mr W presented as an average-weight man who looked his stated age of 35 years. He was neatly dressed and his general hygiene was good. He was mostly pleasant and cooperative but avoided eye contact and became tearful during the parts of the interview related to his recent accident. His speech was soft, with appropriate rate and rhythm. He made prolonged pauses at times. He exhibited no psychomotor activity abnormalities. He had full range of affect and his mood was reported as depressed. His thought process was goal directed and appropriate. He denied any current suicidal or homicidal ideations, intent, or plan, although he admitted to passive wishes of him dying instead of the other man who was thrown out of the car. He denied any delusions, auditory or visual hallucinations, dissociative flashback episodes or obsessions. On the Folstein Mini Mental State Examination he scored 27/30. Two points were subtracted during serial 7's and one during recall. He was future oriented and his insight and judgment were fair.

PERTINENT PHYSICAL FINDINGS

His vital signs were a temperature of 97.7°F, heart rate 100 per minute, blood pressure 140/85 mm Hg, and respiratory rate of 13 per minute. Oxygen saturation on room air was 99.0%. His pupils were equal and reactive to light and accommodation. No jaundice, anemia, or lymphadenopathies were noted. The first and second heart sounds were heard and there was no murmur. The lungs were clear. The abdomen was soft, nontender, and there was no organomegaly. Bowel sounds were heard normally. The extremities showed normal capillary perfusion. The neurological examination was normal. His height was 6′2, and his weight was 180 lb on admission.

LABORATORY DATA

The laboratory data obtained 2 weeks ago from his primary care doctor (PCP) revealed a BUN of 13 mg%, creatinine 0.9 mg%. The HCO_3 was 23.5 mEq/L, with a chloride level of 106 mEq/L. The sodium level was 140 mEq/L, with a level of potassium of 4.0 mEq/L. The white blood cell count was 8,000/cmm. The hemoglobin was 14.8 gm% with a hematocrit of 40%. The platelet count was 250,000/cmm. VDRL was nonreactive. The fasting blood glucose was 80 mg%. TSH level was normal at 3.0 mIU/L.

OUTPATIENT COURSE

During the first diagnostic interview, the patient was educated into the etiology of his symptoms and the diagnosis of PTSD. He was offered trauma-focused psychological treatments but he reported not being interested at the time. Alternatively, he agreed to start paroxetine. His dose was gradually titrated up to a final dose of 40 mg within a 2-month period, with a modest symptom response. This prompted the patient to try psychotherapeutic interventions 3 months later. Mr W was referred to an individual CBT program with emphasis on exposure-based interventions. Mr W met with a therapist weekly for 12 sessions. To encourage the patient to continue the exercises until anxiety was reduced to half, he was given handouts that illustrated the predictable rise and fall of anxiety during exposure.

The first session included a review of the symptoms, diagnosis, and psychoeducation about PTSD. Progressive muscle relaxation was taught on the first session and kept throughout the following meetings. During the second session, the patient was asked to read aloud a written description of the motor vehicle accident (MVA)and discussions of avoidance were started. Subsequent sessions were based mainly on exposure (first imaginal and then in vivo). The last sessions focused on exploring existential issues (concerning mortality), cue-controlled relaxation, and interventions to address estrangement and social isolation. The last session centered on a review of all treatment procedures.

Mr W was taught early during treatment about the principles behind CBT and he showed that he was able to use them to practice in-between treatment sessions and in his own posttreatment homework. As early as 6 weeks after the initiation of treatment, the patient completed a self-report battery and reported significantly lower levels of the initial symptoms, particularly the ones related to avoidance and trauma-related intrusive memories. His participation in social activities and difficulty with work performance were also significantly improved. However, Mr W continues to experience occasional nightmares and a few somatic complaints, such as palpitations.

DISCHARGE MEDICATIONS

Paroxetine 40 mg p.o. daily.

DSM-IV-TR MULTIAXIAL DIAGNOSIS

Axis I. Chronic Post-traumatic Stress Disorder (PTSD)
Axis II. None
Axis III. R/O borderline hypertension
Axis IV. Severity of psychosocial stressor: moderate, recent trauma, problems at work, social isolation.
Axis V. Global assessment of functioning:

At admission: 45; serious impairment in social and occupational functioning, as evidenced by social isolation, avoidance of previously enjoyed daily activities and frequent nightmares and flashbacks.

At discharge: 65; mild symptoms such as occasional nightmares and somatic complaints, no significant impairment in daily functioning.

FORMULATION

A. Diagnostic

This patient meets DSM-IV-TR diagnostic criteria for PTSD. He was involved in a severe motor-vehicle accident in which he responded with horror and helplessness after being trapped in a car for several hours waiting to be rescued. Although he did not experience severe physical injury, he witnessed and was confronted by the death of a passenger in another car. He presents with more than one symptom of reexperiencing the traumatic event, as manifested by the presence of recurrent and intrusive thoughts, images, and nightmares. He also exhibits both psychological distress and physiological reactivity to exposure to internal and external cues that resemble the traumatic experience, such as feelings of extreme fear while driving in the rain, and new onset of palpitations and chest discomfort mainly while starting his car in the morning.

The patient has three symptoms of avoidance of stimuli associated with the trauma. He is unable to remember important aspects of the accident, and seems to have no recollection of the time he lost control of his car. He exhibits clear efforts to avoid thoughts or feelings associated with the day of the accident, as evidenced by him refusing to talk about the event, changing the channel when commercials for snow tires appear, and taking an alternative road when driving home. Finally, he has markedly diminished interest in significant activities including participating in hobbies on the weekends such as golfing, exercising at the gym, and socializing with friends after work.

Mr W exhibits more than two persistent symptoms of increased arousal, as indicated by difficulty concentrating at work and exaggerated startle response. His exaggerated focusing on the environment while driving, causing him marked delays, may be the result of a hypervigilant state.

Finally, Mr W has been experiencing these symptoms for the last 6 months, making them chronic in nature. These symptoms have caused him severe impairment at work, in terms of efficiency, ability to attend important meetings and appointments with clients. He has also withdrawn from his regular social activities and has limited his interactions to work-related encounters.

Diagnostic confusion may result when treating a patient with PTSD, secondary to its comorbidity and overlapping symptoms with major depressive disorder, substance abuse, and other anxiety disorders. Although Mr W admits to depressed mood, its duration does not meet the criteria for depression or dysthymia. Except for intermittent sleep difficulties secondary to nightmares, he denied the presence of other neurovegetative symptoms such as changes in appetite or energy level, which would support the diagnosis of a mood disorder.

This patient does not meet criteria for other Axis I disorders, including other anxiety disorders or substance abuse disorders, which are frequently seen in patients with PTSD. He also does not meet the criteria for a psychotic or cognitive disorder.

B. Etiologic

The patient's symptoms clearly followed the occurrence of a severely traumatic event. It is important to recognize the patient's preexisting biological and psychological risk factors and the events that occurred before and after the trauma. The patient may have a history of childhood trauma after experiencing the death of his father at a very young age, leading to biological and psychological sequelae.

A psychoanalytic model of the disorder suggests that the current trauma has reactivated a yet-unresolved psychological conflict. It would be interesting to further explore the feelings and thoughts the patient had surrounding the loss of his father, and the chronicity and severity of the reported symptoms of sadness, abnormal sleep architecture, and difficulties in school at that time. The support the patient received and the way he coped with painful effects during that time may reveal important information from a psychological perspective.

During the physical exam, he was noted to have borderline hypertension and tachycardia. He also presented with multiple somatic complaints such as palpitations and mild chest discomfort with an otherwise negative medical workup. This suggests evidence for altered function in the noradrenergic system, a common finding in patients with PTSD. There is no particular reason to believe that he has a medical condition that could cause new onset of anxiety symptoms, mood, or personality changes such as cardiac (arrhythmias), respiratory (Chronic Obstructive Pulmonary Disease) or autoimmune problems (Lupus Erythematosus Sclerosus (LES)), infections (HIV, syphilis), endocrine problems (thyroid or adrenocortical abnormalitites), or cancer. Mr W has no cardiac abnormalities, and he does not use illicit substances that may trigger his symptoms. In this case, the new onset of symptoms (not present before the accident) points toward an impaired psychological and physiological response to a traumatic event. Although the patient does not have other psychiatric diagnoses, he has a family history of depression, which could represent a genetic vulnerability for serotonin, noradrenaline, and other neuroendocrine dysregulations.

Patients with PTSD tend to see powerful emotions as a threat that the original trauma will happen again. Therefore, they somatize intense affects, or medicate them by abusing substances. This patient does not use illicit drugs or abuse prescription medications. Nonetheless, this is something that will require careful monitoring during treatment. Oscillations between memory intrusion and memory failure are common in PTSD, as a result of activation of dissociative defenses to maintain painful affects out of awareness. This is evident in the patient's difficulty in remembering important parts of the accident while simultaneously being distressed by intrusive thoughts and recollections of the event.

C. Therapeutic

In vivo or imaginary exposure therapy can be of extreme benefit for the patient given his prominent symptoms of avoidance. In exposure therapy for PTSD, the patient is guided through vivid memories of the trauma until extinction occurs. In this case, the exposure can be done in a graded fashion, as in systematic desensitization. While driving with the patient to the place of the accident, the therapist helps him to confront painful memories and feelings by teaching him relaxation techniques and cognitive approaches to coping with stress. Group therapy may be considered in this patient to reduce isolation and stigma.

The patient is agreeable to taking medications, therefore he may be initiated on an SSRI such as sertraline or paroxetine, which are FDA-approved first-line medications for the treatment of PTSD. Symptoms should continue to be monitored with goals to reduce the core PTSD symptoms, impairment in areas of work and social functioning, and to improve resilience to stress. Continuing comprehensive assessment for comorbid conditions such as major depression and substance abuse is of paramount importance in this patient. The alpha-adrenergic antagonist prazosin could be added for the persistence of nightmares and signs of increased adrenergic reactivity such as palpitations and increased startle response. Other alternatives such as different antidepressants or mood stabilizers should be considered if there is only partial response to initial treatment (after eight weeks), or if comorbid conditions emerge.

D. Prognostic

Mr W's protective factors include having a history of good premorbid functioning, strong social and family support, and the absence of other psychiatric or medical conditions. However, his current social isolation, the possibility of childhood trauma, and the genetic vulnerability for psychiatric illness are associated with more severe and chronic symptoms.

POSTTRAUMATIC STRESS DISORDER

1. Introduction

Posttraumatic stress disorder (PTSD) is an anxiety disorder that develops after an individual has been exposed to a traumatic event outside the range of normal human experience that caused horror and intense fear. The clinical picture follows three specific clusters: reexperiencing the traumatic event, avoidance of reminders of the event, and hyperarousal. It is a common psychiatric disorder that can cause significant morbidity. In severe cases, it can have a devastating effect on the patient's quality of life.

2. Epidemiology

PTSD is the fourth most common psychiatric disorder in the United States and it accounts for significant morbidity and disability. However, this condition may be underdiagnosed, since patients with PTSD are more likely to seek treatment for their symptoms in a primary care setting, than to visit a psychiatrist. Patients are also usually reluctant to talk about their history of trauma or their bothering symptoms without prompting. On the other hand, patients with PTSD frequently suffer from other psychiatric conditions. PTSD is associated with major depressive disorder, substance use disorders, other anxiety disorders, as well as significant medical problems, such as hypertension and chronic pain syndromes.

The lifetime prevalence of PTSD has been estimated to be approximately 5% to 6% for men and 10% to 14% for women. However, 10% to 20% of people exposed to a traumatic event will develop PTSD. The disorder most commonly develops after exposure to a direct traumatic event, but it can also result indirectly, such as in the case of the unwitnessed traumatic death of a loved one, or proximity to a major disaster.

Interpersonal violence is a high predictor of PTSD, as evidenced by the high rates of PTSD among victims of rape. Women have a higher likelihood of developing PTSD, although the increased vulnerability has not been well studied. Fifty percent of cases of PTSD in women are associated with sexual assault.

3. Etiology

Structural alterations in specific brain structures such as the amygdala and hippocampus have been noted in patients with PTSD. The differences found in hippocampal function and the effect on memory may contribute to cognitive impairment and intrusive recollections.

The unique neuroendocrine alterations found in patients with PTSD suggest that this entity could be one specific type of response to extreme stress. Similar to patients suffering depression and chronic stress, PTSD patients also have increased levels of corticotrophin release factor. However, PTSD patients differ by showing decreased levels of circulating cortisol and more abundant and increased responsiveness of the glucocortisol receptor. They exhibit increased sensitivity of the Hypothalamic-pituitary-adrenal axis (HPA) negative feedback inhibition, increased 24-hour urinary excretion of noradrenaline and elevated plasma concentrations of dopamine, noradrenaline and serotonin. These neuroendocrine alterations and the increased reactivity of alpha-2 adrenergic receptors can help explain somatic symptoms in patients with PTSD.

Findings from prospective studies suggest that having a higher degree of activation of the sympathetic nervous system and having been exposed to a traumatic event in the past could be risks factors for PTSD. One of the current hypotheses about the etiology of symptoms in PTSD is based on findings that low cortisol levels combined with adrenergic activation facilitate learning in animals. If this occurs in traumatized people, it will assist the strong encoding of the traumatic memory and its related severe feelings of distress. This could potentially develop into distorted perceptions and thoughts related to the event, which will result in an altered perception of danger and the ability to deal with a threat.

Some preexisting factors are found to be related to the exposure of a traumatic event and the development of PTSD. They include familial psychopathology, demographic factors described below, a history of prior trauma, and the presence of psychopathology prior to the trauma.

Although fear conditioning research in animal models suggests a genetic vulnerability in sensitivity to environmental stress, it appears that unique environmental contributions have a stronger effect than any of the genetic contributions studied to date. Men are more likely to be exposed to a traumatic event throughout their life, but women are more likely to develop PTSD. Among women, no relationship has been found between age and development of symptoms of PTSD. In men, there is a strong correlation between age and PTSD, due to increased exposure to trauma during the life span. Racial or ethnic status does not appear to provide consistent differences in the prevalence of PTSD. Current research suggests that earlier trauma may sensitize people to later trauma. For example, if stress hormones, such as cortisol, stay elevated for prolonged periods of time following a traumatic event, there might be a depletion of these hormones, resulting in an impaired response to exposure to later trauma. It has been hypothesized that prior psychopathology such as substance abuse disorders, conduct disorder, and certain types of personality disorders could lead to increased exposure to traumatic events, adding risk to the development of PTSD.

4. Diagnosis

Patients with PTSD are sometimes ashamed of having a psychiatric disorder, and may experience their PTSD symptoms as more physical in nature. They may describe nonspecific symptoms, such as shortness of breath, tremor, insomnia, and unexplained pain, without associating these with their trauma history. Persons suffering from alexithymia experience only the physiological correlates of the affective state, without registering feelings in the psychological dominion. Most people do not experience PTSD when faced with overwhelming trauma.

The diagnosis of PTSD remains a clinical diagnosis. According to the DSM-IV-TR, this diagnosis can be made if the patient has been exposed to a traumatic event that involves actual or threatened death or injury, and produces intense fear, helplessness, or horror, associated with new onset of symptoms of reexperiencing, avoidance, and increased arousal (Table 3C.2.)

5. Treatments

A. NONPHARMACOLOGICAL TREATMENTS

Cognitive therapy, anxiety management training (AMT), and exposure therapy are treatments that exhibit sufficient empirical support in well-controlled clinical trials among populations of trauma survivors for the treatment of PTSD.

Exposure therapy involves guiding the patient through vivid remembrances of the traumatic event until extinction occurs. Some studies have

TABLE 3C.2 DSM-IV-TR Diagnostic Criteria for Posttraumatic Stress Disorder

A. *The person has been exposed to a traumatic event in which both of the following were present:*
- (1) the person experienced, witnessed, or was confronted with an event or events that involved actual or threatened death or serious injury, or a threat to the physical integrity of self or others
- (2) the person's response involved intense fear, helplessness, or horror. **Note:** In children, this may be expressed instead by disorganized or agitated behavior

B. *The traumatic event is persistently reexperienced in one (or more) of the following ways:*
- (1) recurrent and intrusive distressing recollections of the event, including images, thoughts, or perceptions. **Note:** In young children, repetitive play may occur in which themes or aspects of the trauma are expressed
- (2) recurrent distressing dreams of the event. **Note:** In children, there may be frightening dreams without recognizable content
- (3) acting or feeling as if the traumatic event was recurring (includes a sense of reliving the experience, illusions, hallucinations, and dissociative flashback episodes, including those that occur on awakening or when intoxicated). **Note:** In young children, trauma-specific reenactment may occur
- (4) intense psychological distress at exposure to internal or external cues that symbolize or resemble a n aspect of the traumatic event
- (5) physiological reactivity on exposure to internal or external cues that symbolize or resemble an aspect of the traumatic event

C. *Persistent avoidance of stimuli associated with the trauma and numbing of general responsiveness (not present before the trauma), as indicated by three (or more) of the following:*
- (1) efforts to avoid thoughts, feelings, or conversations associated with the trauma
- (2) efforts to avoid activities, places, or people that arouse recollections of the trauma
- (3) inability to recall an important aspect of the trauma
- (4) markedly diminished interest or participation in significant activities
- (5) feeling of detachment or estrangement from others
- (6) restricted range of affect (e.g., unable to have loving feelings)
- (7) sense of a foreshortened future (e.g., does not expect to have a career, marriage, children, or a normal life span)

D. *Persistent symptoms of increased arousal (not present before the trauma), as indicated by two (or more) of the following:*
- (1) difficulty falling or staying asleep
- (2) irritability or outburst of anger
- (3) difficulty concentrating
- (4) hypervigilance
- (5) exaggerated startle response

E. *Duration of the disturbance (symptoms in Criteria B, C, and D) is more than 1 month.*

F. *The disturbance causes clinically significant distress or impairment in social, occupational, or other important areas of functioning.*

Specify if:
Acute: if duration of symptoms is less than 3 months
Chronic: if duration of symptoms is 3 months or more

Specify if:
With delayed onset: if onset of symptoms is at least 6 months after the stressor

Adapted from American Psychiatric Associati on. Diagnostic and Statistical Manual of Mental Disorders: Text Revision. 4th Ed. Washington, DC: American Psychiatric Association, 2000.

shown that exposure therapy is highly effective at reducing avoidance and at improving general social functioning and negative health perceptions.

AMT uses cognitive and behavioral strategies to teach patients the skills to manage painful emotions associated with PTSD. They include mastering relaxation techniques, breathing retraining, trauma education, cognitive restructuring, and communication skills. A recent study by Taylor et al. (2003) showed that prolonged exposure therapy and AMT-reduced dissociative symptoms, trauma-related guilt and anger, and depressive symptoms at culmination of treatment.

Cognitive processing therapy is an example of combination treatments developed in 1992 by Resick & Schnicke that include elements of cognitive therapy, exposure therapy, and AMT. The cognitive therapy component involves addressing specific cognitive distortions resulting from the trauma, whereas the exposure component involves writing and reading about the event.

B. PHARMACOLOGICAL TREATMENTS

1. Antidepressants

Selective Serotonin Reuptake Inhibitors (SSRIs), monoamine oxydase inhibitors, and tricyclic antidepressants alleviate symptoms of PTSD. SSRIs are at least as effective as other antidepressants but are associated with fewer side effects. For this reason, they are the first-line pharmacological intervention for PTSD. Sertraline and paroxetine are the only FDA-approved medications for the treatment of this disorder. If there is no response to an 8-week trial with an SSRI at adequate doses, some authors recommend that treatment should be switched to venlafaxine or nefazodone. Trazodone is frequently used as an adjunctive treatment for insomnia; mirtazapine was effective in reducing PTSD and general anxiety in one recent controlled trial.

2. Mood Stabilizers

The use of mood stabilizers is derived from "kindling" models of PTSD suggesting that repeated stimulation of limbic structures causes them to become sensitized. According to the Expert Consensus Guidelines on the treatment of PTSD, mood stabilizers such as valproic acid should be added if there is partial response to SSRIs. Some clinicians consider that their potential side effects, added to the limited evidence-based data supporting their effectiveness in this population, make them less favorable options.

3. Anxiolytics

Although benzodiazepines are effective in reducing anxiety in PTSD, they do not have effects in the core symptoms of this disorder such as hyperarousal, intrusive thoughts, and emotional numbness. Clinical studies suggest altered GABAergic function in patients with PTSD. This finding is supported by a recent quantitative PET study that demonstrated reduced binding to the benzodiazepine-GABA A receptor complex in veterans with PTSD, therefore corroborating the lack of effect of benzodiazepines in the treatment of this disorder.

4. Typical Antipsychotics

Typical antipsychotics have not been examined systematically in the treatment of PTSD and are generally not recommended.

5. Atypical Antipsychotics

Small studies have found olanzapine and risperidone to be beneficial in the treatment of patients with PTSD, who were unresponsive to conventional pharmacological treatment, regardless of the presence or absence of psychotic symptoms. These medications could be effective predominantly when excessive hypervigilance, intense anger, or psychotic symptoms are evident. However, more research on the use of these agents in PTSD is warranted.

6. Antiadrenergic Agents

In the central nervous system, alpha(1)-adrenergic receptors are known to have a role in sleep and startle response. Prazosin, an alpha(1)-adrenergic receptor blocker, has shown effect in reducing nightmares and facilitating overall improvement in PTSD symptoms. Preliminary results suggest its efficacy in preventing PTSD symptoms when administered early after the trauma. Clinicians should monitor for orthostatic hypotension, usually seen early in therapy.

6. General Formulation for PTSD

A. DIAGNOSTIC

The diagnosis of PTSD according to the DSM-IV-TR requires the exposure to a traumatic event to which the patient responded in horror. Symptoms that follow this exposure belong to three different clusters: reexperiencing, avoidance, and hyperarousal for at least 1 month.

PTSD is associated with high rates of psychiatric comorbidity, including mood, anxiety, and substance abuse disorders. This high comorbidity could be the result of the direct effect of PTSD, a consequence of potentially shared factors of vulnerability, or trauma-type specific mechanisms. It is crucial to identify preexisting and new psychopathology, as well as new onset of overlapping symptomatology, since this will determine the quality of life, prognosis issues, and treatment decisions in patients with PTSD.

It is common to see somatic complaints accompanying PTSD, usually secondary to activation of primitive defense mechanisms and to neuroendocrine dysregulation. Therefore, it is important to assess and monitor for prescription medication abuse. Denial, minimization, projective disavowal and dissociative defenses, are common defense mechanisms activated in patients with PTSD to cope with painful affective states. Anger and guilt are commonly seen as a defense against more distressed feelings of underlying vulnerability.

B. ETIOLOGIC

Important predisposing risk factors have been identified in PTSD. They include prior history of trauma, presence of a personality disorder, genetic vulnerabilities to psychiatric illness, demographic factors, and history of substance abuse among others.

Psychodynamic theory proposes the presence of a preexisting conflict that is reawakened by the new traumatic event in patients with PTSD. The cognitive model poses that the affected person is incapable of processing the trauma and continues to experience the stress, while attempting to extinguish the trauma through avoidance. Biologic factors related to PTSD include alterations in specific brain regions (amygdala and hippocampus) implicated in fear and memory processes, as well as neurochemical and endocrine changes resulting in altered physiological responses to stress.

C. THERAPEUTIC

Psychotherapy and pharmacotherapy have both been found efficacious, and treatment selection should be tailored to the individual patient. Given that there are no pharmacological agents designed to specifically target the biologic alterations in PTSD, using agents with known efficacy in mood and anxiety disorders is the preferred choice. SSRIs are the first-line medication among which sertraline and paroxetine are the ones approved by the FDA. Mood stabilizers may be added if there is a partial response to SSRIs. Benzodiazepine use should be avoided due to lack of evidence of effectiveness, and the risk of addiction, especially in patients with comorbid alcoholism. Alpha(1)-adrenergic receptor blockers may be used in patients with PTSD experiencing sleep disruption, nightmares, and symptoms suggestive of excessive adrenergic reactivity.

D. PROGNOSTIC

In general, patients with a strong network of social supports are less likely to experience PTSD in its severe forms and are more likely to recover faster. The very young and the very old have more difficulty with traumatic events than those in midlife, probably due to inadequate coping mechanisms to deal with the physical and emotional insults of the trauma. A good prognosis is predicted by rapid onset of symptoms, short duration (less than 6 months), good premorbid functioning, strong social support, and absence of other psychiatric and medical risk factors.

7. Risk Assessment

In a community survey, patients with PTSD were 14.9 times more likely to attempt suicide than subjects without PTSD. The assessment and treatment of comorbidities contribute to the reduction of suicide risk. A child history of trauma and comorbid conditions such as major depression, alcoholism, and cluster B personality disorders, enhance the risk for suicide in patients with PTSD.

KEY POINTS (ABPN Examination)

A. When interviewing a patient with posttraumatic stress disorder

1. Know that given the high prevalence of avoidance symptoms, patients rarely bring up the exposure of a traumatic event without prompting and may present initially with somatic complaints.
2. Do not forget to make a thorough assessment of safety, including suicidal ideations, intent, or plans.
3. Do not forget to ask about any history of prior trauma. Childhood trauma is common in patients with PTSD.
4. Ask about comorbidities, particularly mood disorders, anxiety disorders, and substance abuse disorders, which have a high prevalence among this population.

B. When presenting a patient with posttraumatic stress disorder

1. Acknowledge that symptoms of other psychiatric comorbid conditions such as mood or anxiety disorders may overlap with PTSD or be the result of shared risk factors for vulnerability.
2. If diagnosis is unclear, state that you would use a structured diagnostic interview like SCID-DSM-IV for clarification.

SUGGESTED READINGS

American Psychiatry Association. *Diagnostic and statistical manual of mental disorders (DSM-IV)*. 4th Ed. Washington, DC: American Psychiatry Association, 1994.

Boscarino JA. Posttraumatic stress disorder, exposure to combat, and lower plasma cortisol among Vietnam Veterans: Findings and clinical implications. *Consult Clin Psychol* 1996;64:191–201.

Bremner JD, Licinio J, Darnell A, et al. Elevated CSF corticotrophin-releasing factor concentration in posttraumatic stress disorder. *Am J Psychiatry* 1997;154:624–629.

Breslau N, Davis GC, Andreski P, et al. Traumatic events and posttraumatic stress disorder in an urban population of young adults. *Arch Gen Psychiatry* 1991;48:216–222.

Breslau N, Davis GC, Peterson EL, et al. Psychiatry sequelae of posttraumatic stress disorder in women. *Arch Gen Psychiatry* 1997;54:81–87.

Brunello N, Davidson JRT, Deahl M, et al. Posttraumatic stress disorder: Diagnosis and epidemiology, comorbidity and social consequences, biology and treatment. *Neuropsychobiology* 2001;43:150–162.

Davidson JR, Rothbaum BO, van der Kolk BA, et al. Multicenter, double-blind comparison of sertraline and placebo in the treatment of posttraumatic stress disorder. *Arch Gen Psychiatry* 2001;58:485–492.

Davidson JR. Use of benzodiazepines in social anxiety disorder, generalized anxiety disorder, and posttraumatic stress disorder. *J Clin Psychiatry* 2004;65(suppl 5):29–33.

Davidson JTR, Weisler RH, Butterfield MI, et al. Mirtazapine vs. placebo in posttraumatic stress disorder: A pilot trial. *Biol Psychiatry* 2003;53:188–191.

Deering CG, Glover SG, Ready D, et al. Unique patterns of comorbidity in posttraumatic stress disorder from different sources of trauma. *Compr Psychiatry* 1996;37:336–346.

Foa EB, Davidson JRT, Frances A. The Expert Consensus Guidelines series: Treatment of posttraumatic stress disorder. *J Clin Psychiatry* 1999;60(suppl 16):1–76.

Geuze E, van Berckel BN, Lammertsma AA, et al. Reduced GABAA benzodiazepine receptor binding in veterans with posttraumatic stress disorder. *Mol Psychiatry* 2008 Jan;13(1):74–83.

Hammer MB, Diamond BI. Elevated Plasma Dopamine in posttraumatic stress disorder: A preliminary report. *Biol Psychiatry* 1993;33:304–306.

Keane TM, Marshall AD, Taft CT. Posttraumatic stress disorder: Etiology, epidemiology, and treatment outcome. *Annu Rev Clin Psychol* 2006;2:161–197.

Kessler RC, Sonnega A, Bromet E, et al. Posttraumatic stress disorder in the National Comorbidity Survey. *Arch Gen Psychiatry* 1995;52:1048–1060.

McLeod DS, Koenen KC, Meyer JM, et al. Genetic and environmental influences on the relationship among combat exposure, posttraumatic stress disorder symptoms, and alcohol use. *J Trauma Stress* 2001;14:259–275.

Orquendo M, Brent DA, Birmaher B, et al. Posttraumatic stress disorder comorbid with major depression: Factors mediating the association with suicidal behavior. *Am J Psychiatry* 2005 Mar;162(3):560–566.

Rauch SA, Grunfeld TE, Yardin E, et al. Changes in reported physical health symptoms and social function with prolonged exposure therapy for chronic posttraumatic stress disorder. *Depress Anxiety* 2009;26(8):732–738.

Resnick HS, Kilpatrick DG, Dansky BS, et al. Prevalence of civilian trauma and posttraumatic stress disorder in a representational national sample of women. *J Consult Clin Psychol* 1993;61:984–991.

Shemesh E, Rudnick A, Kaluski E, et al. A prospective study of post-traumatic stress symptoms and nonadherence in survivors of a myocardial infarction (MI). *Gen Hosp Psychiatry* 2001;21:215–222.

Taylor S, Thordason DS, Maxfield, et al. Comparative efficacy of three PTSD treatments: Exposure therapy, EMDR, and relaxation training. *Journal of Consulting and Clinical Psychology*, 2003;71:330–338.

Vaiva G, Thomas P, Ducrocq F, et al. Low Posttrauma GABA plasma levels as a predictive factor in the development of acute posttraumatic stress disorder. *Biol Psychiatry* 2004;55: 250–254.

Wittmann L, Moergeli H, Martin-Soelch C, et al. Comorbidity in posttraumatic stress disorder: A structural equation modelling approach. *Compr Psychiatry* 2008;49:430–440.

Yehuda R, Bierer LM, Schmeidler J, et al. Low cortisol and risk for PTSD in adult offspring of Holocaust survivors. *Am J Psychiatry* 2000; 157:1252–1259.

Yehuda R, Kahana B, Binder-Brynes K, et al. Low urinary cortisol excretion in Holocaust survivors with posttraumatic stress disorder. *Am J Psychiatry* 1995;152:982–986.

Yehuda R, Southwick SM, Krystal JH, et al. Enhanced suppression of cortisol following dexamethasone administration in posttraumatic stress disorder. *Am J Psychiatry* 1993; 159:83–86.

Zatzick DF, Weiss DS, Marmar CR, et al. Posttraumatic stress disorder and functioning and quality of life outcomes in female Vietnam veterans. *Mil Med* 1997;162:661–665.

D. Substance abuse disorders

Natalie Weder, MD, Kirsten M. Wilkins, MD, Gustavo A. Angarita, MD, Robert T. Malison, MD

I. ALCOHOL ABUSE

CASE HISTORY

PRESENT ILLNESS

Mr S is a 21-year-old white male who was brought to the emergency department (ED) by the police after he was found sleeping in a car outside an inner-city bar. Per police report, the patient was incoherent and could not explain what he was doing in his car. His breath alcohol level was 0.2. While the police were interviewing him, Mr S stated that he was "feeling horrible and wanted to die." The police officers brought him to the ED for further evaluation.

Mr S was medically cleared in the ED and then referred for a psychiatric evaluation. The physician on call had to wait 2 hours before being able to interview him, since the patient was initially incoherent and could not stay awake. Two hours later, he was alert and oriented to time, person, and place and could answer questions appropriately. He stated that he is a junior in a local college, and that he was celebrating the end of midterm examinations with friends. He reported drinking approximately four shots of tequila, a martini, and two beers during that night. He had his last drink 1 hour before arriving to the ED. Mr S reported usually drinking alcohol twice a week, with an average of four to five drinks per episode. He had a Driving under the influence (DUI) in the past and has been failing in several subjects in school because he stays up too late to drink and then is unable to finish his school-related work. His parents are concerned with this behavior and recently threatened to stop supporting him financially, unless he stops drinking. However, he denied any history of withdrawal symptoms including seizures or delirium tremens. He stated that he is used to drinking on 2 specific days per week and does not think of drinking during the rest of the week. He also stated that he always drinks the same amount of alcohol, because he enjoys "feeling intoxicated." Mr S denied smoking tobacco or using illicit drugs.

On interview, Mr S denied any distinct periods of depressed or euphoric mood, as well as any neurovegetative signs of a mood disorder. He reported being "happy" most of the time, and consistently denied any suicidal or homicidal ideations, intent, or plans. When questioned about his statement while being interviewed by the police, Mr S stated that he never meant to imply that he was having suicidal thoughts. He stated that he was having "stomachaches" and made that comment in reference to his pain. He also denied any symptoms suggestive of an anxiety, eating, or psychotic disorder.

PSYCHIATRIC HISTORY

Mr S does not carry any past psychiatric disorders. His only contact with a mental health provider was a few months ago when his parents asked him to see a school counselor in regard to his alcohol intake. He had two appointments with this counselor and stopped going, since he does not think he has a problem with alcohol and believes that "drinking is a normal part of college life." He has never been exposed to psychotropic medications, and denied any history of suicide attempts or violence. He had a DUI in the past. He started drinking at age 16, and his drinking habits gradually progressed from one or two drinks per week in high school, to his current intake since he started college. He admitted to trying cannabis once and "hating it" and denied any use of other illicit substances.

FAMILY HISTORY

Mr S's mother has a history of major depressive disorder. There is no other family history of psychiatric illness.

SOCIAL HISTORY

Mr S was born and raised in New York City. He is an only child, and his parents remain together after 30 years of marriage. He graduated high school with average grades and is currently enrolled in a local college, with plans to pursue a career in business. He has had short-lived romantic relationships with heterosexual partners, and stated that he is too young to have a steady relationship and wishes to "enjoy single life as long as possible." He also admitted to having interpersonal problems with his former girlfriends, because they complained about his drinking "habits." He denied any history of physical or sexual abuse. He enjoys playing tennis and spending time with his friends.

PERTINENT MEDICAL HISTORY

Mr S has a history of exercise-induced asthma that has resolved immediately with inhaled albuterol. He has no other active medical problems.

MENTAL STATUS EXAMINATION

Mr S presented as a young white male who appeared younger than his stated age, dressed casually in jeans and a polo shirt. He made good eye contact and was pleasant and cooperative. No abnormal movements were noted. His speech was normal in rate, volume, and rhythm. His mood was reported as "OK, but worried," and his affect was appropriate and mood congruent. His thought process was goal oriented. Mr S denied any suicidal or homicidal ideations, intent, or plans, as well as visual or auditory hallucinations, delusions, or obsessions. His insight was impaired; he was unable to understand how his alcohol intake was causing significant social and school difficulties, as evidenced by the fact that he was currently in an Emergency Department because of his alcohol intake, he is failing in school grades and he has a legal record for a DUI. His judgment was also impaired, as evidenced by the fact that he continues to drink and has no intentions of changing his habits. On the Folstein Mini-Mental State Examination, he scored 30/30, indicating no gross cognitive impairments.

PERTINENT PHYSICAL FINDINGS

The patient's vital signs included a temperature of 97.6°F, heart rate 82 per minute, blood pressure

110/70 mm Hg, and respiratory rate of 14 per minute. Oxygen saturation on room air was 99.0%. His pupils were symmetric and reactive to light. The extraocular muscles were intact, sclerae were anicteric, and mucous membranes were moist. There was no lymphadenopathy or thyromegaly. The first and second heart sounds were heard and there was no murmur. No carotid bruits were heard. The lungs were clear bilaterally. The abdomen was soft and nontender with normal bowel sounds and no organomegaly. The peripheral pulses were intact. The neurological examination was unremarkable.

LABORATORY DATA

Complete blood count (CBC), electrolytes, blood urea nitrogen (BUN), amylase, liver function tests, creatinine, and fasting glucose were within normal limits. The urine drug screen was negative.

COURSE OF ILLNESS

Following this initial evaluation in the ED, Mr S was observed for several hours to rule out any withdrawal symptoms. His vital signs remained within normal limits, and Clinical Institute Withdrawal Assessment for Alcohol-Revised (CIWA-Ar) scores were in the 0 to 2 range. His mood remained stable and he requested to be discharged to his parents' care. Upon discharge, Mr S was offered a referral to the local mental health clinic and was educated about the different pharmacological and psychotherapeutic treatments available for his condition. He stated that he would think about it, but he was not interested in making an appointment at that time. His breath alcohol level at the time of discharge was negative.

DSM-IV-TR MULTIAXIAL DIAGNOSIS

Axis I: Alcohol abuse
Axis II: None
Axis III: Exercise-induced asthma
Axis IV: Severity of psychosocial stressors: moderate; educational, social, and legal problems
Axis V: Global assessment of functioning: 55

FORMULATION

A. Diagnostic

Mr S meets the criteria for alcohol abuse (Table 3D.1). He presents with a maladaptive pattern of alcohol intake that has had an important impact on his daily activities. His school grades are below what is expected from him, and his parents are threatening to withdraw their financial support due to his drinking. In addition, he reported in passing that one of the reasons that he does not have a romantic relationship is that previous partners have complained about his behavior while intoxicated. He had a DUI in the past for drinking while driving, which led to an arrest. He attempted to drive while intoxicated on the night of his evaluation, but he fell asleep in his car and was then found by police. In spite

TABLE 3D.1 Diagnostic Criteria for Alcohol Abuse

1. A maladaptive pattern of alcohol abuse leading to clinically significant impairment or distress, as manifested by one or more of the following, occurring within a 12-month period:
   - Recurrent alcohol use resulting in failure to fulfill major role obligations at work, school, or home (e.g., repeated absences or poor work performance related to substance use; substance-related absences, suspensions or expulsions from school; or neglect of children or household).
   - Recurrent alcohol use in situations in which it is physically hazardous (e.g., driving an automobile or operating a machine).
   - Recurrent alcohol-related legal problems (e.g., arrests for alcohol-related disorderly conduct).
   - Continued alcohol use despite persistent or recurrent social or interpersonal problems caused or exacerbated by the effects of alcohol (e.g., arguments with spouse about consequences of intoxication or physical fights).
2. These symptoms must never have met the criteria for alcohol dependence.

Adapted from American Psychiatric Association. *Diagnostic and Statistical Manual of Mental Disorders: DSM-IV-TR*. Washington, DC: American Psychiatric Association, 2000.

TABLE 3D.2 Diagnostic Criteria for Alcohol Dependence

A maladaptive pattern of alcohol use, leading to clinically significant impairment or distress, as manifested by three or more of the following seven criteria, occurring at any time in the same 12-month period:

1. Tolerance, as defined by either of the following:
   (a) A need for markedly increased amounts of alcohol to achieve intoxication or desired effect.
   (b) Markedly diminished effect with continued use of the same amount of alcohol.
2. Withdrawal, as defined by either of the following:
   (a) The characteristic withdrawal syndrome for alcohol.
   (b) Alcohol is taken to relieve or avoid withdrawal symptoms.
3. Alcohol is often taken in larger amounts or over a longer period than was intended.
4. There is a persistent desire or there are unsuccessful efforts to cut down or control alcohol use.
5. A great deal of time is spent in activities necessary to obtain alcohol, use alcohol, or recover from its effects.
6. Important social, occupational, or recreational activities are given up or reduced because of alcohol use.
7. Alcohol use is continued despite knowledge of having a persistent or recurrent physical or psychological problem that is likely to have been caused or exacerbated by alcohol.

of these difficulties, he continues to drink and stated that he is not interested in seeking help or changing his alcohol intake. He does not meet criteria for other substance use disorders at the present time. On the other hand, Mr S does not meet criteria for alcohol dependence (see Table 3D.2). He does not need to drink more to achieve the same effect and reports obtaining the same effect with his usual four to five drinks, and therefore he does not meet criteria for tolerance to alcohol. In addition, in the first 24 to 48 hours following his alcohol intake, he does not present with signs and symptoms that suggest alcohol withdrawal, such as anxiety, tremulousness, headache, palpitations, insomnia, or more severe symptoms, such as hallucinosis or seizures.

Mr S does not meet criteria for a primary mood disorder, which is highly comorbid with substance abuse. He also denies mood changes or neurovegetative symptoms secondary to his alcohol intake, which would suggest the presence of a substance-induced mood disorder. When evaluating a patient with a substance use disorder, it is highly important to thoroughly evaluate the presence of suicidal or homicidal ideations, since many suicide attempts and acts of violence occur in subjects who are intoxicated at the time. It is not uncommon to see patients who are referred for suicidal ideation while intoxicated. Although some of these statements are only secondary to intoxication, they should always be reassessed by the treating physician or psychiatrist once the patient is sober.

Mr S does not meet criteria for an Axis II disorder. Some personality disorders are associated with substance abuse, particularly antisocial personality disorder (ASPD). Although Mr S has had problems with the law, these problems have only been present when he was intoxicated, and he does not have a long-standing pattern of deceitfulness, aggressive behaviors, consistent irresponsibility, or reckless disregard for his safety or the safety of others.

B. Etiologic

Mr S does not have some of the well-documented risk factors for alcohol abuse, such as family history of substance abuse, history of ASPD or depression, or exposure to traumatic events. However, binge drinking is common in young males. On the other hand, the environmental stress associated with his school's high expectations and the peer pressure in his college may be significant perpetuating factors for his alcohol abuse.

C. Therapeutic

There are several pharmacological and psychotherapeutic interventions that may prove to be helpful for Mr S. Motivational interviewing may help Mr S to increase his motivation to change his behavior toward alcohol intake and move him from a precontemplative stage to a phase of ambivalence and readiness for change. Once, and if, Mr S feels ready to stop drinking, he could benefit from pharmacological treatment to help maintain sobriety. One possibility is an aversive agent such as disulfiram. However, solid commitment and motivation are needed when this agent is chosen, since the risk of side effects is significant. Naltrexone in combination with cognitive behavioral therapy (CBT) or supportive therapy has also shown promising results.

D. Prognostic

Chronic alcohol abuse has been associated with many medical and psychiatric consequences, including several types of cancer, gastrointestinal problems, myocardial infarct, depression, and concomitant use of illicit drugs, among others. Although Mr S does not have the typical risk factors associated with alcohol dependence, such as antisocial personality traits and paternal family history of alcohol dependence, he has continued to drink despite significant social and legal problems and does not show any interest in changing this pattern. His limited insight and lack of ambivalence in regard to the consequences of his alcohol intake are poor prognostic factors for Mr S.

ALCOHOL ABUSE AND DEPENDENCE

1. Introduction

Alcohol is second only to nicotine as the most commonly abused substance today. Alcohol use disorders are among the most common psychiatric disorders in the United States, and they create a significant impact on society in terms of their social, occupational, medical, and legal consequences. Up to 20% of suicides, 80% of homicides, and 50% of fatal motor vehicle accidents involve the use of alcohol. Though there are many alcohol-related disorders listed in the DSM-IV-TR, the two primary alcohol use disorders are alcohol abuse and alcohol dependence. They differ in the severity of physiological and psychosocial consequences of the substance use. Alcohol use disorders are commonly comorbid with other psychiatric disorders, including mood disorders, anxiety disorders, and personality disorders, among others. The prognosis of alcohol and other substance use disorders is poorer when there are other comormid psychiatric illnesses. Treatment of alcohol use disorders may include both pharmacotherapy as well as psychosocial treatments.

2. Epidemiology

Approximately 90% of the United States population has had a drink, whereas 60% to 70% are current drinkers (i.e., they have had a drink in the past 1 to 3 months). The lifetime prevalence of alcohol abuse may be as high as 20% for men and 10% for women. The lifetime risk for alcohol dependence is less: 10% for men and 3% to 5% for women. Rates of drinking vary among different groups of people in the United States. The age of greatest alcohol intake is from the late teens to the mid-20s; however, the age of peak onset of alcohol dependence is in the mid-20s to age 40 years. The earlier the onset of alcohol dependence, the more severe the problem is likely to be and the more likely the patient is to have additional psychiatric comorbidities. Among ethnic groups, there are higher rates of alcohol use disorders among people of Irish and Native American descent. As previously mentioned, alcohol use disorders are often comorbid with other psychiatric illnesses; in particular, Bipolar I Disorder, Schizophrenia, and ASPD.

3. Pharmacology

A drink of an alcoholic beverage contains 10 to 12 g of ethanol (the amount in 12 oz of beer, 4 oz of wine, or 1.5 oz of 80-proof liquor). Alcohol is absorbed into the bloodstream from the small intestine. Rates of absorption from the digestive tract may differ depending on how recently one has eaten. In addition, women have increased bioavailability of alcohol due to lower amounts of gastric alcohol dehydrogenase (ADH) when compared to men. The body metabolizes approximately one drink per hour. Most of the metabolism of alcohol occurs through the action of ADH in the liver, which produces acetaldehyde. Acetaldehyde is then broken down by aldehyde dehydrogenase (ALDH). In the absence of effective ALDH, acetaldehyde builds up, causing flushing, rapid heart rate, hypotension, nausea, and vomiting. This enzyme is important clinically because it may be deficient in certain ethnic groups (10% of Asians lack the efficient form of ALDH and 40% have only low concentrations of the efficient form). Also, one of the pharmacotherapeutic treatments for alcohol dependence, disulfiram, acts to inhibit ALDH.

A central nervous system depressant, alcohol is thought to potentiate the receptor function of inhibitory amino acid gamma-aminobutyric acid (GABA), while inhibiting the receptor function of excitatory amino acid *N*-methyl D-aspartate (NMDA). Alcohol has effects on other neurotransmitters as well, including serotonin, dopamine, and norephinephrine. The effects of alcohol intoxication are often opposite the effects of alcohol withdrawal.

4. Effects of Alcohol on the Body

Alcohol's effect is most notable on the central nervous system. Alcohol intoxication causes mood lability, disinhibition, nystagmus, slurred speech, incoordination, ataxia, and memory impairment (known as "blackouts," wherein the person remains awake while intoxicated, but has no memory of that period of time). At blood alcohol levels of greater than 300, individuals may experience stupor, coma, and possibly death. Alcohol intoxication may help initiate sleep onset, but causes an overall decrease in rapid eye movement sleep and inhibits stage 4 sleep. Chronic alcohol abuse leads to cerebellar degeneration, characterized by ataxia and nystagmus. With regard to the peripheral nervous system, chronic alcohol abuse leads to peripheral neuropathy in about 10% of alcoholics. Alcohol damage to the nervous system is postulated to be secondary to the toxic effects of ethanol and its metabolites, as well as vitamin deficiencies. Thiamine deficiency occurs in up to 80% of alcoholics and contributes to the development of Wernicke's encephalopathy (triad consisting of confusion, ataxia, and ophthalmoplegia).

Alcohol has a notorious effect on the gastrointestinal tract. Alcoholic gastritis and esophageal varices can lead to gastrointestinal bleeding, which, in its most severe form, may be lethal. The liver and pancreas are particularly affected by acute as well as chronic alcohol abuse, leading to alcoholic hepatitis, pancreatitis, fatty liver, and eventually liver cirrhosis and portal hypertension. Severe liver cirrhosis can lead to elevated ammonia level and resulting hepatic encephalopathy.

Chronic alcohol abuse affects the cardiovascular and hematologic systems as well. Patients with alcohol dependence are at increased risk of myocardial infarction (MI) due to the effects of alcohol on blood pressure and cholesterol [elevated low-density lipoprotein (LDL) cholesterol and triglycerides]. The toxic effects of alcohol on the heart muscle can lead to alcoholic cardiomyopathy. Heavy alcohol use decreases production of white blood cells and platelets, and can also increase the mean corpuscular volume of red blood cells. Higher rates of cancer are seen in patients who abuse alcohol; most notably, cancers of the head, neck, esophagus, and stomach. Alcoholics are also at greater risk of developing cancer of the liver, lungs, and colon.

Alcohol is a known teratogen. In high doses, alcohol can produce fetal death and spontaneous abortion. Infants that are born to alcohol-abusing mothers are at risk of fetal alcohol effect, which includes the following symptoms: microcephaly, mental retardation, developmental delays, cardiac defects (i.e., atrial septal defect), and facial abnormalities (absent philtrum, thin upper lip, flattened nasal bridge, and an epicanthal eye fold).

Though alcohol is most commonly associated with negative effects on the body, alcohol may have beneficial effects under certain circumstances. For people without pregnancy, history of alcohol dependence, and certain other medical and psychiatric conditions, alcohol in moderation (i.e., one to two drinks per day, maximum) appears to be associated with a reduced risk of cardiovascular disease. This is postulated to be secondary to an increase in one portion of high-density lipoprotein cholesterol as well as a decrease in platelet adherence.

5. Etiology

Like most psychiatric disorders, the underlying etiology of alcohol use disorders has not been fully elucidated. Alcohol use disorders can be conceptualized as having a complex etiology, incorporating biological, psychological, and social components. Studies suggest a fairly strong genetic component to alcohol use disorders, as close relatives of alcoholics are three to four times more likely to have alcohol problems compared to the general population. The risk of alcohol dependence is increased in offspring of alcoholic parents, in particular alcoholic fathers, even among children who were separated from their parents near birth and adopted into a non–alcohol-abusing family. Other risk factors for alcohol use disorders include history of depression, exposure to trauma, and ASPD.

The reward circuitry of the brain has been postulated to be involved in the development of addictive disorders such as alcohol dependence. This reward circuitry includes the mesolimbic dopamine system: the prefrontal cortex, nucleus accumbens, and the ventral tegmental areas of the brain. Over time, brain receptors which naturally mediate pleasure diminish in number and/or become desensitized to the effects of alcohol. This creates the need for more substance to achieve the same effect (i.e., tolerance). A cycle ensues, wherein the more alcohol the person uses, the more they need.

Psychological theories of alcohol use disorders hypothesize that individuals drink alcohol to reduce psychological distress, tension, and anxiety. Alcohol can cause disinhibition, and individuals may feel more powerful or attractive under the effects of it. Classic psychoanalytic theory postulates that people who abuse alcohol may be fixated at the oral stage of psychosexual development, wherein something taken in by mouth helps soothe frustration. However, such theories are not the focus of treatment-related research for alcohol use disorders at this time. From a behavioral perspective, drinkers may anticipate the pleasurable feelings that alcohol results in and behave in a manner to seek out that "reward." Socially, drinking is a common experience in which the majority of Western culture partakes. It may be more or less acceptable depending upon one's ethnic group, religious group, and environmental setting (e.g., college, where there is an increasing amount of binge drinking).

6. Diagnosis

All mental health clinicians must have a high index of suspicion and screen regularly for alcohol use disorders. Alcohol-related disorders are divided in the DSM-IV-TR into *alcohol use disorders* (i.e., alcohol abuse and alcohol dependence) and *alcohol-induced disorders* (i.e., alcohol intoxication, alcohol withdrawal, and alcohol-induced mood, psychotic, anxiety, and cognitive disorders).

A. ALCOHOL USE DISORDERS

Alcohol abuse includes a maladaptive pattern of recurrent alcohol use over a 12-month period, as manifested by one or more of the following: failure to fulfill major role obligations at work, school, or home; recurrent substance use in which it is physically hazardous; recurrent substance-related legal problems; and continued substance use despite recurrent social or interpersonal problems. See Table 3D.1 for details.

Alcohol dependence includes a maladaptive pattern of alcohol use over a period of 12 months, resulting in three or more of the following: tolerance; withdrawal; alcohol is used in greater amounts or over a longer period than intended; persistent desire/efforts to cut back on alcohol use; great deal of time spent obtaining, using, or recovering from alcohol use; important activities given up due to alcohol; continued use despite physical or psychological consequences. See Table 3D.2 for details. (*Note:* while tolerance and withdrawal are commonly seen in alcohol dependent patients, they are *not* required for the diagnosis of alcohol dependence.)

Various instruments are available to screen for alcohol use disorders. The "CAGE" questions are commonly used and easy to administer. Two or more "yes" answers have specificity for alcohol abuse of around 80%. Note that it does not account for current versus past alcohol use disorders.

CAGE QUESTIONS:

Have you ever felt the need to **cut down** the alcohol use?

Do you get **annoyed** when people criticize your drinking?

Do you feel **guilty** because of something you did while drinking?

Have you ever had alcohol as an **eye opener** to steady your nerves first thing in the morning?

Other screening instruments include the Michigan Alcohol Screening Test (MAST) and the Alcohol Use Disorders Identification Test (AUDIT). The MAST, like the CAGE, does not differentiate between current and past drinking patterns. The AUDIT asks about current frequency and quantity of drinking, which helps to establish the presence of *at-risk drinking* (defined for men as greater than 14 drinks per week or more than 4 drinks on occasion; defined for women or the elderly as greater than seven drinks per week or more than three drinks on occasion). The MAST and AUDIT take longer to perform in clinical practice; hence, some recommend use of the CAGE with follow-up questions for all positive responses (i.e., "Please tell me more about that.").

Establishing the diagnosis of alcohol abuse or dependence requires a thorough history and,

TABLE 3D.3 Diagnostic Criteria for Alcohol Intoxication

A. Recent ingestion of alcohol.

B. Clinically significant maladaptive behavioral or psychological changes (e.g., inappropriate sexual or aggressive behavior, mood lability, impaired judgment, impaired social, or occupational functioning) that developed during, or shortly after, alcohol ingestion.

C. One (or more) of the following signs, developing during, or shortly after, alcohol use:
1. slurred speech
2. incoordination
3. unsteady gait
4. nystagmus
5. impairment in attention or memory
6. stupor or coma

D. The symptoms are not due to a general medical condition and are not better accounted for by another mental disorder.

Adapted from American Psychiatric Association. *Diagnostic and Statistical Manual of Mental Disorders: DSM-IV-TR*. Washington, DC: American Psychiatric Association, 2000.

usually, collateral information from family/friends. However, there are some findings one may observe on physical examination and in the laboratory data of an alcohol-abusing patient. Physical examination findings may include elevated blood pressure, frequent bruising, liver findings (enlarged and smooth in the case of fatty liver; small and nodular in the case of cirrhosis), and, in cases of more advanced liver disease: spider angioma, palmar erythema, jaundice, and fetor hepaticus. One of the most sensitive and specific laboratory markers for recent heavy alcohol use is gamma-glutamyltransferase greater than 30 U/L, which has 60% to 80% sensitivity and specificity. Other laboratory markers of alcohol abuse may include elevated MCV (macrocytic anemia), thrombocytopenia, leukocytosis or leukopenia, elevated liver function tests (LFTs; classic pattern: AST > ALT in a 2:1 ratio), elevated uric acid, hypomagnesemia, and elevated LDL cholesterol and triglycerides. Elevated ammonia level may be found in patients with hepatic encephalopathy. It is important to note that LFTs may be normal in the alcoholic patient with liver "burnout." Note also that not all markers are specific for alcohol abuse nor are all markers found in all alcohol-abusing patients.

B. ALCOHOL-INDUCED DISORDERS

Alcohol intoxication is defined in DSM-IV-TR as clinically significant maladaptive behavioral or psychological changes (e.g., inappropriate behavior, mood lability, impaired judgment, or impaired social/occupational functioning) which occur during or after the ingestion of alcohol. In addition, the individual displays one or more physical signs, including slurred speech, incoordination, unsteady gait, nystagmus, impaired attention or memory, or stupor or coma (Table 3D.3). The symptoms may not be accounted for by a general medical condition or another psychiatric disorder. Most states consider the legal definition of alcohol intoxication to be a blood alcohol content (BAC) of 80 to 100 mg of ethanol per deciliter (mg/dL); however, slowing of psychomotor abilities may occur at levels as low as 20 to 30 mg/dL. When blood alcohol concentration rises to 80 to 200 mg/dL, one can experience increased mood lability, incoordination, and cognitive impairment. Blackouts, nystagmus, and more intensely slurred speech are seen at BAC between 200 and 300. A person with a BAC greater than 300 may experience stupor or coma; a BAC greater than 400 in a nontolerant person may result in respiratory suppression and death.

Alcohol withdrawal includes a spectrum of clinical syndromes, ranging from uncomplicated alcohol withdrawal to alcohol withdrawal delirium. Patients with a history of heavy alcohol use over a long period of time are at risk for alcohol withdrawal upon cessation of (or even just reduction in) alcohol use. The majority of alcohol-dependent patients will experience mild withdrawal symptoms of a self-limiting nature. Symptoms have an onset anywhere from 8 to 36 hours after the last drink

TABLE 3D.4 Diagnostic Criteria for Alcohol Withdrawal

A. Cessation of (or reduction in) alcohol use that has been heavy and prolonged.

B. Two (or more) of the following, developing within several hours to a few days after Criterion A:
1. autonomic hyperactivity (e.g., sweating or pulse rate > 100)
2. increased hand tremor
3. insomnia
4. nausea or vomiting
5. transient tactile, visual, or auditory hallucinations or illusions
6. psychomotor agitation
7. anxiety
8. grand mal seizures

C. The symptoms in Criterion B cause clinically significant distress or impairment in social, occupational, or other important areas of functioning.

D. The symptoms are not due to a general medical condition and are not better accounted for by another mental disorder.

Adapted from American Psychiatric Association. *Diagnostic and Statistical Manual of Mental Disorders: DSM-IV-TR.* Washington, DC: American Psychiatric Association, 2000.

and may include diaphoresis, nausea, vomiting, tremor, elevations in heart rate and blood pressure, anxiety, agitation, insomnia, and transient hallucinations ("alcoholic hallucinosis") (see Table 3D.4). Symptoms of alcohol withdrawal can be quantified and followed by using an instrument such as the CIWA-Ar. Mild uncomplicated alcohol withdrawal usually subsides by day 4 to 5. More severe symptoms of alcohol withdrawal include the development of seizures and delirium. Alcohol withdrawal seizures ("rum fits") typically occur within the first 7 to 38 hours after the last drink and are self-limited. They do not require initiation of routine anticonvulsant therapy. Patients with a history of seizure disorder and metabolic derangements are at greater risk of alcohol withdrawal seizures.

Alcohol withdrawal delirium (delirium tremens or "DTs") is characterized by the onset of confusion, disorientation, inattention, fluctuations in level of alertness, and perceptual disturbances in addition to the physiologic signs of withdrawal discussed above. Autonomic instability may be quite profound, including hypertension, fever, and tachycardia. Seizures may be present. Unlike uncomplicated alcohol withdrawal, alcohol withdrawal delirium will not resolve on its own and is considered a medical emergency which requires inpatient treatment (see below). Patients at greater risk for DTs include those with a prior history of DTs, older patients, and patients with comorbid medical illness (e.g., infection, metabolic derangements, liver disease, and head trauma). Thanks to modern medical treatments, death from DT is now uncommon. However, even treated alcohol withdrawal delirium can continue to wax and wane for weeks. Patients may require the use of sitters and/or restraints to maintain safety and keep intravenous lines intact.

Alcohol-induced mood disorder is diagnosed when there is a prominent and persistent disturbance of mood characterized by either depressed mood (or anhedonia) or expansive (or irritable) mood with evidence from the history, examination, or laboratory findings that the symptoms developed *during, or within a month of*, alcohol intoxication or withdrawal. Similarly, *alcohol-induced anxiety disorder* includes prominent anxiety, panic attacks, obsessions, or compulsions that developed during, or within a month of, alcohol intoxication or withdrawal. These diagnoses are made instead of alcohol intoxication or alcohol withdrawal only when the mood and anxiety symptoms are in excess of those usually associated with those respective syndromes and are severe enough to warrant clinical attention. As alcohol is a central nervous system depressant, depressive symptoms in alcohol-dependent patients are not uncommon. Anxiety is a common symptom of alcohol withdrawal. Hence, clinicians should always ask about the presence of mood and anxiety symptoms in patients who abuse alcohol. If a patient does endorse such symptoms, it can be challenging to determine whether the disorder is primary or secondary to alcohol. Good questions to help determine whether a patient's mood or anxiety symptoms are alcohol-induced are "What is your longest period of sobriety?" followed by, "During that time, did you continue to have [mood or anxiety symptoms]?" In general, alcohol-induced mood and anxiety disorders are treated with abstinence. If symptoms persist after 4 weeks of sobriety, the patient should be reevaluated for the presence of a primary mood or anxiety disorder which may warrant pharmacological treatment and/or psychotherapy.

Alcohol-induced psychotic disorder, also known as "alcoholic hallucinosis," includes the presence of perceptual disturbances (typically vivid auditory hallucinations) that occur within 1 month of the cessation or reduction of heavy alcohol ingestion. In contrast to patients who suffer the perceptual disturbances that accompany alcohol withdrawal delirium, patients with alcoholic hallucinosis have a relatively clear sensorium with few autonomic signs/symptoms. Up to 20% of patients may develop chronic hallucinations, resembling schizophrenia. Though the first-line treatment of alcoholic hallucinosis is abstinence from alcohol, antipsychotic medications have been used with some degree of success for agitated, psychotic patients or those suffering from chronic, persistent hallucinations in the absence of alcohol.

Alcohol-induced cognitive disorders include alcohol-induced persisting amnestic disorder and alcohol-induced persisting dementia. Alcohol-induced persisting amnestic disorder often begins with the onset of confusion, truncal ataxia, and ophthalmoplegia (sixth cranial nerve palsy). This triad is known as Wernicke's encephalopathy and is secondary to thiamine deficiency. Despite treatment with thiamine, the majority of patients who develop Wernicke's encephalopathy will go on to develop a persisting amnestic disorder (known as Korsakoff's psychosis, though it is not a true psychosis). One of the classic characteristics of this illness is confabulation, though this symptom is not invariably present. Alcohol-induced persisting amnestic disorder is primarily a dysfunction of *memory*. By contrast, alcohol-induced persisting dementia is a *global cognitive disorder*, with impairments in memory as well as other cognitive domains (i.e., aphasia, agnosia, apraxia, and executive dysfunction). There are no Food and Drug Administration (FDA)-approved treatments for alcohol-induced cognitive disorders. Treatment is often supportive; like patients with other types of dementia, patients with alcohol-induced cognitive disorders may not be able to safely live independently.

7. Treatments

Like most psychiatric illnesses, the treatment of alcohol use disorders and alcohol-induced disorders should take a biopsychosocial approach, including both pharmacological and nonpharmacological treatment modalities.

A. NONPHARMACOLOGICAL TREATMENT

For those patients who engage in risky alcohol use, but who are not dependent on alcohol, a "brief intervention" can be successful and cost-effective in reducing alcohol intake. Brief interventions can take place in almost any clinical setting, and typically include up to four brief sessions with the patient (5 to 15 minutes each). The focus of the session is reduction in alcohol intake, modifying drinking behaviors, and increasing compliance with therapy. Brief interventions often use techniques of *motivational interviewing*, which is a nonjudgmental, nonconfrontational approach to help patients resolve their ambivalence about changing their drinking behaviors. In motivational interviewing, the clinician asks open-ended questions to assess the impact of drinking on the patient's life and seeks to identify goals and values, which may help motivate the patient for change. The four key principles of motivational interviewing are to express empathy, develop discrepancy, roll with resistance, and support self-efficacy. Techniques used include open-ended questions, affirmations, reflective listening, and summarizing.

While the above techniques may suffice for patients with mild problems with alcohol, patients who have more severe problems with alcohol will often require more intensive treatment. This often comes in the form of *outpatient or intensive outpatient rehabilitation programs*. Intensive outpatient programs often include group and individual meetings several times a week for several weeks. This type of program is best suited for motivated individuals with good social support and may be preferred by patients who are employed.

Programming often includes psychoeducation, group and individual therapy (e.g., CBT), relapse prevention, social skills training, etc.

For patients whose alcohol dependence is severe enough to require medical detoxification, who have minimal social support, or who have failed attempts at outpatient rehabilitation, *inpatient rehabilitation programs* may be of benefit. These programs last anywhere from a week to a year or more, and often begin with a period of medical detoxification (see below for details) followed by intensive inpatient rehabilitation in a residential setting. Programming often includes individual, group, and family therapy.

Alcoholics Anonymous (AA), a 12-step program, offers group support for patients seeking help with a drinking problem. AA meetings are free and are available throughout the United States. The only requirement to join AA is a desire to stop drinking. Al-Anon, a support group for family and loved ones of alcoholics, is often helpful as well.

B. PHARMACOLOGICAL TREATMENTS

1. Alcohol Withdrawal

As described above, alcohol withdrawal includes a spectrum of clinical syndromes, ranging from uncomplicated withdrawal to delirium tremens. The choice of treatment for alcohol withdrawal depends on the severity of symptoms, the stage of withdrawal, psychiatric and medical comorbidities, availability of social support, and the patient's ability to follow instructions and cooperate. Alcohol detoxification can be completed on an outpatient or an inpatient basis, depending on these factors. Patients with more severe withdrawal symptoms, history of alcohol withdrawal seizures or delirium, limited social support, and multiple medical and psychiatric comorbidities are better suited for inpatient detoxification.

In any patient who is undergoing alcohol withdrawal, supportive measures should be instituted. Vital signs should be monitored at least every 4 hours. Patients should be encouraged to take in adequate fluids and nutrition. Nutritional deficiencies should be repleted, including thiamine 100 mg daily, folate 1 mg daily, and a multivitamin daily. Thiamine may be given intramuscularly or intravenously to patients who are unable to tolerate oral intake or who have poor nutritional status. Of note, *intravenous thiamine should be given before glucose* because glucose depletes thiamine stores and may precipitate Wernicke's encephalopathy. Any electrolyte disturbance should be corrected (e.g., hypokalemia and hypomagnesemia). Medications may be required for nausea, vomiting, and insomnia. Scales such as the CIWA-Ar can be used to monitor the severity of withdrawal symptoms and to track the patient's progress during the detoxification period.

Benzodiazepines remain the pharmacological treatment of choice for alcohol withdrawal, due to their efficacy, safety profile, ease of administration, and anticonvulsant properties. Chlordiazepoxide and lorazepam are most commonly used. *Chlordiazepoxide* has the advantage of a long half-life. *Lorazepam*, though shorter-acting, is preferred in patients with liver disease due to its lack of active metabolites. In addition, it is available in oral, intravenous, and intramuscular routes of administration. Benzodiazepines can be given in a symptom-triggered regimen or a structured regimen, tapering to discontinuation over the course of 3 to 5 days. (Table 3D.5 provides a sample alcohol detoxification plan.) Anticonvulsants such as valproate and carbamazepine have been studied in alcohol withdrawal but have not been found to be more effective than benzodiazepines. They may be an alternative if benzodiazepines are contraindicated. Alcohol withdrawal seizures are typically treated with diazepam or lorazepam, and do not usually require initiation of routine anticonvulsant therapy.

For patients who develop *alcohol withdrawal delirium* (or delirium tremens), hospitalization is necessary, often in the intensive care unit where vital signs can be monitored continuously. The treatment of alcohol withdrawal delirium includes administration of intravenous lorazepam, titrated as needed to maintain sedation without obtunding the patient completely. Patients may require a sitter and/or restraints for safety and to maintain intravenous lines, though restraints should be minimized as much as possible. For severe agitation accompanied by psychosis, the use of antipsychotic medication may be necessary. Haloperidol has been the antipsychotic most studied in delirium and is typically used. Though there is concern for lowering the seizure threshold, clinically this is usually not a problem, as the patient is also receiving benzodiazepines. Haloperidol can be given intramuscularly or intravenously. However, recall from the chapter on delirium that intravenous haloperidol is associated with QTc prolongation and risk of

TABLE 3D.5 Sample Alcohol Detoxification Protocol

1. Supportive Measures (a) Monitor vital signs every 4 h (b) Monitor alcohol withdrawal symptoms; consider CIWA-Ar every 4 h
2. Correct Nutritional Deficiencies and Electrolyte Disturbances (a) Thiamine 100 mg daily (b) Folate 1 mg daily (c) Multivitamin daily
3. Lorazepam 2 mg orally every 6 h for 24 h, then 1.5 mg orally every 6 h for 24 h, then 1 mg orally every 6 h for 24 h, then 1 mg orally every 8 h for 24 h, then discontinue lorazepam
4. Lorazepam 2 mg orally every 4 h as needed for breakthrough withdrawal symptoms (CIWA-Ar > 8, blood pressure > 150/90 mm Hg, heart rate > 100 beats/min, temperature > 100.4°F)
5. Trazodone 100 mg orally at bedtime as needed for insomnia

CIWA-Ar, Clinical Institute Withdrawal Assessment for Alcohol-Revised.

cardiac arrhythmias and therefore should be used with caution.

2. Alcohol Abuse and Dependence

Several medications have been studied for relapse prevention in alcohol-dependent patients. Three medications are FDA approved for alcohol dependence: disulfiram, naltrexone, and acamprosate (Table 3D.6).

Disulfiram is an aversive agent which inhibits ALDH. Thus, when a patient taking disulfiram ingests alcohol, he or she suffers severe side effects, including nausea, vomiting, headache, palpitations, and flushing. Patients must be instructed to avoid alcohol in *any* form while taking disulfiram. Common side effects include dermatitis and a garlic-like taste. Disulfiram requires a very motivated patient, and is contraindicated in patients who are pregnant, have heart disease, severe liver disease, and psychosis. The usual dose of disulfiram is 250 mg to 500 mg orally once a day for initiation of treatment (1 to 2 weeks) followed by a maintenance dose of 250 mg daily.

Naltrexone is an opioid antagonist which has been shown to reduce the risk of relapse in alcohol-dependent patients. Side effects include headache, nausea, and constipation. Naltrexone is contraindicated in patients with severe liver disease or in patients taking opioids. The usual dose of oral naltrexone is 50 mg once a day. Naltrexone is also available in a long-acting intramuscular formulation which is administered once a month. The intramuscular dose is 380 mg.

Acamprosate is another oral medication which has been shown to reduce risk of relapse in alcohol-dependent patients. Its exact mechanism of action is not entirely clear, but it is thought to involve an interaction with glutamate and GABA

TABLE 3D.6 FDA-Approved Pharmacological Treatments for Alcohol Dependence

Medication	Mechanism of Action	Dose	Side Effects
Disulfiram	Inhibits ALDH	250–500 mg/day	Aftertaste, fatigue
Naltrexone	Opioid antagonist	50 mg/day	Nausea, headache, constipation
Acamprosate	GABA/glutamate?	666 mg t.i.d.	Nausea, diarrhea, headache

ALDH, aldehyde dehydrogenase; GABA, gamma-aminobutyric acid.

neurotransmitter systems. Common side effects include headache, nausea, abdominal pain, and diarrhea. Acamprosate is contraindicated in patients with severe renal impairment. The usual dose of acamprosate is 666 mg orally three times daily.

The COMBINE study examined the efficacy of medication (naltrexone and acamprosate), behavioral therapies, and their combinations for the treatment of alcohol dependence. This study concluded that patients receiving medical management with naltrexone, cognitive behavioral intervention (CBI), or both fared better on drinking outcomes compared to acamprosate, which showed no evidence of efficacy either with or without CBI.

While not approved by the FDA for treatment of alcohol dependence, *topiramate* has been investigated for the treatment of alcohol dependence. In a 2007 study published in the *Journal of the American Medical Association*, up to 300 mg daily of topiramate combined with a weekly compliance enhancement intervention was more effective than placebo at reducing the percentage of days of heavy drinking from baseline to week 14. Adverse events reported included paresthesia, taste perversion, difficulty concentrating, and anorexia.

8. Prognosis

Chronic alcohol abuse is associated with significant psychosocial and medical consequences, as detailed above. About one third of alcohol-dependent patients stop drinking without formal treatment. Another third reduce drinking with treatment, and the final third never achieve sobriety. Favorable prognostic signs include the absence of ASPD or coexisting substance abuse; employment; family support; and the absence of severe legal difficulties. Similarly, a patient who stays engaged in a program during the initial rehabilitation phase (the first 2 to 4 weeks) has a better chance at maintaining sobriety in the long run. In general, alcohol-dependent patients with comorbid primary psychiatric illness (e.g., schizophrenia or bipolar disorder) tend to run the course of their psychiatric illness. Alcohol abuse does worsen the prognosis for primary psychiatric illnesses and for many medical illnesses. Alcohol has a propensity to reduce inhibitions and increase impulsivity; alcohol abuse is a known risk factor for suicide.

9. General Formulation for Alcohol Abuse and Dependence

A. DIAGNOSTIC

Ensure that the patient meets the DSM-IV-TR criteria for either alcohol abuse or alcohol dependence. Recall that the diagnosis of alcohol abuse generally entails psychosocial, physical, and/or legal consequences of alcohol misuse. Alcohol dependence includes those consequences as well as physiological tolerance and withdrawal (though the latter two symptoms are not required for the diagnosis). In addition, alcohol dependence reflects a pattern of addictive behavior: considerable time spent obtaining, using, or recovering from alcohol; repeated efforts to reduce drinking without success; important activities given up for alcohol; and continued use despite medical or psychosocial consequences. Collateral information may be necessary to establish the diagnosis of an alcohol use disorder, as patients often minimize the impact of their alcohol use. Consider other diagnoses in the differential; in particular, consider mood disorders, anxiety disorders, personality disorders, and other substance use disorders. Keep in mind that in order to diagnose an alcohol-induced mood or anxiety disorder, the symptoms must occur within *1 month* of alcohol intoxication or withdrawal.

B. ETIOLOGIC

From a biological perspective, a family history of alcoholism (in particular, paternal history) or other substance use disorders increases one's risk of developing alcohol dependence. Consider other risk factors such as a personal history of ASPD, depression, or exposure to traumatic events. Consider job or educational setting, cultural factors, and religious factors. If a patient has recently relapsed after a period of sobriety, consider the possibility of an acute life stressor such as divorce, loss of relationship, job loss, or financial stressor.

C. THERAPEUTIC

The patient's readiness for change can be assessed through brief interventions and motivational interviewing. Treatment planning should always take into account the severity of the patient's alcohol abuse and should include biological and psychosocial components. Medical detoxification may be necessary for patients experiencing physiologic withdrawal. Benzodiazepines are the treatment of choice for medical detoxification and for alcohol withdrawal delirium. Long-term treatment options include outpatient, intensive outpatient, or inpatient rehabilitation, all of which are likely to include components of individual, group, and family therapy. Pharmacological treatments are available for alcohol dependence, including disulfiram, naltrexone, and acamprosate. The best results are achieved when such medications are prescribed in conjunction with a psychosocial treatment program aimed at relapse prevention. Twelve-step programs such as AA and Al-Anon (for family members) offer additional support.

D. PROGNOSTIC

Chronic alcohol abuse is associated with significant medical, psychiatric, and psychosocial consequences. While some patients are able to stop drinking without intervention, the majority will require help and unfortunately, some patients will never achieve sobriety. Consider the presence or absence of positive prognostic indicators such as motivation for change, stable employment, family support, and lack of comorbid ASPD or other substance use disorders. Alcohol dependence worsens the prognosis for primary psychiatric illnesses and many medical illnesses as well. Alcohol abuse increases one's risk of suicide.

10. Risk Assessment

All patients with alcohol abuse or dependence must have a careful risk assessment and be evaluated for suicidality and homicidality, as alcohol causes disinhibition and may lead to increased impulsivity. Recall that risk factors for suicide include male gender; white race; divorced, separated, or single status; bisexuality or homosexuality; substance abuse; age more than 45; panic attacks; early loss or separation from parents; family history of suicide; hallucinations; hopelessness; insomnia; lack of future plans; previous suicide attempts; high lethality of previous attempt(s); living alone; low self-esteem; chronic physical illness; severe pain; recent loss; sexual abuse; and unemployment. It is essential to always inquire about suicidal thoughts or plan and perform a risk assessment including questions regarding access to firearms or other potentially lethal methods. In addition to the risk of suicide/homicide, consider the physiologic risk of continued chronic alcohol abuse (gastrointestinal effects, liver disease, dementia, etc.) as well as the worse prognosis with regard to comorbid psychiatric disorders. Also consider the risk of hazardous activities such as driving while intoxicated.

KEY POINTS (ABPN Examination)

A. When interviewing a patient with suspected alcohol abuse or dependence

1. Inquire about past and current patterns of drinking including frequency and quantity.
2. Screen with CAGE questions.
3. Observe for any signs of current withdrawal such as tremor, diaphoresis, anxiety, etc.
4. Screen for comorbid mood, anxiety, personality, and other substance use disorders.
5. Gently, nonconfrontationally assess the patient's motivation for change. Be empathic.
6. Always screen for suicidal or homicidal ideation.

B. When presenting a patient with alcohol abuse or dependence

1. Present the patient's drinking history using DSM-IV-TR criteria.
2. Always consider mood, anxiety, personality, and other substance use disorders in the differential diagnosis.
3. Suggest that you would like to obtain collateral information from family regarding patient's substance abuse history.
4. With regard to treatment, remember to include both nonpharmacological and pharmacological aspects.

SUGGESTED READINGS

American Psychiatric Association. *Diagnostic and Statistical Manual of Mental Disorders: DSM-IV-TR*. Washington, DC: American Psychiatric Association, 2000.

Anderson D, Brachtesende A. Managing alcohol problems, part 2. *Case Manager* 2006;17(6):43–46.

Angres DH, Bettinardi-Anges K. The disease of addiction: Origins, treatment, and recovery. *Dis Mon* 2008;54:696–721.

Anthenelli RM, Smith TL, Irwin MR, et al. A comparative study of criteria for subgrouping alcoholics: The primary/secondary diagnostic scheme versus variations of the type1/type 2criteria. *Am J Psychiatry* 1994;151:1468–1474.

Anton FR, O'Malley SS, Ciraulo DA, et al. Combined pharmacotherapies and behavioral interventions for alcohol dependence. The COMBINE study: A randomized controlled trial. *JAMA* 2006;295:2003–2017.

Berglund M, Thelander S, Salaspuro M, et al. Treatment of alcohol abuse: an evidence-based review. *Alcohol Clin Exp Res* 2003;279(10):1645–1656.

Boniatti M, Diogo LP, Almeida CL, et al. Prevalence and record of alcoholism among emergency department patients. *Clinics* 2009;64(1): 29–34.

Danielson CK, Amstadter AB, Dangelmaier RE, et al. Trauma-related risk factors for substance abuse among male versus female young adults. *Addict Behav* 2008;34(4):395–399.

Franklin, JR, Levenson JL, McCance-Katz EF. Substance-related disorders. In: Levenson JL, ed. *Textbook of Psychosomatic Medicine*. Arlington, VA: American Psychiatric Publishing, 2005: 387–400.

Isaacson JH, Schorling JB. Screening for alcohol problems in primary care. *Med Clin North Am* 1999;83(6):1547–1563.

Johnson BA, Rosenthal N, Capece JA, et al. Topiramate for treating alcohol dependence: A randomized controlled trial. *JAMA* 2007;298(14): 1641–1651.

McRae AL, Brady KT, Sonne SC. Alcohol and substance abuse. *Med Clin North Am* 2001;85(3): 779–801.

Miller WR. Motivational interviewing with problem drinkers. *Behav Psychother* 1983;11:147–172.

Polycarpou A, Papanikolau P, Ioannidis JPA, et al. Anticonvulsants for alcohol withdrawal. Cochrane Database of Systematic Reviews 2005, Issue 3. Art. No. CD005064. DOI: 10.1002/14651858.CD005064.pub2.

Rosenbaum JF, Arana GW, Hyman SE, et al. Drugs for the treatment of addictive disorders. In: Handbook of Psychiatric Drug Therapy. 5th Ed. Philadelphia, PA: Lippincott Williams & Wilkins, 2005:205–242.

Saitz R. Treatment of alcohol and other drug dependence. *Liver Transpl* 2007;13:S59–S64.

Schuckit MA. Alcohol-related disorders. In: Sadock BJ, Sadock VA, eds. *Comprehensive Textbook of Psychiatry*. 7th Ed. Philadelphia: Lippincott Williams & Wilkins, 2000:953–970.

Smith DC, Hall JA, Jang M, et al. Therapist adherence to a motivational-interviewing intervention improves treatment entry for substance misusing adolescents with low problem perception. *J Stud Alcohol Drugs* 2009 Jan;70(1):101–105.

Trevisan LA, Ralevski E, Keegan K, et al. Alcohol detoxification and relapse prevention using valproic acid versus gabapentin in alcohol-dependent patients. *Addict Disord Their Treat* 2008;7:119–128.

II. COCAINE DEPENDENCE

CASE HISTORY

PRESENT ILLNESS

Ms T is a 40-year-old female who was brought to the emergency room by ambulance after she attempted to hit her clinician. Upon admission to the hospital, she was hostile, irritable, guarded, and refused to answer questions. She was observed yelling "That doctor was trying to sell me to the police and that is why she got what she deserved!"

The psychiatry resident on call contacted the patient's clinician and obtained the following information: she has been treated as an outpatient for cocaine dependence, "questionable" bipolar disorder, and antisocial personality disorder (ASPD). Even though her substance of choice is "crack" cocaine, which she smokes on a daily basis (approximately $150 to $200 per week), she also drinks alcohol to "mellow things" (Three 12-oz beers per day) and smokes Tetrahydrocannabinol (THC) to "relax and calm down" (1 to 2 "joints" per day). Her clinician also reports that Ms T has not complained of suicidal ideation, homicidal ideation, depressed mood, appetite disturbances, lack of energy, problems with concentration, insomnia/hypersomnia, obsessions, compulsions, panic attacks, social anxiety, or phobias. She has reported anhedonia and feelings of guilt about her drug use.

She has not been compliant with medications and has never been abstinent while the clinician has seen her. However, Ms T has been very reliable when it comes to making it to her outpatient appointments.

The morning of the patient's admission, her clinician received a phone call from Ms T's significant other. He reported that she had been unusually aggressive, had accused him of giving her "tampered drugs," and had refused to accept any drugs, food, or liquids from him. The clinician was able to contact her and convinced her to come in for an appointment. Upon presentation, she insisted on being seen with the office's door open and displayed paranoid behavior. When the clinician took the phone to call the pharmacist regarding the patient's medications, Ms T stood up and asked her what she was trying to do. The clinician explained her intentions, but Ms T vociferated "You are a liar and you are afraid of me; you are going to call the police!" Immediately thereafter, Ms T jumped in front of her clinician and punched her in the chest.

PSYCHIATRIC HISTORY

Ms T has seen mental health providers since she was 12 years of age. Some of her problematic behaviors as a child included bullying other kids, getting into physical fights, running away from home, stealing from peers and from stores, and disobeying authority figures. She has a long history of sexual abuse by her father, who used to give her drugs before molesting her. She began drinking when she was 10 years old, using THC when she was 13, and using cocaine when she was 14 years old. In spite of her long history of alcohol use, she has never suffered from delirium tremens or from seizures.

A former psychiatrist diagnosed Ms T with bipolar disorder when she was 25 years old and recommended quetiapine, which she has never taken as prescribed. She says that one of the reasons she does not take her medications is because they "make me feel weak and slow." She has had multiple inpatient psychiatric admissions for "mood swings," which have always being while intoxicated with cocaine. As part of these episodes, she has psychomotor agitation, grandiosity, pressured speech, flight of ideas, distractibility, insomnia, and reckless promiscuous behavior. She has never attempted suicide, and she has seen her clinician for the past 3 years.

FAMILY HISTORY

The patient's father has a history of alcohol dependence. Her brother has a history of heroin dependence.

SOCIAL HISTORY

The patient lives with her boyfriend, who is also the person who provides her drugs. She is estranged from her family and has sporadic contact with one of her brothers with whom she "always gets into arguments." She finished seventh grade and is currently unemployed. Ms T was working as a mail carrier when she was incarcerated in 2001 for armed robbery. Once released from jail, she initially had a job as a custodian, which she was not able to keep for more than 3 months, because of her drug use (i.e., arriving late to work, being intoxicated while at work, getting into arguments with customers and supervisors as a result of substance-induced mood changes, etc.). Afterward, she worked as a drug dealer ("I only get out of the house when I need to get money in order to buy cocaine. I learned that the best way of getting drugs is being a drug dealer myself and that is my occupation right now."). As hobbies, she has an interest in crossword puzzles, which has also been progressively decreasing.

PERTINENT MEDICAL HISTORY

Ms T was diagnosed with HIV 5 years ago, which she contracted as a result of practicing unsafe sex (most commonly in the context of cocaine intoxication and efforts to obtain more drug in exchange for sex). She takes efavirenz 600 mg/emtricitabine 200 mg/tenofovir disoproxil fumarate (DF) 300 mg. Her CD4 count is 340 and her viral load is undetectable. She has a history of a laparotomy and resection of one portion of small bowel after an episode of mesenteric ischemia.

MENTAL STATUS EXAMINATION

Ms T remains agitated in spite of being in four-point restraints. Her hair is disheveled, and she is wearing clothes that are not warm enough for the winter. She looks older than her stated age and has a defiant eye contact. She is diaphoretic, and when not talking or yelling, she is clenching her teeth and making tight fists with her hands. Her mood is angry and her affect is congruent with mood. She has flight of ideas, and her thought content is characterized by paranoid and grandiose ideations (e.g., "You people want to give me a hard time because you are envious of me doing whatever I want with my life. You think that I am not aware that you are poisoning my medications in order to make me weak. I have very good connections and will make sure that you all pay for this. I will see you in court and then you will be the ones begging for mercy."). When asked about the presence of perceptual disturbances, she answers: "Do I look crazy to you?—I have none of that and I am not going to play any mind games with you." Three hours later, after receiving an intramuscular injection of haloperidol and lorazepam, she is more cooperative and without alterations in her orientation, memory, or attention. Her insight remains below average (i.e., "What happened had nothing to do with me using crack"), and her judgment is still compromised (i.e., "Tell that doctor that I will get back at her as soon as I contact my lawyers and leave the hospital"). She denies suicidal ideation and when asked about homicidal thoughts, replies "I am smart enough to keep that answer to myself. I have already talked too much."

PERTINENT PHYSICAL FINDINGS

Her vital signs are noted as follows: BP 150/105 mm Hg, HR 105, RR 14, T 97.5. Head is atraumatic; pupils are dilated but reactive to light and accommodation on both sides, and nasal septum is intact. She had poor dental hygiene with evidence of significant dental caries. Heart: mostly rhythmic, though, some ectopic beats are heard. Abdomen has a sagittal scar of former laparotomy. Neurological examination is normal.

LABORATORY DATA

WBC = 6.8, HgB = 12.9, Hct = 39.7, MCV = 95, % N = 67, % L = 24, BUN = 22, Creatinine = 1.1, CO_2 = 22.9, Cl = 103, Na = 135, K = 3.8, AST = 33, ALT = 50, AKP = 90, HIV-1 RNA PCR, Quantitative < 48 copies/mL, CXR WNL. Urine toxicology is positive for cocaine and THC. Brain computerized tomography did not show any acute intracranial pathology. Lumbar puncture was negative for intracranial infections.

HOSPITAL AND OUTPATIENT COURSE

During the first 48 hours Ms T was kept in the ED and she received one intramuscular injection of haloperidol (5 mg) and lorazepam (2 mg) with good control of her agitation. After 48 hours, she was admitted to the inpatient psychiatric unit of a local hospital where she displayed dysphoric mood, hypersomnolence, hyperphagia, anergia, anhedonia, psychomotor retardation, and delusions. These delusions were paranoid (e.g., blaming her clinician of conspiring with the administrative personnel of the hospital in order to hospitalize her), and they significantly improved with haloperidol 5 mg by mouth, per day.

The substance dependence treatment program team was consulted on the fourth day of her psychiatric inpatient admission. By the time they saw her, her psychotic symptoms were under control and she was no longer on haloperidol. They suggested two potential treatment avenues, including both pharmacotherapeutic (e.g., disulfiram or modafinil) and psychotherapeutic (motivational enhancement, contingency management, or CBT) interventions. In support of initiating a course of drug treatment with disulfiram, the treatment team noted that this agent might be beneficial given her comorbid use of both alcohol and cocaine. Alternatively, modafinil was also considered a beneficial option given the patient's symptoms of anergia, anhedonia in the postcocaine period, and the greater tolerability of the latter in comparison to disulfiram. A concern in this case was potential consumption of alcohol or cocaine while on disulfiram, which could lead to potentially harmful cardiovascular or psychiatric side effects (e.g., exacerbation of psychotic symptoms). Given the patient's withdrawal symptoms, such as hypersomnolence, hyperphagia, and dysphoric mood, a decision was made to use modafinil in combination with motivational enhancement therapy for the treatment of her cocaine dependence. She was discharged on the sixth day of her inpatient admission and was referred to an intensive outpatient program. Her abstinence lasted only 1 week after discharge.

DISCHARGE MEDICATIONS

Modafinil 400 mg per day

DSM-IV-TR MULTIAXIAL DIAGNOSIS

Axis I: Cocaine dependence; cocaine intoxication; cocaine withdrawal; substance-induced psychotic disorder, with delusions; rule out posttraumatic stress disorder; and rule out THC abuse/dependence.

Axis II: Antisocial personality disorder

Axis III: HIV, status post laparotomy and resection of portion of small bowel.

Axis IV: Problems with primary support group (estrangement from family members, discord with sibling), problems related to the social environment (inadequate social support), economic problems (inadequate finances), and problems related to interaction with the legal system/crime (history of incarceration).

Axis V: Global assessment of functioning:

At admission: 20; violent and agitated behavior at danger of hurting others. At discharge: 45; serious impairment of social and occupational functioning, but absence of active psychotic symptoms or danger to self or others.

FORMULATION

A. Diagnostic

This patient suffers from a constellation of symptoms that illustrate the diagnosis of cocaine dependence and substance-induced psychotic disorder. Ms T meets criteria for cocaine dependence as evidenced by the following characteristics: presence of withdrawal symptoms, a great deal of time spent in activities necessary to obtain or use the substance, important social/occupational/recreational activities are given up or reduced because of substance use, and the substance use is continued despite having persistent psychological problems caused or exacerbated by it. Her initial presentation suggests the diagnosis of cocaine intoxication given the following constellation of symptoms present at the time of admission: hypervigilance, interpersonal sensitivity, tension, increased alertness, anger, and impaired judgment. In addition to these manifestations, her physical examination revealed tachycardia, high blood pressure, dilated pupils, and psychomotor agitation, all physical signs of stimulant intoxication.

Another condition that must be considered in the differential diagnosis of her initial presentation is "cocaine-excited delirium." Patients suffering from this can have paranoia, agitation, hyperpyrexia, and can worsen to the point of coma and death.

Some of Ms T's presenting symptoms, such as autonomic instability, agitation, and paranoia in someone who has been drinking alcohol, suggest the diagnosis of delirium tremens. However, there is no documentation of alterations in her orientation, memory, and attention, which goes against the diagnosis of delirium tremens.

A diagnosis of cocaine withdrawal is supported due to the fact that within hours after cessation of a heavy and prolonged use, she presented with dysphoric mood, hypersomnia, increased appetite, and psychomotor agitation/retardation.

On the other hand, Ms T was diagnosed with cocaine, or probably THC-induced psychotic disorder because of the prominent delusions that were judged to be due to the direct effects of the drug. The features that differentiate this disorder from cocaine or THC intoxication include the persistence of psychosis beyond the period of acute drug intoxication and the severity of these symptoms, such that they warranted independent clinical intervention. However, her previous clinician confirmed that Ms T did not have a history of psychotic symptoms on the absence of drug use, which rules out the possibility of a primary psychotic disorder.

The presence of psychotic symptoms, for the first time, in someone who is 40 years old does not support the possibility of a new onset primary psychotic disorder. Nevertheless, it does not exclude it either. Another fact against the diagnosis of a primary psychotic disorder is that Ms T's psychotic symptoms did not persist for more than 1 month after being abstinent from cocaine.

New onset psychosis occurs in 0.5% to 15% of HIV positive patients. Psychiatric manifestations could be the result of the HIV infection itself, side effects from the antiretroviral therapy, or opportunistic infections, such as toxoplasmosis, cytomegalovirus, non-Hodgkin's lymphoma, etc. The chronologic association between cocaine use and the patient's symptoms, the negative medical work-up for opportunistic infections, and the resolution of symptoms without any medical interventions other than abstinence from cocaine, support the diagnosis of a cocaine-induced psychotic disorder.

Other important diagnoses in this patient's differential diagnosis include polysubstance dependence, bipolar disorder, posttraumatic stress disorder, primary psychotic disorder, delirium tremens, THC intoxication, THC abuse/dependence, and psychotic disorder due to a general medical condition. This patient does not meet criteria for polysubstance dependence. Her problems associated with cocaine are pervasive enough to justify a diagnosis of cocaine dependence independently of what her pattern of marijuana and alcohol use is. This excludes the diagnosis of polysubstance dependence. At this point, there is not enough evidence to diagnose bipolar disorder given that her mood changes have always been documented in the setting of cocaine intoxication or cocaine withdrawal. Posttraumatic stress disorder is important in the differential given her history of abuse. There is not enough information about symptoms of reexperiencing, avoidance, or increased arousal to confirm or rule out this diagnosis.

This patient's initial symptomatology could be explained by an episode of THC intoxication. It is known that cannabis use can produce maladaptive behavior, psychosis, tachycardia, and hyperphagia, which were symptoms she presented with. However, her positive urine toxicology for THC could have been the result of any use within the past 4 weeks and not necessarily a recent use. Against the possibility of THC intoxication is her report of daily cocaine use, history of manic episodes accompanied by positive urine toxicology screens for cocaine, dilated pupils, and high blood pressure. These findings are more suggestive of the diagnosis of cocaine intoxication.

There is not enough evidence to rule out the diagnosis of THC abuse or dependence. It is unclear if her interpersonal problems and failure to fulfill major obligations are the result of THC use or the result of other problems. In addition, there is no documented evidence of THC use in physically hazardous situations, or of any association between her legal problems and THC use.

This patient meets DSM-IV criteria for ASPD. Since she was 15 years old, she has failed to conform to social rules with respect to lawful behaviors. She has repeatedly performed acts that are ground for arrest such as stealing, getting into physical fights, pursuing illegal occupations, disregarding her safety and the safety of others, repeatedly failuring to sustain consistent work behavior, and showing lack of remorse. In addition, she met the criteria for conduct disorder before she was 15 years old.

B. Etiologic

This patient's history of sexual abuse could have played a significant role in the etiology of her cocaine dependence and ASPD. Some patients report initial and continued use of substances because of the effects of abusive relationships. Several studies have shown associations between self-reported histories of physical and sexual abuse and substance use disorders. The fact that she is single and that her partner is a source of drugs are additional social risk factors for her substance abuse problems. Women seeking treatment for substance use disorders are more likely to be single and to be involved with an addicted partner. Her personality disorder could be one Ms T's additional risk factors for her cocaine dependence. It has been reported that the median prevalence of personality disorders among a population of treated substance use disorder patients can range from 35% to 73%. In fact, it is possible that there are genetic risk factors contributing to both her personality disorder and her substance use disorder.

C. Therapeutic

The initial treatment of Ms T in the phase of acute presentation should be symptom-based, with the goal of initial stabilization. Based on her initial presentation, it is appropriate to consider the use of haloperidol and lorazepam, though some authors would state that the use of neuroleptics should be avoided due to the risk of hyperthermia. Her presentation does not suggest the presence of hyperthermia or a "cocaine-excited delirium"; therefore, there are no contraindications to the use of a neuroleptic. A typical antipsychotic could be effective and safe as long as there is appropriate monitoring for any signs of neuroleptic malignant syndrome. Once the acute phase of agitation and psychosis is controlled, the approach can focus on her withdrawal symptoms, which are most often self-limiting in duration.

Ms T could benefit from a simultaneous treatment of her personality disorder as well as her substance abuse problems. This can take place in a "dual diagnosis" treatment unit, and the appropriate level of care can be determined with different tools, such as The American Society of Addiction Medicine Patient Placement Criteria.

Psychosocial interventions target relapse prevention and enhancement of treatment compliance. She could also benefit from CBT, motivational enhancement therapy, or contingency management (CM). A recent meta-analysis showed high effect sizes in favor of the CBT/CM combined approach for the treatment of substance use disorders. It is also important to keep in mind the availability of other behavioral interventions which could match Ms T's needs (i.e., narcotics anonymous, network therapy, family therapy, and group therapy). In regards to her diagnosis of ASPD, she could be referred to a therapeutic community and other form of group treatments for this condition. These interventions are often considered the treatment of choice for this Axis II disorder. It is thought that in an in-group context, rationalization can be confronted by others who are familiarized with these behaviors. A good prognostic factor for Ms T is the fact that she was engaged in treatment with her clinician. However, it is difficult to predict what will happen with the current working alliance based on the fact that her clinician recommended the inpatient admission and the fact that the patient was very paranoid about her.

Pharmacologically, it is appropriate to consider modafinil or disulfiram to facilitate the abstinence to cocaine. In favor of modafinil are its lack of worrisome side effects and the utility for the treatment of withdrawal symptoms. Another factor in favor of modafinil is its potential role in the treatment of abstinence-related cognitive dysfunction. In favor of disulfiram is its potential benefit for alcohol and cocaine use disorders. If she had been found to be homozygous for the "very low-activity" T allele at the dopamine beta hydroxylase (DBH) gene, the enzyme responsible for the conversion from dopamine to norepinephrine disulfiram, a potent, but nonselective inhibitor of DBH could be tried. Blockage of DBH can lead to higher cocaine aversion facilitate this patient's recovery. However, the effectiveness of this mechanism of action is unclear, and this genetic testing has only been used for research purposes; its utility in clinical settings remains to be established.

D. Prognostic

The use of crack cocaine among HIV-positive women has been associated with immunologic deterioration, failure to suppress the virus, development of AIDS-defining conditions, and mortality due to AIDS-related causes. These findings are even present in those who adhere to the HAART regimens at least 95% of the time. Another negative prognostic factor is the finding that women with cocaine dependence tend to have greater family/socioeconomic problems, more physical/sexual traumas, higher rates of PTSD, and twice the rate of any anxiety disorder, when compared to men. On the Addiction Severity Index, women had more severe scores on nearly every problem area (medical, psychiatric, social, employment). These findings indicate that women have important needs beyond their addiction, perhaps suggesting the need for more comprehensive services.

Ms T's lower educational level and unemployment status are factors that have been associated with poorer treatment retention. On the other hand, concurrent use of cocaine and alcohol produces cocaethylene, a transesterified metabolite associated with more lethality than cocaine alone.

The presence of ASPD in this patient can be considered another poor prognostic factor for treatment retention and continued cocaine abuse. On the other hand, a good prognostic factor for Ms T is her relative compliance with outpatient appointments.

COCAINE DEPENDENCE

1. Introduction

Cocaine's behavioral effects are mediated primarily by its binding to the dopamine transporter and inhibiting the reuptake of synaptic dopamine. Given that reuptake is the primary mechanism of terminating dopamine transmission, cocaine administration results in dose-dependent increases in extracellular levels of dopamine. Cocaine also blocks the reuptake of norepinephrine and serotonin. The robust reinforcing effects of cocaine are thought to result from their effects on the mesolimbic/mesocortical dopaminergic neuronal systems, including the ventral tegmental area (VTA), nucleus accumbens, ventral pallidum, and medial prefrontal cortex. The magnitude of the self-reported "high" in humans correlates with the occupancy of the dopamine transporter by cocaine, and the time course for these ratings parallels cocaine concentrations in the striatum. Neither norepinephrine nor serotonin appear to specifically mediate the reinforcing effects of cocaine. Other neurotransmitter systems may also play a role by modulating dopamine. For instance, glutamate projects to dopaminergic neurons in the nucleus accumbens, and injections of selective NMDA receptor antagonists into the nucleus accumbens block both the dopaminergic effects of psychostimulants and their reinforcing effects in laboratory animals. The inhibitory neurotransmitter γ-aminobutyric acid (GABA) also interacts with dopamine neurons in the nucleus accumbens and the VTA, and pharmacological manipulation of GABA alters both dopamine activity and cocaine self-administration.

In addition to its acute reinforcing effects, cocaine can produce several neurochemical and physiological impairments following chronic use. Studies show decreased postsynaptic dopamine receptors, reduced dopamine function, increases in dopamine transporter in acutely abstinent cocaine abusers relative to control subjects (SPET and PET studies), decreases in dopamine D2 receptor binding in detoxified cocaine abusers relative to control subjects, and reduced cerebral blood flow and cortical perfusion among chronic cocaine users.

2. Epidemiology

Cocaine use has declined relative to its extremely widespread use in the 1980s to early 1990s. Based on the Substance Abuse and Mental Health Services Administration's (SAMHSA's) Treatment Episode Data Set (TEDS), admission rates for primary cocaine treatment have decreased nationally by 24% between 1992 and 2002, from 133 admissions to 101 admissions per 100,000 persons 12 years of age or older. Nonetheless, the number of cocaine-related arrests, drug treatment records, and emergency room mentions demonstrate that cocaine remains a major public health problem. In 2006, 6 million Americans aged 12 years and older had abused cocaine in some form and 1.5 million had abused crack at least once in the year prior to being surveyed.

In the United States, cocaine is used primarily by young male users who outnumber female users by 2 to 1. Black and Hispanic Americans have prevalence rates of cocaine use approximately twice that of whites. Even though cocaine users who ingest cocaine by routes other than smoking are more likely to be white (47%) and male (65%), environmental factors account for the risk of cocaine use considerably more than race or ethnicity.

Certain populations are more vulnerable to cocaine-induced toxicity, primarily due to their inefficient capacity for metabolism and clearance of the drug. They include infants, elderly, fetuses, pregnant women, and patients with liver disease. Other factors that influence individual variation in susceptibility to toxicity include age, sex, body mass, hepatic and renal function, drug-drug interactions, and genetic variability. Black American users are more likely than non-black users to experience rhabdomyolysis, excited delirium, and changes in cardiac rhythm.

Gender differences in the effects of cocaine have also been observed. Men who use cocaine experience higher blood concentration levels, and women are more sensitive to the cardiovascular effects than men. Women presenting for treatment of cocaine dependence are more likely than males to be severely dependent, to abuse other drugs, to have a briefer period of abstinence, and to have childhood histories of physical or sexual abuse. Gender differences in comorbidity have also been found, with female cocaine abusers more likely to have major depression and male cocaine abusers more likely to have ASPD.

The rates of comorbid psychiatric disorders in stimulant abusers are significantly higher than community rates of depression, attention-deficit hyperactivity disorder (ADHD), and ASPDs.

3. Etiology

In order to describe the etiology of cocaine dependence, it is important to review the important genetic and sociocultural factors, learning/conditioning effects, and pharmacological factors related to this drug. The most convincing evidence to date of a genetic influence on cocaine dependence comes from studies of twins. Monozygotic twins have higher concordance rates for stimulant dependence (cocaine, amphetamines, and amphetamine-like drugs) than dizygotic twins. Analyses indicate that genetic factors and unique (unshared) environmental factors contribute about equally to the development of stimulant dependence. There are genetic risk factors with strong loadings on alcohol and drug abuse or dependence. In addition, there is evidence documenting that some of these genetic risks are disorder-specific for substance use disorders.

Common mental disorders are often correlated with each other, co-occurring at greater than chance rates in clinical and epidemiological samples. Some authors, such as Krueger, have proposed that this phenomenon may result from common mental disorders acting as reliable indicators of latent factors, or hypothetical core psychopathological processes, that underlie putatively separate disorders. A number of twin studies have begun to point to common genetic factors linking antisocial behavior and substance use disorders. One study modeled genetic and environmental contributions to latent factor linking symptoms of conduct disorder, attention-deficit hyperactivity disorder, substance experimentation (number of substances used on more than five occasions), and the personality trait of novelty seeking in 334 twin pairs aged 12 to 18 years. The majority of the variance in the latent factor (84%) was attributed to genetic factors.

Social, cultural, and economic factors are powerful determinants of initial use, continuing use, and relapse. Increased use is more likely in countries where cocaine is readily available. Learning and conditioning are also considered important in perpetuating cocaine use. Each inhalation or injection of cocaine yields a euphoric experience that reinforces the antecedent drug-taking behavior. In addition, the environmental cues associated with substance use become associated with the euphoric state so that long after a period of cessation, such cues can elicit memories of the euphoric state and reawaken craving. Lastly, cocaine can produce a sense of alertness, euphoria, and well-being. It may decrease hunger and the need for sleep, and it may improve fatigue-induced performance impaired by fatigue.

4. Diagnosis and Clinical/Medical Complications

Table 3D.7 provides the diagnostic criteria for substance dependence according to the DSM-IV-TR.

Cocaine use can have serious medical complications. These complications can be respiratory, cardiovascular, neurologic, metabolic, and psychiatric, among others. Smoking crack cocaine can lead to thermal injury of the pharynx and airways, haemoptysis, pneumothorax, pneumomediastinum, pneumopericardium, and hemothorax. The Valsalva maneuver that is used to increase the absorption and effects of the drug can lead to alveolar rupture, barotraumas, and bullous emphysema. Subacute pulmonary complications can include interstitial pneumonitis, pulmonary edema, "crack lung" (acute dyspnea and hypoxemia, with fever, hemoptysis, and respiratory failure following crack cocaine use), and bronchiolitis obliterans with organizing pneumonia.

Cocaine use is the most common cause of chest pain in young adults presenting to EDs, and it is also a common cause of MIs in people under 45 years of age. An electrocardiogram interpretation in these instances is extremely difficult and

TABLE 3D.7 Diagnostic Criteria for Substance Dependence

A person meets the criteria for substance dependence when he/she meets three of the following criteria, in the previous year:

– Tolerance (marked increase in amount; marked decrease in effect)

– Characteristic withdrawal symptoms; substance taken to relieve withdrawal

– Substance taken in larger amount and for longer periods than intended

– Persistent desire or repeated unsuccessful attempts to quit

Much time/activity to obtain, use, recover

– Important social, occupational, or recreational activities given up or reduced

– Use continues despite knowledge of adverse consequences (e.g., failure to fulfill role obligation, use when physically hazardous)

In using the DSM-IV criteria, one should specify whether substance dependence is with physiologic dependence (i.e., there is evidence of tolerance or withdrawal) or without physiologic dependence (i.e., no evidence of tolerance or withdrawal)

Adapted from American Psychiatric Association. *Diagnostic and Statistical Manual of Mental Disorders: DSM-IV-TR*. Washington, DC: American Psychiatric Association, 2000.

often ineffective in confirming MI. Enzymes such as creatine kinase and myocardial creatine kinase may well be elevated in the absence of MI, due to increased motor activity, hyperthermia, and skeletal muscle injury. Therefore, cardiac troponins are much more reliable in this respect. The cocaine-related infarction is related to coronary spasm, promotion of platelet aggregation, acceleration of atherosclerosis, and left ventricular hypertrophy, rather than thrombosis. A clear consensus exists against the use of β-blockers, which have been shown to potentiate cocaine-induced chest pain via unopposed alpha adrenergic stimulation.

This drug may also cause seizures and cerebrovascular events. The presence of a thrombotic stroke is more likely with cocaine use than with use of amphetamines, while the presence of a hemorrhagic stroke is more likely with amphetamines.

Excessive cocaine use can result in hallucinations, agitation, hyperthermia, cocaine-excited delirium (hyperthermia, sweating, agitated and paranoid behavior, which may progress to collapse, respiratory arrest, and death). Risk factors for fatal cocaine-excited delirium are Afro-Caribbean race, male gender, and administration of cocaine by smoking or injection.

5. Treatments

A. NONPHARMACOLOGICAL TREATMENTS

Behavioral treatments form the platform for any pharmacotherapy by engaging the patient and facilitating more long-term changes, including prevention of relapse. A specific behavioral approach using positive contingencies to initiate abstinence and prevent relapse has been quite successful for helping individuals who abuse cocaine. The goal of this approach is to decrease behaviors maintained by drug reinforcers and increase behaviors maintained by nondrug reinforcers. This is done by presenting rewards contingent upon documented drug abstinence (positive contingencies) and withdrawing privileges contingent upon documented drug use (negative contingencies). In a 24-week study, cocaine-dependent individuals randomized to behavioral treatment with incentives (i.e., vouchers exchangeable for goods and services or $1.00 lottery tickets after every drug-free urine test) showed greater treatment retention and longer duration of abstinence than the group not receiving incentives.

Another efficacious intervention for the treatment of stimulant abuse is CBT. One study compared CBT alone versus CBT and disulfiram, or CBT and naltrexone. Even though the subjects receiving combined treatments achieved significantly greater reductions in cocaine-positive urinalysis, CBT-treated subjects remained in treatment for a longer time.

B. PHARMACOLOGICAL TREATMENTS

In spite of the fact that more than 60 medications have been investigated for the treatment of stimulant abuse, at present there are no proven pharmacotherapies for cocaine addiction. Certain medications that modulate GABAergic, dopaminergic, and glutamatergic systems, as well as immunotherapy, have shown promise in the treatment of cocaine addiction. Among these medications, topiramate, tiagabine, baclofen, vigabatrin, modafinil, disulfiram, and methylphenidate seem to be the most promising in treatment of cocaine dependence. Propranolol may be effective especially among cocaine-addicted individuals with high withdrawal severity. The results from trials of first- and second-generation neuroleptics are largely negative. Aripiprazole, a partial dopaminergic agonist that may modulate the serotonergic system, shows some promise.

Disulfiram has an indirect action on dopamine through inhibition of the enzyme DBH, which converts dopamine to norepinephrine. The inhibition of DBH can increase dopamine release from noradrenergic nerve endings. This increase in dopaminergic stimulation can relieve a relative dopamine deficiency, which has been associated with chronic cocaine use. This relief may explain the effectiveness of disulfiram for cocaine abuse. Interestingly, it is postulated that a single nucleotide polymorphism (SNP)-1021 C > T accounts for around 50% of the variation in plasma levels of DBH. The T allele is associated with twofold to fourfold lower levels of circulating DBH. Whether this SNP is associated with clinical response to disulfiram in cocaine users is currently being examined in prospective clinical trials.

Given the high comorbidity between cocaine dependence and other psychiatric disorders, in addition to the fact that those disorders may increase the risk for drug use, an integral treatment needs to address both the stimulant addiction and the comorbid disorder. Some examples of this approach are positive trials in which the utilization of antidepressants reduced depressive symptoms, cocaine use, and craving in depressed cocaine-addicted individuals. Also, methylphenidate has been reported to be effective in subjects with comorbid cocaine use and ADHD.

In terms of preventive measures, preliminary results of human studies with anti-cocaine vaccine (which slows entry of cocaine into the brain), *N*-acetylcysteine, and ondansetron are promising, as are several other compounds in preclinical development.

6. Prognosis

There are only a few variables that have been useful in predicting outcomes for cocaine abusers. A high number of days of cocaine use in the month before treatment has been related with poor outcomes. Baseline positive urine toxicologies predict poor retention and outcome rates. On the other hand, low withdrawal severity can predict better response to GABAergic medications while high withdrawal severity can predict better response to β-blockers such as propanolol.

Comorbid depression and alcohol use should be considered risk factors for relapse, while impulsivity and similar personality traits may predict treatment response. Future studies are needed to examine biological markers as predictors of cocaine dependence outcomes, but some preliminary results suggest that stress response and brain activation to cocaine cues may serve as biological markers in the future.

7. General Formulation for Cocaine Dependence

A. DIAGNOSTIC

The disorders associated with the use of cocaine need to be distinguished from both primary mental disorders (i.e., major depressive disorder, schizophrenia paranoid type, bipolar disorder, generalized anxiety disorder, and panic attacks) and disorders induced by other classes of substances or present in the context of a general medical condition (i.e., amphetamine intoxication, phencyclidine intoxication, neuropsychiatric manifestations of systemic lupus erythematosus, etc.). A history of substance ingestion is important in making those distinctions. However, given the unreliability of self-reports, laboratory testing for drugs and collateral information are important. Patients with this disorder exhibit the criteria listed on Table 3D.1. In addition, they can present with a wide variety of symptoms/signs ranging from excessive talkativeness, decreased need for sleep sometimes associated with irritability, inappropriate optimism, euphoria, expansiveness, financial difficulties, and a drug-related legal history.

B. ETIOLOGIC

The etiology of cocaine dependence can be explained by genetic (i.e., monozygotic twins have higher concordance rates for stimulant dependence than dizygotic twins and some studies have shown heritability rates going from 0.65 to 0.79; there are genetic factors that are specific to stimulants), sociocultural (e.g., excessive use is far more likely in countries where cocaine is readily available), learning/conditioning (e.g., each inhalation or injection of cocaine yields a "rush" and a euphoric experience that reinforce the antecedent drug-taking behavior), and pharmacological factors (e.g., cocaine can produce a sense of alertness, euphoria, well-being; it may decrease hunger and the need for sleep, as well as improve performance impaired by fatigue).

C. THERAPEUTIC

There are behavioral and pharmacological treatments for the treatment of cocaine dependence that have been studied in several trials and have provided some positive outcomes. Behavioral treatments form the platform for any pharmacotherapy by engaging patients and facilitating more long-term changes, including prevention of relapse. Some of these treatments include using positive contingencies for negative urine toxicology screenings, decreasing behavior maintained by drug reinforcers, and increasing behavior maintained by nondrug reinforcers. Another efficacious intervention for the treatment of stimulant abuse is CBT, which has been shown to retain the patients in treatment for a longer time.

Among the pharmacological treatments, more than 60 medications have been investigated for the treatment of stimulant abuse, but there are no proven pharmacotherapies for cocaine. Medications such as topiramate, tiagabine, baclofen, vigabatrin, modafinil, disulfiram, and methylphenidate seem to be the most promising in the treatment of cocaine dependence. Preliminary results of human studies with anti-cocaine vaccine (which slows entry of cocaine into the brain) are promising.

D. PROGNOSTIC

The following factors are important in the prognosis of cocaine dependence: gender (women with this condition have shown more severity on the medical, psychiatric, social, and employment areas), level of education and employment status (lower level of education and unemployment have been associated with poorer treatment retention), concurrent use of alcohol (this comorbidity has been associated with more lethality than cocaine alone) and ASPD (which has been related with poor treatment retention and continued cocaine abuse).

8. Risk Assessment

Risk assessment in cocaine dependence should include the risk for medical complications (e.g., barotraumas, pulmonary edema, MIs, hyperthermia, seizures, and cerebrovascular events) and psychiatric complications (e.g., hallucinations, agitation, cocaine–excited delirium with agitation and paranoid behavior, suicidality during the withdrawal, and homicidal behaviors).

KEY POINTS (ABPN Examination)

A. When interviewing a patient with cocaine dependence

1. Patients can present with paranoia, agitation, and mood lability, which can be easily mistaken for a mood disorder.
2. Do not forget to make a thorough assessment of safety, including suicidal ideations (more likely during the initial stage of the withdrawal).
3. Inquire about common complications of cocaine use, such as myocardial infarction, cerebrovascular events, HIV/AIDS, seizures, psychosis, and excited delirium.
4. Gather demographic information that will facilitate the case formulation (e.g., gender, level of education, and employment status)
5. Do not forget to ask about any history of other substance abuse problems, which could alter the prognosis (e.g., alcohol), as well as other comorbid psychiatric conditions (e.g., ASPD), which are common among this population.
6. Take into account the route of administration and its implications on severity of dependence (e.g., intravenous and inhaled forms of administration are more likely to lead to dependence than the snorted one).

B. When presenting a patient with cocaine dependence

1. Acknowledge the importance of differentiating between a primary psychiatric disorder (e.g., mood or psychotic disorder) vs. a substance-induced disorder. This can be facilitated by recommending following up on patient's condition 4 weeks after his/her last day of drug use.
2. Acknowledge that the diagnosis of a personality disorder cannot be made during an acute crisis, unless there is clear evidence of a more pervasive and long- standing behavioral pattern.
3. If diagnosis is unclear, state that you would use a structured diagnostic interview like SCID-DSM-IV for clarification.

Suggested Readings

Angarita G, Reif S, Pirard S, et al. No-show for treatment in substance abuse patients with comorbid symptomatology: Validity results from a controlled trial of the ASAM patient placement criteria. *J Addict Med* 2007;1: 79–87.

Arendt G, de Nocker D, von Giesen HJ, et al. Neuropsychiatric side effects of efavirenz therapy. *Expert Opin Drug Saf* 2007;6:147–154.

Brownlow HA, Pappachan J. Pathophysiology of cocaine abuse. *Eur J Anaesthesiol* 2002;19:395–414.

Carroll KM, Fenton LR, Ball SA, et al. Efficacy of disulfiram and cognitive behavior therapy in cocaine-dependent outpatients: A randomized placebo-controlled trial. *Arch Gen Psychiatry* 2004;61:264–272.

Carroll KM, Nich C, Ball SA, et al. Treatment of cocaine and alcohol dependence with psychotherapy and disulfiram. *Addiction* 1998;93: 713–727.

Cook JA, Burke-Miller JK, Cohen MH, et al. Crack cocaine, disease progression, and mortality in a multicenter cohort of HIV-1 positive women. *AIDS* 2008;22:1355–1363.

Cornish JW, O'Brien CP. Crack cocaine abuse: An epidemic with many public health consequences. *Ann Rev Public Health* 1996;17:259–273.

Cubells JF, Kranzler HR, McCance-Katz E, et al. A haplotype at the DBH locus, associated with low plasma dopamine beta-hydroxylase activity, also associates with cocaine-induced paranoia. *Mol Psychiatry* 2000;5:56–63.

Dackis CA, Kampman KM, Lynch KG, et al. A double-blind, placebo-controlled trial of modafinil for cocaine dependence. *Neuropsychopharmacology* 2005;1:205–211.

Dackis CA, Lynch KG, Yu E, et al. Modafinil and cocaine: A double-blind, placebo-controlled drug interaction study. *Drug Alcohol Depend* 2003;70:29–37.

Devlin RJ, Henry JA. Clinical review: Major consequences of illicit drug consumption. *Crit Care* 2008;12:202.

Dickerson TJ, Janda KD. Recent advances for the treatment of cocaine abuse: Central nervous system immunopharmacotherapy. *AAPS J* 2005;7:E579–E586.

Dutra L, Stathopoulou G, Basden SL, et al. A meta-analytic review of psychosocial interventions for substance use disorders. *Am J Psychiatry* 2008;165:179–187.

Ebert M, Loosen P. *Current Diagnosis & Treatment Psychiatry*: New York: McGraw Hill, 2008.

Forrester JM, Steele AW, Waldron JA, et al. Crack lung: An acute pulmonary syndrome with a spectrum of clinical and histopathologic findings. *Am Rev Respir Dis* 1990;142:462–467.

Galanter M, Kleber HD. *The American Psychiatric Publishing Textbook of Substance Abuse Treatment*. Washington, DC: American Psychiatric Publishing, Inc., 2004.

Galanter M, Kleber HD. *The American Psychiatric Publishing Textbook of Substance Abuse Treatment*. Washington, DC: American Psychiatric Publishing, Inc., 2008.

Gelernter J, Panhuysen C, Weiss R, et al. Genomewide linkage scan for cocaine dependence and related traits: Significant linkages for a cocaine-related trait and cocaine-induced paranoia. *Am J Med Genet B Neuropsychiatr Genet* 2005;136B:45–52.

Grassi MC, Cioce AM, Giudici FD, et al. Short-term efficacy of disulfiram or naltrexone in reducing positive urinalysis for both cocaine and cocaethylene in cocaine abusers: A pilot study. *Pharmacol Res* 2007;55:117–121.

Higgins ST, Budney AJ, Bickel WK, et al. Incentives improve outcome in outpatient behavioral treatment of cocaine dependence. *Arch Gen Psychiatry* 1994;51:568–576.

Hollander JE. The management of cocaine-associated myocardial ischemia. *N Engl J Med* 1995;333:1267–1272.

Howington JU, Kutz SC, Wilding GE, et al. Cocaine use as a predictor of outcome in aneurysmal subarachnoid hemorrhage. *J Neurosurg* 2003;99:271–275.

Kalayasiri R, Sughondhabirom A, Gueorguieva R, et al. Dopamine beta-hydroxylase gene (DbetaH) -1021C–>T influences self-reported paranoia during cocaine self-administration. *Biol Psychiatry* 2007;61:1310–1313.

Karila L, Gorelick D, Weinstein A, et al. New treatments for cocaine dependence: A focused review. *Int J Neuropsychopharmacol* 2008;11:425–438.

Karila L, Weinstein A, Benyamina A, et al. Current pharmacotherapies and immunotherapy in cocaine addiction. *Presse Med* 2008;37:689–698.

Kendler KS, Karkowski LM, Neale MC, et al. Illicit psychoactive substance use, heavy use, abuse, and dependence in a US population-based sample of male twins. *Arch Gen Psychiatry* 2000;57:261–269.

Kendler KS, Prescott CA. Cocaine use, abuse and dependence in a population-based sample of female twins. *Br J Psychiatry* 1998;173:345–350.

Kendler KS, Prescott CA, Myers J, et al. The structure of genetic and environmental risk factors for common psychiatric and substance use disorders in men and women. *Arch Gen Psychiatry* 2003;60:929–937.

Khantzian EJ, Gawin F, Kleber HD, et al. Methylphenidate (Ritalin) treatment of cocaine dependence—a preliminary report. *J Subst Abuse Treat* 1984;1:107–112.

Koe BK. Molecular geometry of inhibitors of the uptake of catecholamines and serotonin in synaptosomal preparations of rat brain. *J Pharmacol Exp Ther* 1976;199:649–661.

Koob GF, Caine SB, Parsons L, et al. Opponent process model and psychostimulant addiction. *Pharmacol Biochem Behav* 1997;57:513–521.

Krueger RF, Hicks BM, Patrick CJ, et al. Etiologic connections among substance dependence, antisocial behavior, and personality: Modeling the externalizing spectrum. *J Abnorm Psychol* 2002;111:411–424.

Lange RA, Cigarroa RG, Yancy CW Jr, et al. Cocaine-induced coronary-artery vasoconstriction. *N Engl J Med* 1989;321:1557–1562.

Leal J, Ziedonis D, Kosten T. Antisocial personality disorder as a prognostic factor for pharmacotherapy of cocaine dependence. *Drug Alcohol Depend* 1994;35:31–35.

Malison RT, Best SE, van Dyck CH, et al. Elevated striatal dopamine transporters during acute cocaine abstinence as measured by [^{123}I] beta-CIT SPECT. *Am J Psychiatry* 1998;155: 832–834.

Maurer HH, Sauer C, Theobald DS. Toxicokinetics of drugs of abuse: Current knowledge of the isoenzymes involved in the human metabolism of tetrahydrocannabinol, cocaine, heroin, morphine, and codeine. *Ther Drug Monit* 2006;28:447–453.

Najavits LM, Lester KM. Gender differences in cocaine dependence. *Drug Alcohol Depend* 2008;97:190–194.

Nelson EC, Heath AC, Lynskey MT, et al. Childhood sexual abuse and risks for licit and illicit drug-related outcomes: a twin study. *Psychol Med* 2006;36:1473–1483.

NIDA. NIDA InfoFacts: Methamphetamine. Last accessed March 27, 2008.

O'Brien MS, Anthony JC. Risk of becoming cocaine dependent: Epidemiological estimates for the United States, 2000–2001. 2005;30:1006–1018.

Pap A, Bradberry CW. Excitatory amino acid antagonists attenuate the effects of cocaine on extracellular dopamine in the nucleus accumbens. *J Pharmacol Exp Ther* 1995;274:127–133.

Pennings EJ, Leccese AP, Wolff FA. Effects of concurrent use of alcohol and cocaine. *Addiction* 2002;97:773–783.

Petrakis IL, Carroll KM, Nich C, et al. Disulfiram treatment for cocaine dependence in methadone-maintained opioid addicts. *Addiction* 2000;95:219–228.

Poling J, Kosten TR, Sofuoglu M. Treatment outcome predictors for cocaine dependence. *Am J Drug Alcohol Abuse* 2007;33:191–206.

Prakash A, Das G. Cocaine and the nervous system. *Int J Clin Pharmacol Ther Toxicol* 1993;31:575–581.

Preti A. New developments in the pharmacotherapy of cocaine abuse. *Addict Biol* 2007;12:133–151.

Ritz MC, Lamb RJ, Goldberg SR, et al. Cocaine receptors on dopamine transporters are related to self-administration of cocaine. *Science* 1987;237:1219–1223.

Roberts DC, Andrews MM, Vickers GJ. Baclofen attenuates the reinforcing effects of cocaine in rats. *Neuropsychopharmacology* 1996;15: 417–423.

Rothman RB, Baumann MH. Therapeutic potential of monoamine transporter substrates. *Current Top Med Chem* 2006;6:1845–1859.

Rounsaville BJ, Anton SF, Carroll K, et al. Psychiatric diagnoses of treatment-seeking cocaine abusers. *Arch Gen Psychiatry* 1991;48:43–51.

Ruttenber AJ, Lawler-Heavner J, Yin M, et al. Fatal excited delirium following cocaine use: epidemiologic findings provide new evidence for mechanisms of cocaine toxicity. *J Forensic Sci* 1997;42:25–31.

Sadock BS, Sadock VA. *Kaplan & Sadock's Synopsis of Psychiatry*. 10th Ed. Philadelphia, PA: Lippincott Williams & Wilkins, 2007.

SAMHSA. National Survey on Drug Use and Health, 2008.

Sinha R, Garcia M, Paliwal P, et al. Stress-induced cocaine craving and hypothalamic-pituitary-adrenal responses are predictive of cocaine relapse outcomes. *Arch Gen Psychiatry* 2006;63: 324–331.

Siqueland L, Crits-Christoph P, Gallop R, et al. Retention in psychosocial treatment of cocaine dependence: predictors and impact on outcome. *Am J Addict* 2002;11:24–40.

Sofuoglu M, Kosten TR. Emerging pharmacological strategies in the fight against cocaine addiction. *Expert Opin Emerg Drugs* 2006;11:91–98.

Tsuang MT, Lyons MJ, Eisen SA, et al. Genetic influences on DSM-III-R drug abuse and dependence: a study of 3,372 twin pairs. *Am J Med Gen* 1996;67:473–477.

Volkow ND, Fowler JS, Gatley SJ, et al. PET evaluation of the dopamine system of the human brain. *J Nucl Med* 1996;37:1242–1256.

Volkow ND, Wang GJ, Fischman MW, et al. Relationship between subjective effects of cocaine and dopamine transporter occupancy. *Nature* 1997;386:827–830.

Weinstock J, Alessi SM, Petry NM. Regardless of psychiatric severity the addition of contingency management to standard treatment improves retention and drug use outcomes. *Drug Alcohol Depend*. 2007;87:288–296.

Withers NW, Pulvirenti L, Koob GF, et al. Cocaine abuse and dependence. *J Clin Psychopharmacol* 1995;15:63–78.

Young SE, Stallings MC, Corley RP, et al. Genetic and environmental influences on behavioral disinhibition. *Am J Med Genet* 2000;96:684–695.

Ziedonis DM, Kosten TR. Depression as a prognostic factor for pharmacological treatment of cocaine dependence. *Psychopharmacol Bull* 1991;27: 337–343.

E. Cognitive disorders

Gauri P. Khatkhate, MD, Kirsten M. Wilkins, MD

I. DEMENTIA

CASE HISTORY

PRESENT ILLNESS

Mr S is an 86-year-old widowed white male brought to the geropsychiatry clinic by his son for evaluation of Mr S's "memory problems." The son states that he first noticed these changes about a year ago, when his father would occasionally forget to pay bills or have trouble keeping appointments. Over the last few months, these lapses became more frequent, to the point where Mr S's son took over the management of his father's finances, and his daughter started filling pillboxes weekly with medications and taking him to doctor's visits. The son also notes that his father now tends to forget recent conversations and seems to have trouble finding the right words. Mr S has hired a maid to help with the household chores and upkeep since the death of his wife 4 years ago. He is able to care for his own grooming and hygiene, and continues to drive and do some basic shopping. Per his son, Mr S seems to enjoy family gatherings, but has gradually stopped other activities, such as visiting the senior center and playing cards with his friends. The family has not noticed Mr S to be particularly sad, but at times he seems disinterested, has been losing weight, and complains that he does not sleep well. They have not noticed any paranoia, hallucinations, or behavioral problems. Today's visit was prompted by an episode a few weeks ago in which Mr S got lost driving to his local grocery store, was found by police miles away and confused, and was escorted home. Since then, the family has been increasingly concerned about Mr S's ability to drive and to live independently, so they brought him in for an evaluation.

On the interview, Mr S states that he is not sure why he is there. He agrees that he has "a little" trouble with his memory, but does not consider it a serious problem and is not bothered by it. He reports that his mood is "fine" and denies having any thoughts of harming himself, though he does sometimes wish he were in heaven with his wife. Mr S endorses difficulty sleeping through the night, but notes that he naps frequently during the day. He looks forward to seeing his family on weekends, and spends his days reading the paper and watching television. He denies feeling anxious or suspicious, and denies any auditory or visual hallucinations.

PSYCHIATRIC HISTORY

Mr S had no history of psychiatric problems till 3 years ago, about a year after the death of his wife. At that time, he began experiencing sadness, crying spells, low appetite, anergia, and hopelessness. He lost interest in all activities, and rarely left the house. He began expressing vague suicidal ideation. Mr S was placed on citalopram 20 mg by his PCP, and 2 months later his acute depressive symptoms had resolved. The citalopram was tapered off last year. Mr S has no history of suicide attempts. He currently drinks an occasional glass of wine, but has no history of alcohol or illicit drug abuse. He has a 40-pack year smoking history, but quit over 20 years ago.

FAMILY HISTORY

Mr S's father had dementia and died at the age of 90. His daughter was treated for depression in her 50s. There is no other family history of psychiatric illness.

SOCIAL HISTORY

Mr S was born and raised in Pittsburgh, PA. He graduated high school and joined the Army, where he served in World War II (WWII). He had some combat experience, but rarely speaks of it. After the war, Mr S went to college and graduated with a degree in accounting. He worked in this field for many years, and eventually ran his own business. Mr S married at the age of 24 and had 2 children, a son and a daughter. He has three grandchildren and seven great grandchildren. Several family members, including his son and daughter, live nearby and are helpful. Mr S retired at the age of 66, and spent the next few years traveling widely with his wife. His wife died four years ago after 58 years of marriage. Mr S lived alone after this in the same house, but 8 months ago moved into a condominium in a different neighborhood to be closer to his children.

PERTINENT MEDICAL HISTORY

Hypertension, hyperlipidemia, Benign Prostatic Hypertrophy (BPH), and cataracts. He takes Atenolol, Simvastatin, Terazosin, aspirin (ASA), and multivitamins on a daily basis.

MENTAL STATUS EXAMINATION

Mr S presented as an elderly white male who appears his stated age. He is casually dressed and well groomed, makes fair eye contact, and is pleasant and cooperative. He has a mild bilateral postural tremor, no rigidity, and a gait that is somewhat slowed but otherwise normal. His speech is notable for paucity of content and word finding difficulty. His mood was reported as "fine," and his affect is euthymic but superficial and constricted in range. Thought process is circumstantial. Mr S denies any suicidal or homicidal ideation, intent, or plans and has no evident delusions. He denies auditory and visual hallucinations. His insight is impaired; he is unable to accurately report his recent memory problems and the change in his ability to function independently. His judgment is fair. On the Folstein Mini-Mental State Examination (MMSE), he scored 18/30 indicating a moderate level of impairment. He scored 5/10 points on orientation, 3/3 on registration, 2/5 on serial 7s, 1/3 on delayed recall, 0/1 on repetition, 2/2 on naming, 3/3 on 3-step command, 1/1 on reading, 1/1 on writing, and 0/1 on copying intersecting pentagons.

PERTINENT PHYSICAL FINDINGS

His vital signs were a temperature of 98.2°F, heart rate of 64 per minute, blood pressure of 140/90 mm Hg, and respiratory rate of 16 per minute. Oxygen saturation on room air was 97.0%. His pupils were somewhat small with evidence of clouding from cataracts. The extraocular muscles were intact, sclerae were anicteric, and mucous membranes were moist. There was no lymphadenopathy or thyromegaly. The first and second heart sounds were heard, and there was no murmur. Carotid bruit was heard on the left side. The lungs were clear bilaterally. The abdomen was soft and nontender with normal bowel sounds and no organomegaly. The peripheral pulses were intact. The neurological examination was notable for symmetrically hypoactive reflexes, decreased sensation in the bilateral lower extremities, and equivocal Babinski.

LABORATORY DATA

Complete blood count (CBC), electrolytes, blood urea nitrogen (BUN), creatinine, fasting glucose, and thyroid stimulating hormone (TSH) were within normal limits. Rapid plasma reagin (RPR) was nonreactive. The B_{12} levels were mildly decreased, and the folate levels were normal.

COURSE OF ILLNESS

Following his initial evaluation, Mr S was started on donepezil 5 mg, which he tolerated well. At 1 month follow-up, the dose was increased to 10 mg, and memantine was later added and titrated to 10 mg b.i.d. Over the next year, Mr S continued to live independently in his condo, though the family began coming in more often. After much coaxing, Mr S agreed to stop driving, and his children took him on shopping trips and outings. His MMSE score remained essentially stable over this period, as did his level of function. Gradually, Mr S's memory and function began to decline, and he needed increasing help with day-to-day activities. After an episode in which Mr S left the stove on while making coffee, setting off the fire alarm in his building, Mr S's children decided that it was no longer safe for him to live alone. Mr S moved in with his daughter and her husband. He began waking up at night and wandering about the house, disrupting the sleep of other family members. He was prescribed 50 mg of trazodone, and his sleep improved. About 3 years after his initial evaluation, Mr S's daughter brought him to clinic reporting that he was having periods of agitation and aggression, and was accusing family members of stealing from him. Mr S showed some improvement with 0.5 mg b.i.d. of risperidone, but the behaviors did not fully resolve. Eventually, Mr S required significant assistance with such activities as bathing and toileting, and his daughter no longer felt able to care for him at home. Mr S was admitted to a nursing home, and his cognition continued to decline. Ultimately, he needed help for all his basic activities of daily living, and became essentially mute. He stopped eating and drinking adequately but did not appear to be in any physical distress, and the family decided against invasive interventions. Mr S passed away of likely respiratory failure at the age of 92, 6 years after his initial diagnosis.

DISCHARGE MEDICATIONS

Donepezil, 5 mg PO daily; memantine 10 mg PO b.i.d.; risperidone 0.5 mg PO b.i.d.

DSM-IV-TR MULTIAXIAL DIAGNOSIS (AT INITIAL EVALUATION)

Axis I. Dementia of the Alzheimer's type, with late onset, without behavioral disturbance

Major depressive disorder, single, severe, in remission

Axis II. None

Axis III. Hypertension, hyperlipidemia, BPH, cataracts

Axis IV. Severity of psychosocial stressors: moderate—widowed, living alone

Axis V. Global assessment of functioning: 40—major impairment in several areas such as work, judgment, thinking

FORMULATION

A. Diagnostic

Mr S meets DSM-IV-TR criteria for dementia. At this initial evaluation, he has the requisite memory impairment, as evidenced by his forgetfulness. He also has impairment in other cognitive domains such as aphasia, seen in his word finding difficulty, and executive dysfunction. By the time of presentation, these deficits are impairing his functioning to the point that he needs family assistance with finances, medications, and keeping appointments. The deficits are a decline from a previously higher level of functioning, when Mr S was an accountant running his own business. Per the family report, Mr S's course has been gradual and progressive, which is required for the diagnosis of dementia of the Alzheimer's type. There is nothing in his presentation to suggest delirium, and he does not seem to be experiencing another acute Axis I condition. Based on his clinical history, physical examination, and laboratory data, another illness causing memory impairments seems less likely.

Though Mr S's case seems most consistent with Alzheimer's, there are several other conditions that need to be considered and ruled out. First, Mr S has several risk factors and physical findings for vascular disease, thus raising the possibility of vascular dementia (VaD). In order to make this diagnosis, Mr S would need either focal neurological findings, which are not present, or laboratory evidence of cerebrovascular disease such as infarctions on head computerized tomography (CT) or magnetic resonance imaging (MRI). Dementia with Lewy bodies (DLB) is another consideration given Mr S's gradual onset and continuing decline, but is less likely given the absence of the core features of this illness—fluctuating cognition, visual hallucinations, and parkinsonian symptoms. Mr S does not have the early personality changes that would indicate frontotemporal dementia (FTD), and does not have physical or laboratory findings suggestive of other causes of dementia such as normal pressure hydrocephalus or hypothyroidism. When evaluating an elderly patient for memory changes, normal aging or mild cognitive impairment (MCI) are also considerations, but Mr S's impairments are clearly more severe. An important diagnostic consideration to keep in mind for

Mr S is depression. Though his current symptoms of weight loss, sleep changes, and decreased social activity may be related to aging or to his dementia, they could also be indicative of residual depressive symptoms and this needs to be assessed further, as depression can alter performance on cognitive testing and decrease quality of life.

B. Etiologic

Mr S has several risk factors that predispose him to dementia. The most important of these is his advanced age, especially age over 85. Mr S also has a first-degree relative who had dementia, which increases his risk of developing the illness. Though he is not likely to have pure VaD, Mr S's vascular risk factors increase his risk of a cerebrovascular event, which can worsen Alzheimer's symptoms. While it is difficult to talk of precipitating events in Alzheimer's disease, it is possible that the change of environment when he moved into a new home and neighborhood helped to uncover and heighten Mr S's cognitive deficits.

C. Therapeutic

The medical treatments for the cognitive deficits in dementia are cholinesterase inhibitors and memantine. There is evidence that memantine in combination with donepezil is better than donepezil alone. Mr S, during the course of his treatment, was placed on both agents. His cognition stayed stable for nearly a year and then declined after that, which is consistent with the important but limited benefits these drugs provide. Mr S also developed delusions and behavioral disturbances during his illness. These can be treated with medication, including antidepressants, anticonvulsants, and antipsychotics, though there is no FDA-approved treatment for these distressing symptoms. In Mr S's case, trazodone and risperidone provided some benefit. Other nonpharmacological interventions might have been helpful as well, including a calm and consistent environment, an effort to understand and address the source of the behaviors, and redirection of attention. Keeping Mr S's vascular risk factors such as hypertension and hyperlipidemia under good control would also have been important in order to prevent the additive effects of a cerebrovascular insult.

D. Prognostic

The progression of Alzheimer's disease is inexorable, but factors such as older age, delirium, falls, concurrent physical illness, and behavioral disturbances can hasten the course.

DEMENTIA

1. Introduction

Dementia is not a single entity, but rather a syndrome characterized, as per the DSM-IV-TR criteria, by impairment in memory and at least one other cognitive domain. These include aphasia (language disturbance), apraxia (impaired ability to carry out motor activities despite intact motor function), agnosia (inability to identify objects despite intact sensory function), and executive dysfunction (impairment in planning, organizing, sequencing, abstracting). The impairments must represent a change from a previous level of functioning, cause significant social or occupational impairment, and cannot occur exclusively during an episode of delirium. There are a number of specific diseases that cause dementia via a loss of neurons or structural brain damage. These specific dementias have differences in clinical presentations and physical findings that help distinguish them from one another. Dementia is a devastating illness that affects millions of people, and the number of cases is expected to rise dramatically as the population ages. As dementia progresses, patients require increasing help and supervision, and the course is often complicated by behavioral disturbances such as wandering, agitation, sleep disruption, and paranoia. Caring for a patient with dementia places an enormous financial, physical, and emotional burden on the caregiver, and the evaluation and treatment of the patient with dementia must include assistance, education, and support for the caregiver as well.

2. Epidemiology

The prevalence of dementia is estimated to be approximately 3% to 11% among community dwelling elderly over the age of 65. Age is the strongest risk factor for dementia, and prevalence rises to 20% to 50% in those older than 85. Alzheimer's disease is the most common form of dementia, accounting for over 60% of cases. According to a report from the Alzheimer's Association, an estimated 5.2 million Americans had Alzheimer's disease in 2008. This number is expected to increase dramatically as the population ages. VaD is the second most common type of dementia, accounting for 5% to 20% of cases. Other forms of dementia, including Lewy body dementia and FTD, account for the rest.

3. Etiology

There are multiple possible causes of dementia, and this brief review will focus on a few of the more commonly seen types.

A. DEMENTIA OF THE ALZHEIMER'S TYPE

Though a definitive diagnosis of Alzheimer's Dementia (AD) can only be made at autopsy, a clinical presentation of gradual onset of cognitive deficits and continuing cognitive decline is most characteristic of AD and is included in the DSM-IV-TR criteria for the diagnosis. AD generally begins with difficulty with recent memory that worsens over time. Eventually, deficits in other cognitive domains become apparent. A fluent aphasia often manifests as trouble with naming and word finding. Apraxia may lead to problems with dressing or feeding oneself. Personality changes may occur including apathy and irritability, and patients may also develop behavioral disturbances such as agitation, psychosis, and wandering (Table 3E.1).

Gross pathological findings in AD include cortical atrophy and enlargement of the ventricles. On a histological level, B-amyloid plaques and neurofibrillary tangles are classic findings, though it is important to note that these may also be present in other conditions and in normal aging. B-amyloid is derived from the cleavage of amyloid precursor protein (APP), and accumulates in the brain, surrounded by abnormal axons and dendrites, to form the extracellular plaques seen in AD. Neurofibrillary tangles are intracellular filaments composed of abnormally phosphorylated tau protein, and their density correlates with the severity of the dementia. A characteristic feature of AD is the loss of presynaptic cholinergic neurons in the basal nucleus of Meynert, resulting in a decrease in cerebral cholinergic activity.

TABLE 3E.1 Diagnostic Criteria for Dementia of the Alzheimer's Type

A. The development of multiple cognitive deficits manifested by both (1) memory impairment (impaired ability to learn new information or to recall previously learned information) (2) one (or more) of the following cognitive disturbances: (a) aphasia (language disturbance) (b) apraxia (impaired ability to carry out motor activities despite intact motor function) (c) agnosia (failure to recognize or identify objects despite intact sensory function) (d) disturbance in executive functioning (i.e., planning, organizing, sequencing, abstracting)
B. The cognitive deficits in Criteria A1 and A2 each cause significant impairment in social or occupational functioning and represent a significant decline from a previous level of functioning.
C. The course is characterized by gradual onset and continuing cognitive decline.
D. The cognitive deficits in criteria A1 and A2 are not due to any of the following: (1) other central nervous system conditions that cause progressive deficits in memory and cognition (e.g., cerebrovascular disease, Parkinson's disease, Huntington's disease, subdural hematoma, normal-pressure hydrocephalus, brain tumor) (2) systemic conditions that are known to cause dementia (e.g., hypothyroidism, vitamin B_{12} or folic acid deficiency, niacin deficiency, hypercalcemia, neurosyphillis, HIV infection) (3) substance-induced conditions
E. The deficits do not occur exclusively during the course of a delirium.
F. The disturbance is not better accounted for by another Axis I disorder (e.g., major depressive disorder, schizophrenia).

Adapted from American Psychiatric Association. *Diagnostic and Statistical Manual of Mental Disorders: DSM-IV-TR*. American Psychiatric Association, 2000.

There have been many risk factors proposed for the development of AD including age, apolipoprotein E (ApoE) status, and family history. Advanced age is the strongest risk factor. *ApoE*, a cholesterol-carrying protein that binds to B-amyloid is coded by a gene with three alleles, E2, E3, and E4. Having two E4 alleles significantly increases the risk of developing AD, as does having one E4 allele, though to a lesser extent. However, E4 is neither necessary nor sufficient for the development of AD, and routine genetic testing is not recommended. Family history also plays a role; having a first-degree relative with AD increases risk by fourfold over the general population. Some cases of AD show a clear familial pattern with autosomal dominant inheritance, a younger age of onset, and a more rapid course. Chromosome 14, which contains the presenilin I gene, chromosome 19, which contains the gene for ApoE, and chromosome 1, which contains the gene for presenilin II, have all been implicated in this familial form. A mutation on chromosome 21, which codes for APP, has also been implicated. It is noteworthy that a majority of patients with Down's syndrome develop an Alzheimer's like dementia by age 40.

B. VASCULAR DEMENTIA

VaD is the second most common form of dementia, and is diagnosed, per DSM-IV-TR, when an individual meets the general criteria for dementia (impairment in memory and at least one other cognitive domain, decline in function and social and occupational impairment) and also has focal neurological signs and symptoms or laboratory evidence of cerebrovascular disease. The clinical presentation of VaD differs from AD in that onset may be more sudden with subsequent stepwise decline if further vascular events occur. In practice, however, this stepwise progression is less common and patients have a more gradually progressive course as in AD. The deficits in VaD tend to be patchy, depending on the location of the vascular insult, rather than following a relatively predictable sequence. Memory may be only mildly affected, whereas there is a more early and severe decline in executive function. Patients are more likely to have aphasia and gait disturbance. Medical history may reveal strokes, transient ischemic attacks, or vascular risk factors such as hypertension. Other systemic illnesses that can cause cerebrovascular disease and lead to VaD include atherosclerosis, diabetes, hyperlipidemia, cardiac embolism, autoimmune and infectious vasculitis, and vasculopathies.

VaD may be caused by lesions that are hemorrhagic, ischemic, or both, and can be related to large- or small-vessel disease. Risk factors for the development of VaD include older age, lower educational and income level, lower blood pressure or orthostatic hypotension, larger lesions, recurrent strokes, and left hemispheric stroke. The assessment for VaD must include tests that measure executive function, such as the clock-drawing task, the Executive Interview, and the Trail-Making Test. Physical examination may reveal neurological findings such as hyperreflexia, extensor plantar reflex, and focal motor or sensory deficits. Neuroimaging with CT or MRI may show vascular lesions. Oftentimes, VaD is not pure but seen in combination with AD, the so-called "mixed" dementia. In these cases, infarcts as well as plaques and tangles may be seen.

C. DEMENTIA WITH LEWY BODIES

DLB, sometimes considered a variant of AD, may account for 10% of all dementia cases, and up to 30% of cases diagnosed as AD. Like AD, DLB shows progressive cognitive decline. However, fluctuating cognition, visual hallucinations, and parkinsonism are unique features. Patients may present with recurrent episodes of confusion with variable attention and alertness in the context of gradually worsening cognitive deficits. Visual hallucinations are relatively common and tend to be well formed and detailed. Patients also may have parkinsonian symptoms such as rigidity, bradykinesia, gait impairment, and postural instability. These symptoms are less responsive to L-dopa than they are in patients with Parkinson's disease. Neuropsychiatric symptoms, including visual hallucinations, delusions, apathy, and anxiety may appear early in the course.

DLB must be distinguished from the dementia that develops in 20% to 40% of patients with Parkinson's disease. This is generally accomplished by looking at the time course of the onset of the cognitive symptoms in relation to the parkinsonian ones. A proposed rough guideline is that if dementia and motor symptoms develop within a year of each other, then DLB is more likely, whereas if dementia develops more than a year after the motor symptoms, then the patient may have Parkinson's disease with dementia. The Lewy bodies from which DLB gets its name are cytoplasmic inclusions composed of alpha-synuclein, a normal synaptic protein that accumulates in an insoluble form. In Parkinson's disease, these Lewy bodies are present in the substantia nigra, whereas they are also seen in limbic and neocortical areas in DLB, and their concentration may correlate with the dementia. In addition to Lewy bodies, plaques and tangles are also seen in DLB.

D. FRONTOTEMPORAL DEMENTIA

The term FTD refers to a group of neuropsychiatric diseases characterized by progressive dementia with memory loss, executive dysfunction, and changes in personality and behavior. The executive dysfunction and personality changes can manifest as poor judgment, impulsivity, perseveration, apathy, aggression, disinhibition, hyperorality, compulsive behaviors, and inappropriate social behavior. These symptoms occur early in the course, when memory is only mildly impaired, and may be the presenting complaint. Pick's disease refers to similar presentations in which argentophilic inclusions ("Pick bodies") are found in neurons. Another group of FTD disorders, including primary progressive aphasia, presents with disruption of language as its primary feature. FTD may account for approximately 15% of dementia cases. These disorders may develop sporadically, though they often are seen in families. The age of onset is younger than for other dementias, generally between 35 and 75, and rarely seen after that. On imaging, frontal and anterior temporal atrophy may be evident. Abnormal tau protein has been implicated, and FTD has been linked to chromosome 17.

4. Diagnosis

As in most other aspects of medicine, a good history is the key to the diagnosis of dementia. History should be obtained not only from the patient but also from the family members or other reliable sources of collateral information. The time course and nature of the patient's deficits and physical examination findings, as noted above, can help to make a diagnosis of dementia and also to differentiate the most likely etiology. When taking a history, it is also important to ask about changes in function, safety issues, and changes in behavior and personality, as these all play an important role in the evaluation and treatment of the patient with dementia. Changes in function may begin as a gradual loss of the ability to manage household tasks and finances, and progress to difficulties with self-care tasks such as bathing, dressing, toileting, and feeding. Understanding a patient's functional status is a way to monitor the progression of the illness and allows the thorough assessment of the patient's and family's needs and referral to appropriate resources. As a patient's functional capacity changes, safety issues also arise and must be investigated. Patients and their families should be asked about driving ability, fire risks such as leaving a stove or other appliance on and unattended, and wandering and getting lost. Personality and behavior changes are among the most distressing symptoms for the families. These may include apathy, impulsivity and disinhibition, agitation, aggression, changes in the sleep-wake cycle, and psychotic symptoms such as paranoia and hallucinations. Patients with dementia should also be assessed for depression, as depression is common early in the course of dementia and is especially prominent in VaD.

While a thorough history is most important in the diagnosis of dementia, other tools contribute as well. The MMSE is commonly used to detect impairment, establish a baseline, and follow change over time. A score of less than 24 has generally been accepted as abnormal, though it may be more useful to use ranges or values that have been corrected for age and education. While valuable and widely accepted, the MMSE has its limitations. For example, patients with high levels of education may score within the normal range despite problems, and the MMSE cannot measure progression in severe dementia or detect executive dysfunction. In cases where the diagnosis is unclear, neuropsychological testing may be helpful but it is not part of the routine diagnostic workup.

Physical examination findings can also be helpful in the evaluation of dementia. In AD, the examination will most likely be normal, or primitive reflexes such as the glabellar, grasp, and snout reflexes may be evident. The examination in VaD may reveal focal neurological findings or physical evidence of vascular disease. Lewy body dementia is notable for tremor, rigidity, or gait disturbance. Normal pressure hydrocephalus, an uncommon but potentially reversible cause of dementia, presents with a classic triad of memory impairment, gait disturbance, and incontinence. Cognitive deficits accompanied by impaired position and vibration sense, ataxia, nystagmus, and parasthesias, especially with a history of substance abuse, should raise the possibility of a substance-induced dementia, particularly alcohol-related dementia. A rapidly progressive dementia in a younger patient accompanied by myoclonus may indicate the presence of a prion disease. Findings consistent with immunosuppression should prompt concern for human immunodeficiency virus (HIV) dementia.

Laboratory data in the evaluation of dementia are used to look for treatable or reversible causes such as hypothyroidism or cerebrovasculitis, though these are not often found. Commonly ordered tests include B_{12}, folic acid, RPR, CBC, chemistry, erythrocyte sedimentation rate (ESR), and TSH. Tests such as HIV and antinuclear antibody (ANA) may be ordered if clinically indicated. The use of routine neuroimaging is controversial. Imaging in AD is often normal, or may show atrophy in the medial and temporal lobes and enlarged ventricles. White matter hyperintensities are common and also found in healthy adults. As it is of limited utility in the diagnosis and treatment of the majority of cases of dementia, imaging is best reserved for patients with early or otherwise atypical presentations. Electroencephalogram (EEG) and lumbar puncture (LP), likewise, are recommended in unusual cases and are not part of the routine workup.

When evaluating a patient for dementia, three important differential diagnoses to keep in mind are delirium, depression, and MCI. Both delirium and dementia show cognitive impairment, but the impairments in delirium tend to be more acute in onset, and are marked by inattention, altered arousal, and fluctuation in mental status, which are generally not seen in dementia. Older patients with depression may present with complaints of cognitive changes and perform worse than expected on cognitive testing. In contrast to patients with dementia, however, they are more likely to have a prior history of depression, to be inattentive, show psychomotor changes, and have poor motivation, and to improve with encouragement and additional time. Of note, patients with pseudodementia develop dementia at a rate up to six times that of the general population. MCI is a term used to indicate memory changes that are beyond those seen in normal aging (i.e., slowed retrieval time), with affected individuals performing 1.5 standard deviations below age-appropriate norms. In the most common type, the amnestic type, only memory is impaired and other cognitive domains remain intact. Patients with MCI progress to AD at a rate of 10% to 15% per year.

5. Treatments

A. NONPHARMACOLOGICAL TREATMENTS

1. Cognitive Impairment

Strategies such as keeping the patients in familiar environments, frequent cues, and writing things down may help decrease confusion and improve functioning in patients with dementia. In addition, several studies have examined the efficacy of specific cognitive interventions in improving or preserving cognitive function. In a randomized, placebo-controlled study, Davis et al. at the University of Texas looked at three specific interventions—spaced retrieval, training in face-name associations, and cognitive stimulation. In the spaced retrieval intervention, subjects were asked to recall information over progressively longer time periods. In the face-name associations training, subjects were taught techniques to help remember staff members' names. In the cognitive stimulation intervention, subjects were given a variety of attention-based tasks. At the end of the 5-week study period, subjects showed an improved ability to recall personal information and face-name associations as compared to the control group. However, these gains did not translate into other areas of cognitive functioning and did not appear to improve quality of life.

2. Behavioral and Psychiatric Symptoms

Behavioral and psychiatric problems in dementia are common and include agitation, aggression, wandering, hallucinations, delusions, depression, anxiety, and sleep disturbances. These symptoms are often more distressing for the patient and caregiver than the memory loss. They also predict caregiver stress, functional decline, and eventual need for nursing home placement. Anxiety and agitation are the most common symptoms, with agitation occurring in 50% of patients at some point during their illness. Families and caregivers must be reassured that these disturbances are common and are not their fault or to be taken personally. They must also be educated that patients cannot control their behavior as they did in the past and that reasoning, arguing, or punishing the patient will not work. The first step in the management of behavioral symptoms is to assess for any possible medical cause, delirium, or discomfort. The next step is to look for patterns or triggers. Understanding the source of the behavior may allow treatment of the underlying problem by modifying the environment, providing reassurance, etc. Calm settings and familiar routines may help prevent behavioral problems, as might clear and simple communication. Redirecting attention to pleasant activities can also be a helpful technique. There has been some evidence that aromatherapy, exercise, music therapy, and pet therapy can be beneficial as well.

B. PHARMACOLOGICAL TREATMENTS

1. Cognitive Impairment

The mainstays of the treatment for cognitive impairment are the cholinesterase inhibitors and memantine. There are currently three widely used cholinesterase inhibitors—rivastigmine, galantamine, and donepezil. These medications work by inhibiting the enzyme acetylcholinesterase, thus increasing the amount of acetylcholine available in the synapse and maximizing cholinergic transmission. They are not able to stop or reverse the dementia process, but have been shown to slow progression and loss of function. All three have similar efficacy and are approved for the treatment of mild to moderate AD, though donepezil is also approved for the treatment of severe AD. Studies show that these drugs are also effective in the treatment of VaD and DLB. The main side effects of cholinesterase inhibitors are nausea, vomiting, and diarrhea, related to peripheral cholinergic effects, and insomnia. Donepezil seems to be the best tolerated of the three. Memantine is an extrapyramidal symptoms N-methyl-D-aspartic acid (NMDA) receptor antagonist that blocks the binding of glutamate, an excitatory neurotransmitter, and the subsequent influx of calcium. The NMDA receptor is involved in learning and memory, but excessive stimulation is toxic and leads to cell death. It is thought that memantine may have a neuroprotective effect. Like the cholinesterase inhibitors, however, memantine can slow but not halt the progression of dementia. Memantine is FDA-approved for moderate to severe AD, and there is evidence for its use in VaD as well. Common side effects are headache, dizziness, hypertension, and constipation. Studies have shown that the combination of memantine and donepezil is more effective than donepezil plus placebo.

2. Behavioral and Psychiatric Symptoms

Medications can sometimes be a useful adjunct to nonpharmacological therapy of behavioral and psychiatric symptoms in dementia. While evidence regarding the efficacy of antipsychotics for these symptoms is limited, antipsychotics, mainly high potency typical neuroleptics such as haloperidol and the atypical agents, are frequently used for the treatment of psychosis and agitation. Many practitioners and families find these medications to be a helpful and important treatment tool. It must be noted, however, that there are no FDA-approved treatments for the behavioral disturbances in dementia and that atypical antipsychotics as a class carry an FDA black box warning due to an increased risk of death with the use of atypical antipsychotics in the elderly with dementia. A meta-analysis published in the *Journal of the American Medical Association*, which looked at published and unpublished trials, noted a small increased risk of death, consistent with the FDA findings. It is not clear how much of this increase is related to the use of antipsychotics versus patient characteristics. A careful discussion with family members regarding the risks and benefits of these medications is vital prior to beginning the treatment. These medications must also be used with caution as the elderly are at higher risk for extrapyramidal symptoms (EPS) and sedation. Patients with DLB are particularly sensitive to EPS, so risperidone and typical antipsychotics should be avoided. In DLB, there is a greater cholinergic deficit, and cholinesterase inhibitors may be helpful for the prominent visual hallucinations. SSRIs, particularly citalopram, may also improve agitation, and all are useful in the treatment of depression. Data on the effectiveness of anticonvulsants such as valproic acid and carbamazepine are mixed. Trazodone may be beneficial, especially in the context of sleep disturbances. Medications that are highly anticholinergic can worsen confusion and should not be used. Benzodiazepines may have a role in the setting of acute time-limited anxiety, but as they carry the risk of sedation, gait impairment, and worsened cognition, their use should be minimized.

6. Prognosis

There is some variation in data between studies estimating survival in dementia. One study from 2005 found a median survival of 10.5 years from onset and 5.7 years from diagnosis. Most studies show survival between 4 and 10 years after diagnosis. Several factors appear to influence mortality, including advanced age, physical illness, severity of dementia, delirium, wandering, falls, and behavioral problems.

7. General Formulation for Dementia

A. DIAGNOSTIC

A definitive diagnosis of dementia can generally be made only at autopsy. In practice, a presumptive diagnosis is made based largely on history with additional information from physical examination and laboratory data. The DSM specifies that dementia involves impairment in memory as well as impairment in one other cognitive domain. When only memory impairment is present, a diagnosis of amnestic syndrome is made. The cognitive deficits must also represent a decline from a previous level of functioning, thus a person with mental retardation, for example, cannot be diagnosed with dementia unless there has been a change in their cognition (as happens with many patients with Down's syndrome after the age of 40). Other possible diagnoses that present with cognitive changes must be considered as well, before the diagnosis of dementia can be made. These include normal aging, Mild Cognitive Impairment (MCI), delirium, and depression.

Normal aging is associated with cognitive changes including decrease in fluid reasoning, impaired novel problem solving, and slowed processing and retrieval time. However, these changes, while they can be aggravating, do not interfere with function. If functional impairment is present, the possibility of dementia should be considered. MCI refers to performance that is 1.5 standard deviations below age-adjusted norms on cognitive testing. If the impairment is in memory alone, it is described as amnestic type, though MCI can affect any cognitive domain. Because the impairments are relatively mild, functional changes are minor. Patients with MCI must be monitored closely as they progress to dementia at a rate of 10% to 15% per year. Delirium is another illness that presents with cognitive impairment, but unlike in dementia, the onset tends to be relatively sudden and there is marked fluctuation in arousal and attention. Delirium should always be considered in the differential of cognitive changes, however, as it represents a medical emergency. The term pseudodementia has often been used to describe the cognitive changes seen in some older patient with depression. Unlike patients with dementia, these patients tend to show poor attention and effort and perform better with more time and encouragement. They are also more likely to have other signs and symptoms of depression. Of note, patients who display cognitive impairment in the setting of depression have an elevated rate of developing dementia in the future.

B. ETIOLOGIC

There are multiple possible etiologies of dementia that must be considered once the diagnosis is made. These include neurodegenerative diseases (i.e., Alzheimer's disease, FTD, Lewy body dementia, Parkinson's disease, Huntington's disease), vascular diseases, infectious causes (i.e., HIV, Creuzfeldt-Jakob disease), trauma, hydrocephalus, and toxic-metabolic conditions (i.e., alcoholism, hypothyroidism). Age is the major predisposing risk factor for dementia. Family history and genetics also play a role, though genetic screening is not recommended at this time. Vascular risk factors are important in the development of VaD, and can also worsen the course of Alzheimer's disease. Higher educational level and certain genetic variants (i.e., ApoE2) may be protective factors.

C. THERAPEUTIC

The treatment of dementia involves addressing both the cognitive impairment and the frequently associated neuropsychiatric symptoms including depression, agitation, paranoia, hallucinations, disinhibition, and sleep changes. Nonpharmacological approaches to treatment include careful assessment for underlying causes of behavioral changes (i.e., pain, delirium or other medical illness, fear) as well as attempts to address these when possible, providing a calm, familiar, and consistent environment, and redirection of attention with pleasant activities. Ensuring that communication is clear, including consideration of hearing and visual deficits, can be helpful, as can caregiver education about these often distressing symptoms. There are no FDA-approved pharmacological treatments for the behavioral disturbances of dementia, but antipsychotics, mood stabilizers, and antidepressants are often used. Because elderly patients, especially those with cognitive impairment, are more sensitive to side effects, care should be taken to use the lowest effective doses for the least amount of time. Benzodiazepines and highly anticholinergic medications should be avoided because of the potential for delirium. A thorough risk-benefit discussion with the medical decision maker is vital when using these medications, as uses are often off-label and atypical antipsychotics, though commonly used, carry an FDA warning for increased risk of death. Pharmacological treatment for the cognitive impairments consists of the cholinesterase inhibitors such as donepezil, which is approved for mild, moderate, and severe dementia, and the NMDA receptor antagonist memantine, which is approved for moderate and severe dementia. It is important to note that while these medications slow progression, none can reverse or halt the dementia process. When treating a patient with dementia, it is also important to ensure that the patient is in a safe environment. Resources such as adult day care centers and respites can provide patients with stimulation and socialization while also giving caregivers a much needed rest. Ultimately, placement in a nursing home may be necessary.

D. PROGNOSTIC

The prognosis of dementia depends on the etiology. Neurodegenerative diseases result in a progressive illness, though the rates of progression vary. Survival times of between 4 and 10 years have been noted in various studies. There are factors that can influence survival. These include age, comorbid medical illness, presence of delirium, and falls, among others.

8. Risk Assessment

There are several safety issues that must be considered in the patient with dementia. Ability to drive is a common and often very sensitive topic. As dementia progresses, patients experience deficits in visuospatial abilities, judgment, and memory. This increases their risk of having an accident, but many patients are not fully aware of their deficits and are afraid of losing their independence. Patients should be routinely asked about driving, and if there are any concerns, they should be referred to the local Department of Motor Vehicles for a formal evaluation. Wandering is a commonly seen behavior in dementia, which places patients in unfamiliar surroundings and possibly in harm's way. Safe Return bracelets, which have contact information, are one tool that may be helpful when wandering is a concern. Cooking is another activity that may prove hazardous in the setting of cognitive impairment. Leaving stoves or other appliances on and then forgetting about them, for example, can cause fires that are dangerous for the patient and others in the area. Use of a microwave or food delivery services may be ways to help with this issue. Aggression and impulsivity, as previously noted, are behavioral disturbances seen in dementia, and can cause harm to both the patient and the caregiver. Caregivers may be reluctant to spontaneously disclose these behaviors, and should be encouraged to report them so that they can be treated and to call 911 if they feel acutely threatened. Elderly patients, particularly those with physical or cognitive impairments, are extremely vulnerable and at risk of abuse. Assessment for physical, emotional, and financial abuse should be part of the standard evaluation. Finally, the care of patients with dementia can be exhausting and frustrating, and caregivers are at increased risk for depression and health problems. For patients with dementia to receive the best possible treatment, caregivers must be provided with support and resources, including information about respite care and referral to support groups.

KEY POINTS (ABPN Examination)

A. When interviewing a patient with suspected dementia

1. Remember that a thorough history is key to diagnosis, including the onset and course of the cognitive impairment.
2. Look for any obvious physical signs such as parkinsonism or focal neurological findings that may help point to the etiology.

B. When presenting a patient with suspected dementia

1. Acknowledge that patients with cognitive impairments may not be able to provide accurate history, and that collateral information is vital for the assessment.
2. Always consider the possibility of delirium in the differential diagnosis of dementia.

(*continued*)

KEY POINTS (ABPN Examination) (Continued)

3. Be aware of any impairments in hearing or vision that may interfere with communication, and compensate if possible.
4. Test the patient's cognition using MMSE and the clock-drawing task if possible. Pay special attention to patient's level of alertness.
5. Ask about changes in function including Instrument Activities of Daily Living (iADLs) and Basic Activities of Daily Living (bADLs).
6. Ask about safety-related issues such as driving, taking medications, getting lost.
7. Assess for the presence of behavioral and psychiatric symptoms including hallucinations, paranoia, agitation, depression, and anxiety.

3. Remember to discuss issues related to functional status and safety.
4. Note that there are no FDA-approved treatments for the behavioral disturbances of dementia, and that risk vs. benefit discussions are key.
5. With regard to management, remember to include both nonpharmacological and pharmacological aspects.
6. Mention the importance of assessing burden and providing assistance to the caregiver.

SUGGESTED READINGS

Blazer DG, Steffens DC, Busse EW. *Essentials of Geriatric Psychiatry*. Arlington, VA: American Psychiatric Publishing, Inc., 2007.

Boustani M, Peterson B, Hanson L, et al. *Screening for Dementia in Primary Care: A summary of the evidence for the U.S. Preventive Services Task Force*. *Ann Intern Med* 2003 June 3;138(11):927–937.

Davis RN, Massman PJ, Doody RS. Cognitive intervention in Alzheimer disease: A randomized placebo-controlled study. *Alzheimer Dis Assoc Disord* 2001;15(1):1–9.

Fleming KC, Adams AC, Petersen RC. Dementia: Diagnosis and evaluation. *Mayo Clin Proc* 1995;70:1093–1107.

Kaufman, DM. *Clinical Neurology for Psychiatrists*. 5th Ed. Philadelphia, PA: W. B. Saunders, 2001.

McKeith I, Mintzer J, Aarsland D, et al. Dementia with Lewy bodies. *Lancet Neurol* 2004; 3: 19–28.

McKhann GM, Albert MS, Grossman M, et al. Clinical and pathological diagnosis of frontotemporal dementia. *Arch Neurol* 2001;58:1803–1809.

Roman GC. Vascular dementia: Distinguishing characteristics, treatment, and prevention. *J Am Geriatr Soc* 2003;51:S296–S304.

Schneider LS, Dagerman K, Insel, PS. Efficacy and adverse effects of atypical antipsychotics for dementia: meta-analysis of randomised, placebo-controlled trials. *Am J Geriatr Psychiatry* 2006;14(3):191–210.

Schneider LS, Dagerman KS, Insel, P. Risk of death with atypical antipsychotic drug treatment for dementia. *JAMA* 2005;294(15):1934–1943.

Shigeta M, Homma A. Survival and risk factors for mortality in elderly patients with dementia. *Curr Opin Psychiatry* 2002;15(4):423–426.

Waring SC, Doody RS, Pavlik VN, et al. Survival among patients with dementia from a large multi-ethnic population. *Alzheimer Dis Assoc Disord* 2005;19(4):178–183.

II. DELIRIUM

CASE HISTORY

PRESENT ILLNESS

Mrs J, an 85-year-old woman with Alzheimer's disease, was brought to the emergency department by her husband who reported she had been increasingly confused over the past week or so. He reported no known precipitant to this change in mental status. He stated the patient was becoming increasingly disoriented. She kept insisting she was "at work" and that she needed to "go home," and she started calling him by her sister's name. She was sleeping more during the day and less at night. Her appetite had been poor. At night, she appeared to have distressing visions of seeing an intruder at the bedroom door. The patient's husband thought maybe this was "just her Alzheimer's getting worse," but the change worried him so he brought her in. He denied any recent change in mood, sleep, appetite, interests, or energy prior to the change in mental status. He denied any aggressive behavior or threats to harm self or others. The patient was a poor historian due to drowsiness and was unable to provide any useful information.

Mr J reported his wife had been diagnosed with Alzheimer's disease 6 years prior. She had experienced a gradual decline in cognitive and functional abilities. She required assistance with all instrumental activities of daily living as well as some basic activities of daily living. She was able to feed herself and ambulate independently, although she was intermittently incontinent. The family hired a home health aid who came 3 days per week to help with bathing and other ADLs. Mrs J also attended adult day care. She had no history of aggression, though she had been paranoid recently that the home health aid was "stealing" from them.

PSYCHIATRIC HISTORY

Mrs J had been diagnosed with Alzheimer's disease, as above. She had no history of psychiatric hospitalizations, other psychiatric illnesses, suicide attempts, or violence. No history of substance abuse or dependence.

FAMILY HISTORY

The patient's brother also had Alzheimer's disease.

SOCIAL HISTORY

Mrs J had a college education and had formerly worked as a schoolteacher. She had been married for 55 years and had two adult children who lived nearby. Her one brother was deceased, due to complications from dementia. Her sister was alive and in good health. Mrs J formerly enjoyed gardening, sewing, and church activities, though these had substantially decreased as her cognition declined.

PERTINENT MEDICAL HISTORY

The patient's medical history was significant for hypertension, osteoarthritis, macular degeneration, and hyperlipidemia. She had no known drug allergies. Her daily medications included Atenolol 50 mg daily, Donepezil 10 mg daily, and Simvastatin 40 mg each evening. In addition, Mr J reported he had been giving her a few "Tylenol PM" each night since she started having insomnia.

MENTAL STATUS EXAMINATION

Mrs J was an 85-year-old white female who appeared her stated age. She appeared thin but not frail, and was dressed in a hospital gown. She was mildly disheveled. She was sleeping on a hospital bed and was arousable when her name was called. She often nodded off during the interview. Her speech was often muffled. She was not agitated or combative. She was unable to properly describe her mood, and her affect was flat. There was no evidence of suicidal/homicidal ideation nor auditory/visual/tactile hallucinations, though her ability to answer such questions was limited. There was no evidence of delusions or paranoia. Her thought processing was disorganized with word salad. Her recent and remote memory were impaired. She was oriented to self only. She could not participate in full cognitive testing due to decreased level of alertness. Insight and judgment were clearly poor.

PERTINENT PHYSICAL FINDINGS

Vital signs were a temperature of 100°F, sitting heart rate of 75 per minute, sitting blood pressure of 120/80 mm Hg, and respiratory rate of 16 per minute. Standing heart rate was 100 per minute with a standing blood pressure of 90/60. Oxygen saturation on room air was 97.0%. She was lethargic and poorly attentive. Her body habitus was thin but not emaciated. The pupils were equal and reactive to light and accommodation. The oropharynx was dry. No jaundice, rash, or lymphadenopathy was noted. The heart and lung examinations were unremarkable. The abdomen was soft. There was no organomegaly. The bowel sounds were heard normally. Extremities were without cyanosis, clubbing, or edema. Neurological examination was limited by the patient's poor cooperation but did not reveal any focal deficits.

LABORATORY DATA

The laboratory data obtained at intake were remarkable for BUN of 30 and creatinine 1.4. CBC was notable for a white blood cell count of 14,000/cm^3 with a left shift. Urinalysis revealed cloudy urine, 3+ bacteria, 15 white blood cells/high-power field, and positive leukocyte esterase. Other laboratory tests done were negative or within normal limits, including electrolytes, liver function tests, Venereal Disease Research Laboratory (VDRL), TSH, serum and urine toxicology screen, ammonia, B_{12}, and folate levels. Chest x-ray was negative. A CT scan of the brain without contrast showed cortical volume loss and periventricular white matter disease without evidence of acute intracranial abnormality. An electrocardiogram (ECG) revealed normal sinus rhythm.

HOSPITAL COURSE

Mrs J was admitted to the medicine ward where she was given intravenous (IV) fluids and treated with antibiotics. Urine culture grew more than 10^5 *Escherichia coli* bacteria per mL. Blood cultures were negative. Initially in the hospitalization, nursing staff noted waxing and waning of her level of alertness, disorientation, and reversal of sleep-wake cycle. She was managed behaviorally with frequent reorientation, environmental modification, and sleep hygiene. Her husband was frequently at her bedside. She did not become agitated or combative and did not require any psychotropic medication for management of her symptoms while in the hospital. Her mental status gradually improved, though she had not yet returned to her baseline per her husband. She was discharged once she was able to take oral antibiotics and adequate nutrition and fluids.

DISCHARGE MEDICATIONS

Atenolol 50 mg daily, donepezil 10 mg daily, simvastatin 40 mg each evening, and amoxicillin-clavulanate 875 mg twice daily for one week.

DSM-IV-TR MULTIAXIAL DIAGNOSIS

Axis I. Delirium due to multiple etiologies (urinary tract infection, dehydration, medications)
Dementia due to Alzheimer's disease, moderate
Axis II. None
Axis III. Urinary tract infection, hypertension, dehydration, and hyperlipidemia
Axis IV. Severity of psychosocial stressor: severe; medical, cognitive and functional decline and lack of social support
Axis V. Global assessment of functioning at the time of discharge: 40

FORMULATION

A. Diagnostic

This patient meets all four of the DSM-IV-TR criteria for delirium due to multiple etiologies. She had a disturbance of consciousness with reduced clarity of awareness of the environment and reduced ability to focus, sustain, or shift attention. She exhibited a change in cognition compared to her baseline, including disorientation and new onset perceptual disturbances. Her change in mental status developed abruptly, over a period of days to weeks, and had a fluctuating quality to it. Finally, there was evidence from the history and laboratory data that the delirium had multiple etiologies.

The distinction between delirium and dementia can be challenging, and these two disorders commonly coexist. Mrs J had a 6-year history of dementia, as evidenced by a gradual, progressive decline in cognitive and functional abilities. Dementia and delirium may both present with impaired memory, disorientation, impaired thinking, sleep-wake cycle disruption, and perceptual disturbances. The onset and course of the cognitive impairment are two key features of delirium which help differentiate it from dementia. In delirium, the onset is typically acute or subacute, occurring over hours to days. In dementia, the onset of cognitive deficits is typically gradual and insidious. In addition, there is a fluctuating level of alertness and attention in delirium, which is not typically seen in dementia (DLB is one exception). Mrs J clearly met criteria for both dementia and delirium.

Also important to rule out in this case is a mood disorder such as major depressive disorder, which may present with worsening attention/concentration, poor appetite, and impaired sleep. However, there was no history of anhedonia, sad mood, feelings of worthlessness, excessive guilt, or hopelessness. In addition, the onset of the patient's change in mental status was fairly abrupt, more so than one would expect with a mood disorder. Similarly, one could consider the possibility of a primary psychotic disorder given the patient's paranoia, persecutory delusions, and visual hallucinations. However, a new-onset primary psychotic disorder at age 85 would be very unusual. Finally, one could consider a substance use disorder. However, there was no recent history of abuse of substances, and the patient's toxicology screens were negative. It is important to note in this case that there was no past psychiatric history to suggest a mood disorder, substance use disorder, or psychotic disorder, and that the patient's symptoms are best explained by another Axis I diagnosis (delirium).

B. Etiologic

From a biological perspective, her age, her visual impairment, and her underlying dementia place her at risk for developing delirium. She also has a family history of cognitive disorders, which may have genetically predisposed her to developing dementia. Mrs J suffered from an underlying infectious process and dehydration, and had been given anticholinergic medication (i.e., diphenhydramine), all of which likely contributed to the change in her mental status. Insomnia and sleep deprivation may also be contributing. Psychologically, there are no clear etiologic factors contributing to the patient's presentation. It is noteworthy that she began to ask to "go home" and began to call her husband by her sister's name. During a time of stress, some patients with cognitive impairment may cry out for "home," or other familiar, comforting images. When hospitalized in unfamiliar surroundings, patients with cognitive impairment may experience psychological distress and fear which may manifest as agitation. Socially, the patient has had to move from the comfort of her own home and previously enjoyed activities to the unfamiliar environment of the hospital where she is essentially confined to her room all day. Medical personnel (virtual strangers to the patient) now come to her day and night, asking questions, drawing blood, and providing medications. These changes may further exacerbate her disorientation and confusion. Her social network has become increasingly limited. She has lost a brother and likely has lost several friends at this age, as well. She appears to have good social support from her husband, adult day care, and home health, though it is unclear whether this support is adequate, given the extent of her care needs.

C. Therapeutic

The treatment of delirium is first and foremost the identification and treatment of the underlying etiology. In this case, the patient received antibiotics for a urinary tract infection, IV fluids for dehydration, and stopped receiving diphenhydramine. The patient received beneficial nonpharmacological interventions including frequent reorientation, sleep hygiene, environmental modification, and frequent family visits, which are often helpful in the treatment of delirium. In this case, the patient did not require any psychiatric medications to help manage the behavioral symptoms of delirium. It will be important to educate the patient's husband on the proper use of over-the-counter medications (i.e., avoid the use of Tylenol PM) at home. With regard to her dementia, she is taking donepezil, a cholinesterase inhibitor approved for the treatment of mild, moderate, and severe Alzheimer's disease. She may benefit from the addition of memantine, an NMDA antagonist which is approved for the treatment of moderate to severe Alzheimer's disease. In Mrs J's case, it would be advisable to postpone the addition of any new psychotropic medications until her mental status has returned to baseline and her stage of dementia can be more accurately assessed.

D. Prognostic

In general, delirium is associated with significant morbidity and mortality. Positive prognostic indicators for Mrs J include her relatively short duration of illness, relatively little medical comorbidity, and a rapid evaluation and treatment. It is important to remember that full recovery of mental function may not occur for days to even months after the underlying etiology of delirium is addressed. Mrs J has underlying dementia of the Alzheimer's type, an illness which will eventually progress to a stage of severity in which she will require total care. In this sense, her prognosis is poor. As above, she is taking a cholinesterase inhibitor which may provide some delay in the progression of her illness, though will not halt its progression altogether.

DELIRIUM

1. Introduction

Delirium is a common neuropsychiatric syndrome, which is seen in all health care settings. Patients with delirium typically exhibit an altered level of consciousness, impairment in attention and orientation, as well as disturbances of perception, behavior, sleep-wake cycle, and affect. Delirium most commonly presents acutely, over hours to days, and typically has a waxing and waning symptom course. It may present as one of three subtypes: hyperactive, hypoactive, or mixed. By definition, delirium is attributable to an underlying medical condition or substance intoxication or withdrawal. Delirium contributes significantly to patient morbidity and mortality as well as patient and caregiver distress. It contributes to increased hospital lengths of stay, increased rates of institutionalization, and reduced level of overall functioning.

2. Epidemiology

Delirium affects 10% to 30% of all medically ill, hospitalized patients. Up to 60% of nursing home residents aged 65 years and older may have delirium. Elderly patients are at particular risk for delirium, given the age-related changes of the brain, decreased cholinergic functioning, and co-occurrence of central nervous system disorders such as dementia and cerebrovascular disease. Additional risk factors for delirium include young age (i.e., children), sensory deprivation, HIV infection, burns, postsurgical status (i.e., cardiac, hip, transplant), dialysis, sleep deprivation, multiple medications, malnourishment, abrupt discontinuation of alcohol or drugs, and terminal illness, among others.

3. Etiology

By definition, delirium is secondary to an underlying medical condition or substance intoxication or withdrawal. The potential etiologies of delirium are numerous. The cornerstone of treatment of delirium is reversal of the underlying etiology; hence, the etiology (or etiologies) must be identified in order to properly treat delirium. Multiple medical conditions have been implicated, including infection, cardiac illness, metabolic and endocrine abnormalities, trauma, neoplastic illness, autoimmune disease, cerebrovascular disease, and others. Polypharmacy and drug intoxication and withdrawal are very common etiologies of delirium. Medication classes which are frequently associated with delirium include opiates, benzodiazepines, and medications with anticholinergic properties (e.g., antihistamines, benztropine, tricyclics, and antispasmodics). Often, multiple etiologies converge together to produce delirium.

The neuropathogenesis of delirium is hypothesized to involve certain neural circuits and neurotransmitters. Functional neuroimaging studies have shown reduced blood flow in both cortical and subcortical regions. Reduced cholinergic activity is the best established neurotransmitter dysfunction in delirium. Disruptions in the functioning of other neurotransmitters, including dopamine, serotonin, and gamma-aminobutyric acid have also been implicated in the pathogenesis of delirium. Other proposed etiologies of delirium include glial dysfunction, increased blood-brain barrier permeability, and immune activation.

4. Diagnosis

Delirium is commonly missed in the clinical setting, and undetected delirium portends a poorer outcome. In order to diagnose delirium, the DSM-IV-TR requires that the patient has an altered level of consciousness, impaired attention, and cognitive deficits or perceptual disturbances, which are not better accounted for by a preexisting dementia (Table 3E.2). Symptoms develop over a short period of time (i.e., hours to days) and exhibit a fluctuating course. In addition, there must be evidence from the history, physical examination, or laboratory findings that the change in mental status is directly related to a general medical condition or substance.

Since delirium has a variety of clinical presentations, it complicates the accurate and timely diagnosis of this column. Three subtypes of delirium which are commonly described in the literature include the following: *hyperactive*, characterized by agitation, disorientation, and psychotic features; *hypoactive*, characterized by somnolence, withdrawal, and apathy; or *mixed*, consisting of fluctuations between hyperactive and hypoactive subtypes. The hyperactive and mixed types may be misdiagnosed as mania, an anxiety disorder or psychotic disorder, such as schizophrenia; whereas, the quiet, hypoactive type may be mistaken for depression or may not raise clinical concern at all.

The differential diagnosis for delirium includes not only mood, anxiety, and psychotic disorders, but also other cognitive disorders. Most notable among the differential diagnoses is dementia. Dementia and delirium share several key features, including cognitive deficits (memory impairment, disorientation, language disturbance) and perceptual disturbances. Helping to distinguish between the two are the onset and course of illness. Delirium typically presents over a short period of time, hours to days, whereas dementia has a more insidious onset. Delirium waxes and wanes over time, whereas the course of dementia is typically

TABLE 3E.2 Diagnostic Criteria for Delirium

A.	Disturbance of consciousness (i.e., reduced clarity of awareness of the environment) with reduced ability to focus, sustain, or shift attention.
B.	A change in cognition (such as memory deficit, disorientation, language disturbance) or the development of a perceptual disturbance that is not better accounted for by a preexisting, established, or evolving dementia.
C.	The disturbance develops over a short period of time (usually hours to days) and tends to fluctuate during the course of the day.
D.	There is evidence from the history, physical examination, or laboratory findings that the disturbance is caused by the direct physiological consequences of a general medication condition or substance (intoxication or withdrawal).

Adapted from American Psychiatric Association. *Diagnostic and Statistical Manual of Mental Disorders: DSM-IV-TR.* American Psychiatric Association, 2000

progressive. (One exception is DLB, which may present similarly to delirium with fluctuating cognition, hallucinations, and impaired attention.) Another notable distinguishing feature is level of consciousness and attention, both of which are impaired in delirium but not in dementia (until perhaps late stages and in the case of DLB).

Delirium is often the initial harbinger of underlying illness; as such, timely diagnosis and investigation for causes are essential. A complete history and physical examination, as well as mental status examination and cognitive testing, are indicated. The most commonly used and recognized screening tool to assess cognition is the Folstein MMSE. A brief, 30-item test, the MMSE can be easily administered at the bedside and is familiar to most, if not all, practitioners. Cognitive domains tested include orientation, immediate/recent memory, language, attention, and concentration. Serial MMSEs may be helpful in monitoring the patient's mental status over time. Other screening tools which may be utilized in the diagnosis of delirium include the Confusion Assessment Method, the Cognitive Test for Delirium, the Delirium Rating Scale, and the clock-drawing test. Neither the MMSE nor the clock-drawing test reliably distinguishes between delirium and dementia.

Additional investigation of delirium includes a thorough medication inventory (both prescription and over-the-counter medications), arterial blood gases or oxygen saturation, laboratory testing (CBC, basic metabolic panel, calcium, magnesium, phosphate, liver function tests, urinalysis, urine and serum toxicology screens, TSH, B_{12}, others as clinically indicated), ECG, chest x-ray, and often neuroimaging. Though not routinely used for the diagnosis of delirium, EEG may be helpful in certain cases. EEG can help clarify the diagnosis when seizures are suspected. In addition, the diffuse slowing of the background rhythm seen in patients with delirium is not typically seen in patients with early dementia, depression, or schizophrenia.

5. Treatments

It cannot be overemphasized that the "first-line treatment" of delirium is the identification and reversal of the suspected underlying cause. While this is taking place, however, additional nonpharmacological and pharmacological treatment interventions may be indicated.

A. NONPHARMACOLOGICAL TREATMENT

Though insufficient to reverse delirium on their own, several psychosocial and environmental interventions have been suggested to reduce the agitation, confusion, and disorientation of the patient suffering from delirium. Orientation cues, such as verbal reorientation by staff, calendars, and appropriate day/night lighting should be utilized. The patient should have sensory impairments minimized by the use of corrective lenses or hearing aids as needed. Familiarity in the form of consistent staff members, family visits, or pictures may be comforting. Television or radio may provide a nice, relaxing distraction or help the patient maintain contact with the outside world; however, excess noise should be avoided. Given that sleep deprivation may worsen delirium, treatment interventions should be scheduled such that uninterrupted sleep at night is maximized. Patients should be allowed to participate in their own self-care and treatment when possible.

B. PHARMACOLOGICAL TREATMENTS

There are no medications that are approved by the U.S. Food and Drug Administration for the treatment of delirium, and there is a paucity of randomized, controlled trials of medications for this purpose. However, some patients suffering from delirium may require medications to treat significant agitation or psychotic symptoms, which compromise their safe care in the hospital. All psychotropic medications carry their own risks of side effects, so the risks must be carefully weighed against the need for symptom control in an individual patient.

The first-generation antipsychotic haloperidol is the medication most commonly used for symptomatic treatment of delirium. Generally considered safe in the medically ill, haloperidol has a rapid onset of action and can be administered orally, intramuscularly, or intravenously. Haloperidol has less orthostasis, less sedation, and less anticholinergic effects compared to other first-generation antipsychotics. Antipsychotics such as haloperidol do carry the risk of EPS, though this risk is reduced when the medication is given intravenously. IV use of haloperidol has, however, been associated with risk of torsades de pointes. The American Psychiatric Association advises that patients who have QTc prolongation greater than 450 milliseconds or greater than a 25% increase in QTc from baseline should be placed on telemetry with consideration given to discontinuation of haloperidol or cardiology consultation. It should be noted that IV use of haloperidol constitutes "off-label" use and given the cardiac risks, some hospitals discourage this form of administration. When dosing haloperidol in the delirious patient, one should start low (i.e., 0.25 to 0.5 mg every 4 hours as needed in the elderly; 1 to 2 mg in younger adults) and frequently reassess the need for the medication. Gradual tapering of antipsychotics is preferred over abrupt discontinuation.

Second-generation antipsychotics have also been studied for use in the treatment of delirium. Medications such as risperidone, quetiapine, and olanzapine have small studies and case reports suggesting their efficacy. However, randomized, controlled trials are lacking and none of these medications has been shown consistently to be superior to haloperidol. These medications may represent reasonable alternatives to haloperidol in certain patient populations. Choice of antipsychotic medication may be based on several individual factors, including desired side effects (e.g., sedation), lack of side effects (e.g., EPS), drug-drug interactions, cardiac comorbidities, etc.

Benzodiazepines are sometimes used for their sedative and anxiolytic effects. They are first-line treatment for delirium secondary to alcohol or sedative-hypnotic withdrawal. However, they are not recommended for routine use in delirium due to other etiologies, given their sedative effects as well as their potential for paradoxical disinhibition and worsening of cognitive impairment.

6. Prognosis

Delirium is a negative prognostic sign, associated with increased morbidity and mortality. Delirium contributes to longer postoperative recuperation periods, increased hospital lengths of stay, increased rates of institutionalization, and reduced level of overall functioning. Delirious patients are at greater risk of medical complications, such as pneumonia or decubitus ulcers. Reported mortality rates among hospitalized elderly patients with delirium range from 22% to 76%. The exact mechanism by which the increase in mortality occurs is not fully known, but this increased risk persists in the months following discharge from the hospital. Full cognitive recovery from delirium may take weeks to months, lagging behind the reversal of the underlying medical condition.

7. General Formulation for Delirium

A. DIAGNOSTIC

Ensure that the patient meets the DSM-IV-TR criteria for delirium due to multiple etiologies (Table 3E.2). Consider other diagnoses in the differential, in particular, dementia, depression, psychotic disorders, and substance use disorders. The distinction between delirium and dementia can be challenging, and these two disorders commonly coexist. Dementia and delirium may both present with impaired memory, disorientation, impaired thinking, sleep-wake cycle disruption, and perceptual disturbances. The onset and course of the cognitive impairment are two key distinguishing features. In delirium, the onset is typically acute or subacute, occurring over hours to days. In dementia, the onset of cognitive deficits is typically gradual and insidious. In addition, there is a fluctuating level of alertness and attention in delirium, which is not typically seen in dementia (DLB is one exception).

Always consider the possibility of a mood disorder such as a major depressive episode (MDE) or a manic episode, both of which may also present with impaired attention/concentration, agitation, poor appetite, impaired sleep, and in severe cases, psychosis. However, with an MDE, one would expect to also see symptoms such as anhedonia, sad mood, feelings of worthlessness, excessive guilt, or hopelessness. In a manic episode, one would expect to see irritable or euphoric mood, flight of ideas, grandiosity, and pressured speech. In addition, the onset of delirium is fairly abrupt with a fluctuating course, more so than one would expect with a mood episode. Past psychiatric history may provide helpful clues in making these distinctions.

Similarly, one could consider the possibility of a primary psychotic disorder if symptoms such as paranoia, persecutory delusions, visual hallucinations, and disorganized thinking were present. However, if this were the case, the patient's past history would likely reveal a prior diagnosis of psychotic disorder. Typically, patients with psychotic disorders do not have a waxing and waning attentional deficit or decreased level of consciousness. In addition, a new-onset primary psychotic disorder in an elderly patient would be very unusual. Finally, one should consider whether a substance use disorder is also present. Both substance intoxication and withdrawal may present with delirium. In these cases, the patient's past psychiatric and substance abuse history (with collateral information from family and friends) as well as toxicology screens would be helpful in making this diagnosis.

B. ETIOLOGIC

From a biological perspective, certain factors place one at risk for development of delirium: age (elderly and children), central nervous system disorders such as dementia and cerebrovascular disease, sensory impairment, HIV infection, burns, postsurgical status (i.e., cardiac, hip, transplant), dialysis, sleep deprivation, multiple medications, malnourishment, abrupt discontinuation of alcohol or drugs, and terminal illness, among others. Certain medications should always be considered in the etiology of delirium: anticholinergics (including antihistamines, antiparkinsonian medications, tricyclic antidepressants, and antispasmodic agents), opiates, and benzodiazepines. The list of potential medications contributing to delirium is extensive. Consider common etiologies of delirium, including hypoxia, hypoglycemia, metabolic derangement, infection, and alcohol or sedative-hypnotic withdrawal. Consider the impact of pain and pain management, particularly in the postoperative patient. Psychologically, patients with cognitive impairment may experience psychological distress and fear in an unfamiliar environment. This distress and fear may manifest as agitation, calling out for loved ones, or suspiciousness of medical staff. Socially, patients with delirium have been removed from their families, the comfort of their home, and their previously enjoyed work and leisure activities. The new, unfamiliar environment of the hospital with its sterile atmosphere and similar environment regardless of time of day may be disorienting and frightening for the delirious patient. Both overstimulation and understimulation of the patient's senses may be problematic. Family members may be unable to visit regularly during a patient's prolonged hospitalization, due to their own familial and occupational obligations. Lack of familiarity and comfort from familiar faces may further contribute to disorientation and agitation.

C. THERAPEUTIC

Appropriate treatment of delirium begins with identification and reversal of the underlying cause. Treatment should include both nonpharmacological and pharmacological approaches. As described above, nonpharmacological treatment should be geared toward restoring sensory impairments, frequent reorientation, providing adequate lighting and noise, and encouraging familiarity through family visits or comforting objects from home. Pharmacological therapy should take into account target symptoms (i.e., psychosis, agitation, insomnia, combativeness, etc.) as well as the patient's medical comorbidities and potential for drug-drug interactions. Antipsychotic medications, in particular, haloperidol, have been the agents most studied in the treatment of behavioral disturbances of delirium. Benzodiazepines are best avoided in the delirious patient due to risk of worsening of cognitive impairment and paradoxical disinhibition; the exception is the patient withdrawing from alcohol or sedative-hypnotics. Careful consideration must be given to the risk-benefit ratio as well as the side effect profile of any psychotropic medication used in a delirious patient. Also, patients with delirium are not likely to possess the capacity to make their own medical decisions. Hence, identification of a surrogate decision maker is prudent. This person is usually a spouse or other close family member or, if one has been previously designated, a durable power of attorney.

D. PROGNOSTIC

Delirium is a negative prognostic sign, associated with prolonged hospitalization, increased rate of medical complications, and increased rate of institutionalization. It is important to note that cognitive recovery often lags behind correction of the underlying medical etiology. Full recovery from delirium is less likely in the elderly and in patients with AIDS. If untreated, delirium may progress to seizures, stupor, coma, or death. Delirium is associated with increased mortality both during hospitalization and in the months following discharge.

8. Risk Assessment

One of the biggest risks in delirium is lack of timely diagnosis and evaluation for underlying causes. As soon as delirium is suspected, the workup should begin. The sooner the etiology can be identified and corrected, the better. Patients with delirium may be disoriented, agitated, and combative, thereby posing a risk of danger to self or others. They may pose an indirect risk to themselves when their agitation and behavioral disturbances compromise safe and timely medical treatment (i.e., pulling out IV lines, etc.). The use of psychotropic medications, sitters, and/or physical restraints may be necessary to keep the patient and staff safe and allow necessary medical care. Except in cases of emergency, restraints are typically used as a last resort, following failure of nonpharmacological management of behavioral disturbances. Restraints themselves may be confusing and distressing to delirious patients. Hence, the need for restraints should be reevaluated regularly according to hospital policy and discontinued as soon as possible.

KEY POINTS (ABPN EXAMINATION)

A. When interviewing a patient with suspected delirium

1. Remember that mental status may fluctuate.
2. Take a thorough past medical history as well as medication inventory, including over-the-counter medications.
3. Take a thorough substance abuse history. If substance withdrawal is suspected, look for other outward signs such as tremor, diaphoresis, anxiety, etc.
4. Do not forget to test cognition. At a minimum, test the patient's orientation, short term recall, naming, attention, and concentration. If time allows, perform the MMSE.
5. Assess for the presence of perceptual disturbances (illusions, hallucinations), paranoia, etc.

B. When presenting a patient with suspected delirium

1. Acknowledge that mental status in the delirious patient may fluctuate, so the brief interview may not have captured the overall pattern of mental status change.
2. Always consider the possibility of dementia in the differential diagnosis of delirium, particularly in elderly patients.
3. Suggest that you would like to obtain collateral information from family and staff regarding patient's baseline mental status, noted changes in mental status, and current behavioral issues.
4. Remember the first-line treatment of delirium is reversal of the underlying cause.
5. With regard to behavioral management, remember to include both nonpharmacological and pharmacological aspects.

Suggested Readings

American Psychiatric Association. *Diagnostic and Statistical Manual of Mental Disorders: DSM-IV-TR*. Washington, DC: American Psychiatric Association, 2000.

American Psychiatric Association. Practice guideline for the treatment of patients with delirium. *Am J Pyschiatry* 1999;156(suppl 5):1–20.

Folstein MF, Folstein SE, McHugh PR. "Mini-mental state." A practical method for grading the cognitive state of patients for the clinician. *J Psychiatry Res* 1975;12:189–198.

Francis J, Kapoor WN. Delirium in hospitalized elderly. *J Gen Intern Med* 1990;5:65–79.

Gleason, OG. Delirium. *Am Fam Physician* 2003;67(5):1027–1034.

Hart RP, Levenson JL, Sessler CN, et al. Validation of a cognitive test for delirium in medical ICU patients. *Psychosomatics* 1996;37:533–546.

Inouye SK. Delirium in Older persons. *N Engl J Med* 2006;354:1157–1165.

Inouye SK, van Dyck CH, Alessi CA, et al. Clarifying confusion: The confusion assessment method. A new method for the detection of delirium. *Ann Intern Med* 1990;113:941–948.

Kakuma R, du Fort GG, Arsenault L, et al. Delirium in older emergency department patients discharged home: Effect on survival. *J Am Geriatr Soc* 1992;51:443–450.

Meagher DJ. Delirium: Optimising management. *BMJ* 2001;322:144–149.

Rockwood K. The occurrence and duration of symptoms in elderly patients with delirium. *J Gerontol* 1993;48:M162–M166.

Seitz DP, Gill SS, van Zyl LT. Antipsychotics in the treatment of delirium: A systematic review. *J Clin Psychiatry* 2007;68:11–21.

Trzepacz PT. Anticholinergic model for delirium. *Semin Clin Neuropsychiatry* 1996;1: 294–303.

Trzepacz PT, Baker RW, Greenhouse J. A symptom rating scale for delirium. *Psychiatry Res* 1988;23:89–97.

Trzepacz PT, Meagher DJ. Delirium. In: Levenson JL, ed. *Textbook of Psychosomatic Medicine*. Arlington, VA: American Psychiatric Publishing, 2005:91–130.

Vaurio LE, Sands LP, Wang Y, et al. Postoperative delirium: The importance of pain and pain management. *Anesth Analg* 2006;102: 1267–1273.

F. Personality disorders

Natalie Weder, MD

I. BORDERLINE PERSONALITY DISORDER

CASE HISTORY

PRESENT ILLNESS

Ms O is a 34-year-old single Hispanic woman who was admitted to the inpatient unit as a voluntary patient after taking 10 Tylenol tablets in an attempt to overdose and then calling her mother asking for help. She had taken the tablets after having an argument with her landlord, who had called to inform her of a raise in the rent. She had spent her rent money buying clothes and found herself unable to pay it. She denied having planned the overdose and stated that she took them impulsively after feeling so overwhelmed with anxiety about how to manage her expenses and feeling "stupid" for not being able to negotiate a "reasonable raise" with her landlord. However, soon after taking the Tylenol tablets, she felt "more relaxed and under control."

When asked about depressive symptoms, she denied any periods of consistent depressed mood that lasted more than a day but stated that she had frequent mood swings which lasted from minutes to an hour and that in a single day, she could go from feeling "happy and relaxed" to feeling "hopeless and overcome with sadness," especially if something did not go as planned. She frequently feels "empty and lonely" and has few friends. She had also a difficult time describing herself and noted that she would frequently think that she does not know who she "really is." She has had close relationships in the past, but she soon discovered that people were not "as nice as they initially seemed." and she then chose not to have them in her life. She has also struggled to stay in the same job for long, mostly because of feeling very incompetent and overwhelmed when her boss questions her or has a complaint, and she impulsively decides to leave. The patient denied any episodes of hypomania or mania, as well as any neurovegetative symptoms of depression. She also denied any suicidal or homicidal ideations, intent, or plan at the time of admission to the inpatient unit, as well as any presence of psychotic symptoms.

PSYCHIATRIC HISTORY

The patient's first contact with a mental health treatment provider was in her early teens when she was sent to the school counselor for "anger problems," which she reports that she continues to have. She had one previous inpatient admission for a similar overdose after a breakup with her boyfriend, but she continues to have "minor overdoses" when she feels "overwhelmed," where she takes "a few extra doses" of her medication to "deal with her anger." She is currently on fluoxetine (Prozac) 40 mg PO daily. She had a trial of valproic acid several years ago, which was stopped due to weight gain. She denied any history of physical violence, but she had frequent anger outbursts, during which she would hit the wall and scream at "whoever is around." She currently sees a therapist weekly and a psychiatrist for medication management every 3 months. She denied any history of childhood physical or sexual abuse, as well as any history of alcohol or illicit drug abuse. However, she described her parents as being "careless" and not very involved in the care of their children. She also denied any involvement with the legal system.

FAMILY HISTORY

The patient's mother was diagnosed with major depressive disorder in her 30s.

SOCIAL HISTORY

Ms O was born in Dallas, Texas, and was the second child of an intact family. Her father worked as a truck driver and spent long periods of time away from home. Her mother was a housewife. Ms O finished high school and took two semesters of college, but she quit school because she found college to be too "overwhelming." She currently works three times a week in retail, selling clothes at the local mall.

PERTINENT MEDICAL HISTORY

Patient denied any history of serious medical problems.

MENTAL STATUS EXAMINATION

Ms O presented as a slightly overweight Hispanic woman who looked her stated age of 34 years. She was casually dressed and her general hygiene was good. She was pleasant and cooperative but avoided eye contact.

Her speech was slowed, with appropriate volume and rhythm. Her psychomotor activity was normal. She had a full range of affect and her mood appeared depressed. Her thought process was goal oriented and appropriate. She denied any suicidal or homicidal ideations, intent, or plan, as well as any delusions, auditory or visual hallucinations, or obsessions. On the Folstein Mini-Mental State Examination, she scored 30/30 indicating that she had good cognitive functioning. Her insight was fair; she could not think of any other way of dealing with her "overwhelming feelings" that did not involve overdosing and she was unable to assess the negative consequences and risks of her action. Her judgment was poor.

PERTINENT PHYSICAL FINDINGS

Her vital signs included a temperature of 97.9°F, heart rate 74 per minute, blood pressure 100/80 mm Hg, and respiratory rate of 12 per minute. Oxygen saturation on room air was 99.0%. Her pupils were equal and reactive to light and accommodation. No jaundice, anemia, or lymphadenopathy was noted. The first and second heart sounds were heard and there was no murmur. Lungs were clear.

Abdomen was soft and nontender and there was no organomegaly. Bowel sounds were heard normally. Extremities showed normal capillary perfusion. Neurological examination was normal. She weighed 170 lb on admission.

LABORATORY DATA

The laboratory data obtained at admission revealed a BUN of 12 mg% and creatinine 0.7 mg%. HCO_3 was 23.7 mEq/L, with a chloride level of 105 mEq/L. The sodium level was 135 mEq/L, with a potassium level of 3.5 mEq/L. The white blood cells count was 6,500/cmm. Hemoglobin was 14.8 gm%, with a hematocrit of 40%. The platelet count was 300,000/cmm. VDRL was nonreactive. The fasting blood glucose was 90 mg%. TSH level was normal at 3.0 mIU/L.

HOSPITAL COURSE

Ms O was continued on fluoxetine 40 mg PO daily, since both the patient and her outpatient provider reported that the medication was helpful in controlling her anger outbursts and irritability. The treatment team considered starting a mood stabilizer to target her impulsivity and mood swings; however, after reviewing the risks and benefits of these medications, the patient decided against taking them. She was very concerned about weight gain and did not like to have the blood levels drawn.

During her hospital stay, she presented with calm and appropriate mood. She reported enjoying the "quiet environment and supportive staff in the hospital," although there was one particular nurse whom she disliked and refused to take medications from. She consistently denied any suicidal or homicidal ideations, intent, or plan as well as any urges to overdose or harm herself throughout her admission. A meeting with Ms O's outpatient treatment providers was held to decide the best treatment option for her. Both her psychiatrist and current therapist felt that the patient would benefit from a more comprehensive and intensive treatment modality. They also worried about the reinforcing effects of this admission and were concerned about the fact that the patient was "in no hurry to leave and go back to life." The treatment team contacted a local center that provided dialectical behavioral therapy (DBT) and discussed this option with Ms O. She was particularly looking forward to having the option of calling her therapist for "coaching sessions" on an as-needed basis and having particular sessions to learn skills. During her admission, the patient worked on identifying the triggers that made her take impulsive decisions and on coping skills to handle her emotional dysregulation in a more effective way. Several meetings with the patient's family members and the hospital's social worker were held to help her find options in the community and to help her with her financial concerns.

She was discharged after a 5-day inpatient admission. No signs of depressive, hypomanic, or manic episodes were noticed during her stay at the hospital. She was scheduled for an intake admission to start the DBT the day after her admission, and her current therapist agreed to continue meeting with her during this transition.

DISCHARGE MEDICATIONS

Fluoxetine 40 mg PO daily.

DSM-IV-TR MULTIAXIAL DIAGNOSIS

Axis I. None
Axis II. Borderline personality disorder (BPD)
Axis III. None
Axis IV. Severity of psychosocial stressor: moderate, problems at work and lack of social support
Axis V. Global assessment of functioning:

At admission: 30; significant mood lability and impulsivity, recent suicidal behavior, unable to function at home

At discharge: 55; moderate symptoms (occasional anger outbursts, housing instability, inability to find and keep social relationships)

FORMULATION

A. Diagnostic

This patient meets six out of the nine DSM-IV-TR criteria for BPD. She has a history of unstable relationships which she ends abruptly after devaluating them, chronic feelings of loneliness, impulsivity in quitting her job and spending money (unable to pay rent), recurrent thoughts of self-harm, marked reactivity to mood, and an unstable sense of self.

The distinction between BPD and several mood disorders can be challenging, and these two disorders commonly coexist. Important mood disorders to rule out in this case include a major depressive disorder, bipolar disorder, cyclothymia, and dysthymia. The duration of her depressed mood does not meet the criteria for either a major depressive disorder or dysthymia. In addition, she denied any neurovegetative signs of depression, such as fatigue, poor concentration, or changes in her appetite or sleep patterns. She also does not meet the criteria for a manic or hypomanic episode. Ruling out cyclothymia in patients with BPD can be particularly difficult. This patient presents with a long-standing history of frequent mood swings and impulsivity, which are common in cyclothymia. However, her mood swings are very short lived and seem to only appear in reaction to a particular stressor. She also does not present with grandiose mood, pressured speech, racing thoughts, or psychomotor agitation, which would point to a hypomanic episode. Her mood swings and impulsivity are better explained by her underlying personality disorder and her emotional dysregulation. One will also need to rule out mood disorder due to a medical condition and a substance-induced mood disorder. This patient denies any history of substance abuse and is not taking any medications known to induce mood symptoms. There are no particular reasons to believe that she has a condition that could cause mood symptoms, such as pregnancy, endocrine problems (e.g., thyroid or parathyroid problems, adrenocortical problems), vitamin B_{12} deficiency, neurological conditions (e.g., multiple sclerosis), autoimmune conditions (e.g., systemic lupus erythematosus), infections (e.g., HIV infection, mononucleosis), or cancers. However, routine laboratory tests to rule out a mood disorder due to a medical condition should include thyroid function tests and vitamin B_{12} and folate levels, among others.

This patient does not meet the criteria for other Axis I disorders, including anxiety disorders or substance abuse disorders, which are frequently seen in patients with BPD. She also does not meet the criteria for a psychotic or cognitive disorder.

Important Axis II disorders to rule out in patients with BPD include narcissistic personality disorder and dependent personality disorder. However, this patient is not showing any signs of needing others to make decisions for her or to give her continuous reassurance and support. On the contrary, she seems to make frequent impulsive decisions without being able to think before acting or getting advice from important people in her life. She also does not present with an arrogant attitude, a grandiose sense of self-importance, and does not seem to be focusing on success or needing to feel "special," which is characteristic of people with narcissistic features. Some of her behaviors could raise the diagnostic suspicion of antisocial personality disorder (ASPD) (e.g., her impulsivity, irritability, and failure to save money for her rent). However, there is no evidence of a history of conduct disorder during her childhood, she does not show any disregard to others, and she does not seem to lack remorse response. Therefore, this patient's primary diagnosis is BPD.

B. Etiologic

This patient denied a history of childhood sexual, physical, or emotional abuse, which is commonly encountered in patients with this illness. According to DBT, many adults with BPD have a predisposing emotional vulnerability and are raised in an environment experienced as "invalidating," in which a child's expression of emotions is met with erratic and sometimes extreme responses. Ms O described her parents as "careless" and "not involved in their children's care," which makes it important to rule out the presence of neglect and an environment lacking in nurture and warmth. The precipitating event for this patient's overdose and subsequent admission was the lack of money to pay the rent and the feelings of anger and frustration at not being able to negotiate a lower raise in the rent with her landlord. It will be important to identify in detail what this patient's usual triggers are for increased emotional dysregulation to be able to prevent further self-harm behaviors. On the other hand, this would also allow the treatment team to identify perpetuating factors that can lead to more suicide attempts or self-harm behaviors, as well as impulsive behaviors that significantly diminish this patient's quality of life.

C. Therapeutic

This patient has had a moderate response to treatment with a selective serotonin reuptake inhibitor (SSRI), which has shown to be helpful for depression, anxiety, and rejection sensitivity in patients with BPD. However, an important target in this patient's pharmacological treatment would be to reduce her impulsivity and mood lability. Some of the medications that have shown to be helpful for this goal include mood stabilizers and olanzapine. However, when starting a patient on a new psychotropic medication, it is of paramount importance, in addition to carefully reviewing the medication's side effect profile as well as the risks, benefits, and alternative treatments, to assess the patient's agreement with the treatment plan and compliance with medications. This patient was very firm in refusing to take either a mood stabilizer or an antipsychotic medication, and the chances of her complying with that recommendation were scarce. It will be important to communicate this to Ms O's outpatient provider, who would have a longer period of time to establish a therapeutic alliance with her and discuss the possibility of trying one of these medications.

Ms O presents with significant self-harm behavior and has had two suicide attempts. The treatment modality that has maximum evidence for effectiveness in treating suicidal behavior is DBT. She also would benefit from learning skills to help with her emotional dysregulation and from coaching calls to effectively deal with the episodes of anger and impulsivity that have led to important problems in her life. Another option to consider is psychodynamic psychotherapy, which has also shown to be effective in this population.

D. Prognostic

Ms O has some important positive prognostic factors, such as the lack of narcissistic entitlement, absence of substance abuse disorder, mood disorders or other psychiatric illnesses, and the absence of parental divorce. She has also been compliant with treatment in the past, which is another good prognostic factor. Although it was previously thought that BPD was a lifelong illness, current research has shown some remarkable remission rates across several years in this population. However, the presence of suicidality and self-harm behaviors highly raises the chance of a fatal incident in Ms O's presentation.

BORDERLINE PERSONALITY DISORDER

1. Introduction

Patients with BPD suffer from affective instability, unstable and sometimes enmeshed interpersonal relationships, problems with impulsivity, and suicidal or self-harming behaviors. Most researchers think that the core problem in BPD stems from a pervasive emotional dysregulation, secondary to genetic vulnerability, environmental stressors, and dysfunctional behavior. In many instances, it is a severe psychiatric illness associated with maladaptive functioning in several aspects of daily living, disability, high utilization of health resources, and a high suicide rate.

2. Epidemiology

This disorder affects approximately 1% to 1.5% of the adult population. The female-male ratio is 2:1 and it occurs up to five times more frequently among first degree relatives. Patients with BPD have been estimated to represent 6% of primary care outpatients, 15% of psychiatric outpatients, and 25% of psychiatric inpatients.

Both chronic and acute suicidality are important problems in patients with this disorder. The estimated rate of completed suicide in this population is approximately 10%. Rates of suicide peak between ages 18 and 30 years, and around 25% of subjects who completed suicide met the criteria for BPD. Important risk factors for completed suicide include the presence of comorbid substance abuse or major depressive disorder and the number of previous suicide attempts.

Comorbid psychiatric diagnoses are quite common among patients with this disorder. Commonly encountered comorbidities include mood disorders (36%), anxiety disorders (16%), and substance abuse disorders (40%). Patients with comorbid psychiatric diagnoses have lower rates of response to treatment.

3. Etiology

BPD is the personality disorder with the most extensive research behind it. Different theories have been developed over time to try to elucidate the pathophysiology of this illness. Otto Kernberg described patients with this disorder as suffering from severe character pathology, who were neither neurotic nor psychotic and who had unstable identities. They also used primitive defenses, such as splitting and projective identification, and lacked object constancy in their relationships.

Marsha Linehan, the creator of a therapeutic intervention for patients with BPD and self-harming behavior, used the biosocial theory to further understand the development of this disorder. She hypothesized that BPD is primarily a dysfunction of the emotion regulation system. Children with a preexistent emotional vulnerability are placed in an "invalidating environment," which supports and promotes emotional dysregulation. She described an "invalidating environment" as one in which communication of private experiences or feelings is usually met with erratic, inappropriate, or extreme responses. Interestingly, some studies have shown that patients with BPD have increased rates of soft neurological signs, attention deficit disorder, and abnormal EEG findings.

Risk factors associated with the development of BPD include an unstable family environment, family history of psychopathology, and childhood abuse. Child maltreatment has consistently been associated with the later development of BPD. In particular, children with a history of sexual abuse have four times more likelihood of developing BPD when compared with children without a history of sexual abuse. Studies have shown that the age of onset of the sexual abuse and its severity and chronicity are important in conferring risk for this personality disorder. BPD has also been associated with specific heritable traits such as impulsivity, neuroticism, and affective lability.

4. Diagnosis

Patients with BPD frequently complain of chronic feelings of emptiness and have a difficult time sustaining stable interpersonal relationships. Many of them engage in self-harm or suicidal behaviors and appear to live in a state of crisis. The diagnosis of BPD remains a clinical diagnosis.

According to the DSM-IV-TR, this diagnosis can be made in early adulthood if a patient meets at least five out of the nine described criteria (Table 3F.1). Patients with BPD interpret real or perceived abandonment as a personal rejection and the fear of being alone makes them engage in efforts to avoid this abandonment. They also have significant problems with object constancy; they usually can only have an image of the person who is in front of them based on that current interaction. They tend to idealize persons only to later devaluate them if they find any aspect of that person not meeting the patient's idealized image. Patients also have a very difficult time describing or keeping a stable, reliable self-image and thus feel "empty inside." The marked impulsivity seen in BPD can sometimes be confused with hypomanic or manic episodes since patients act in an impulsive, sometimes reckless, manner. They also have significant mood lability, which can change in a matter of hours; patients can report feeling depressed only to feel happy and optimistic a few hours afterward.

TABLE 3F.1 Diagnostic Criteria for Borderline Personality Disorder

A pervasive pattern of instability of interpersonal relationships, self-image, and affects and a marked impulsivity beginning by early adulthood and present in a variety of contexts, as indicated by at least five of the following:

1. Frantic efforts to avoid real or imagined abandonment (without including suicidal or self-mutilating behavior covered in Criterion 5)
2. A pattern of unstable and intense interpersonal relationships characterized by alternating between extremes of idealization and devaluation
3. Identity disturbance: markedly and persistently unstable self-image or sense of self
4. Impulsivity in at least two areas that are potentially self-damaging (e.g., spending, sex, substance abuse, reckless driving, binge eating)
5. Recurrent suicidal behavior, gestures, or threats or self-mutilating behavior
6. Affective instability due to a marked reactivity of mood (e.g., episodic dysphoria, irritability, or anxiety usually lasting a few hours and only rarely more than a few days)
7. Chronic feelings of emptiness
8. Inappropriate, intense anger or difficulty controlling anger (e.g., frequent displays of temper, constant anger, recurrent physical fights)
9. Transient, stress-related paranoid ideation or severe dissociative symptoms

Adapted from American Psychiatric Association. *Diagnostic and Statistical Manual of Mental Disorders: Text Revision.* Washington, DC: American Psychiatric Association, 2000.

TABLE 3F.2 Behavioral Patterns in Borderline Personality Disorder According to Marsha Linehan

1. *Emotional vulnerability*: Difficulties in regulating negative emotions
2. *Self-invalidation*: Failure to recognize one's own emotional responses
3. *Unrelenting crises*: Frequent negative environmental episodes
4. *Inhibited grieving*: Tendency to overcontrol negative emotional responses
5. *Active passivity*: Failure to solve one's own problems and instead engage others in solving problems
6. *Apparent competence*: Tendency to appear more competent than one actually is

Adapted from Linehan M. *Cognitive Behavioral Treatment of Borderline Personality Disorder*. New York, NY: The Guilford Press, 1993:10.

Another important aspect of BPD is the short-lived psychotic episodes (also referred to as micropsychotic episodes). Marsha Linehan described specific behavioral patterns that are common in BPD (Table 3F.2). One of the most severe problems encountered in patients with BPD is the suicidal and self-harming behaviors. Patients may superficially cut their wrists, burn themselves with a cigarette, or overdose on their medications. Even though the ratio of suicide attempts to committed suicides is high, the mortality rate in BPD reaches 10%, which is similar to that of schizophrenia. Although all normal individuals have some of these characteristics, these must be long-standing and intense for the diagnosis of BPD to be made.

5. Treatment

A. NONPHARMACOLOGICAL TREATMENTS

Different psychotherapeutic approaches with psychodynamic, cognitive, or behavioral orientations have been used for the treatment of BPD. Although there is no consensus in the field of what the best psychotherapy for this population is, the two treatments with maximum research to support their efficacy are psychodynamic psychotherapy and DBT. DBT has shown promising results, particularly in decreasing suicidal and self-harm behaviors. A recent study comparing DBT with nonbehavioral psychotherapy provided by experts showed that patients who received the former were half as likely to make a suicide attempt, required few hospitalizations for suicidal ideations, and had lower suicide risk across all suicide attempts and self-injurious behaviors. They also had lower rates of hospitalizations, lesser number of emergency visits, and fewer dropout rates. On the other hand, transference-focused psychotherapy has also shown to reduce suicidality in this disorder, as well as anger, irritability, and impulsivity, and in one study, it showed more efficacy than DBT in decreasing anger and irritability. Research seems to suggest that patients with BPD require prolonged treatments and seem to benefit from structured settings.

B. PHARMACOLOGICAL TREATMENTS

Although the primary treatment of BPD is considered to be psychotherapy, there has been a growing interest in finding effective medications to treat the core symptoms of BPD. Several different classes of psychotropic medications have been studied in patients with BPD. However, many of these studies have not been double-blind randomized, controlled trials and have had limited power due to a small sample size and a high frequency of comorbidities among the studied subjects. The two classes of medications with the maximum evidence-based support are SSRIs and the atypical antipsychotic olanzapine.

1. Antidepressants

SSRIs are considered by many experts to be the gold standard of pharmacological treatment in patients with BPD. Some of the randomized, controlled trials looking at SSRIs have found them to be beneficial in improving depression and anger ratings. A study comparing fluoxetine and placebo found that the SSRI was helpful in improving depression and anger ratings, although the improvement was never more than 20% of the baseline assessments. Another study found that patients on fluoxetine reported improvements in problems with aggression, with improvements noticed most consistently at the end of the second month of treatment. On the other hand, fluvoxamine was shown to reduce the symptoms of mood swings, but not aggressive or impulsive symptoms.

MAOIs have shown some positive results in the treatment of this condition. Tranylcypromine was studied in one double-blind placebo controlled study and was found to be of benefit in treating depression, anxiety, and rejection sensitivity, but it was not helpful in treating emotional dysregulation. Phenelzine has also shown to decrease symptomatology as measured by the Buss-Durkee Hostility Inventory. On the other hand, studies looking at the use of tricyclic antidepressants have not shown substantial positive reports of efficacy of these medications in the treatment of BPD. In addition, due to the low therapeutic window of this class of medications, one should be particularly careful in using tricyclics in patients with a history of self-harm behaviors.

2. Mood Stabilizers

Many studies examining the role of mood stabilizers in the treatment of BPD have focused on mood lability and anger problems. Depakote has been shown to reduce interpersonal sensitivity, anger, hostility, and impulsive aggression when compared to placebo in patients with BPD. There are also a few studies demonstrating the efficacy of topiramate and lamotrigine in the treatment of anger in BPD. The findings for carbamazepine have been mixed. One study showed dramatic results in reducing behavioral dyscontrol, as well as anger and anxiety, while another study did not find any significant effects of carbamazepine in the treatment of BPD. On the other hand, lithium has not shown to be consistently beneficial in the treatment of BPD.

3. Anxiolytics

Interestingly, it has been reported that patients with BPD who were taking alprazolam reported increased ratings of suicidality and behavioral dyscontrol. To date, there are no randomized, controlled trials showing that benzodiazepines are effective in the treatment of this condition.

4. Typical Antipsychotics

Typical antipsychotics, such as haloperidol, trifluoperazine, and thiothixene, have been shown to be helpful in treating depressive symptoms, interpersonal sensitivity, illusions, ideas of reference and psychoticism, hostility, and global functioning in patients with BPD. Another study found that patients on flupenthixol decanoate administered every 4 weeks had significantly fewer suicide attempts when compared with placebo.

5. Atypical Antipsychotics

The only atypical antipsychotic that has been studied in several randomized, controlled trials is olanzapine and the results have been consistently positive. This medication has been shown to be helpful in treating anxiety, paranoia, anger, and interpersonal sensitivity in patients with BPD. However, the side effect profile of this medication, including weight gain and the metabolic syndrome, should be carefully considered when prescribing olanzapine to patients with BPD.

6. Prognosis

Even though BPD is considered to be a psychiatric illness with a prolonged course of action, some newer studies suggest that the diagnosis is not as stable over time as previously thought. One study found that after a 6-year follow-up, approximately 75% of patients with BPD had achieved remission, and only 6% of these had a later recurrence. Poor prognostic factors include severity of affective instability, family history of mental illness, particularly maternal psychopathology, and history of childhood abuse.

7. General Formulation for BPD

A. DIAGNOSTIC

BPD is a Cluster B personality disorder that can be easily confounded with other psychiatric illness. When establishing the diagnosis, it is of paramount importance to consider several conditions in the differential diagnosis. The most common mood disorders in the differential diagnosis include major depressive disorder and bipolar disorder. Some key differences are the duration of depressive and hypomanic/manic symptoms, which usually last a few minutes or hours in patients with BPD in comparison with mood disorders, which have a more prolonged and defined duration of mood symptoms. On the other hand, mood disorders tend to present in more circumscribed episodes which usually remit, whereas BPD presents with more pervasive mood lability. Patients with mood disorders usually have more stable relationships and a clearer sense of self.

Narcissistic personality disorder, dependent personality disorder, and histrionic personality disorder are all important in the differential diagnosis of BPD. People with narcissistic personality disorder have a relatively more stable sense of self-image, less impulsivity, and less self-harming behavior, and they are more preoccupied with the feelings of value, worth, and respect. Patients with histrionic personality disorder also have difficulties with intimacy, but anger, self-harming behavior, and impulsivity are not core features of the disease. On the other hand, dependent personality disorder is also characterized by fear of abandonment, but relationships are more stable and there is less mood instability and less self-harm behavior.

One should also carefully rule out frequent comorbidities, such as anxiety, mood, and substance-induced disorders.

B. ETIOLOGIC

Important predisposing factors in BPD include biological factors, such as a family history of BPD, as well as psychological and social factors, such as a history of physical and sexual abuse or neglect. It is especially important to be aware of precipitating factors associated with suicide in patients with BPD. Although studies looking at this issue are scarce, some precipitating factors associated with suicide include recent losses or humiliating life events, affect instability, and presence of comorbidities, such as substance abuse or major depressive disorder.

C. THERAPEUTIC

Appropriate treatment should include both nonpharmacological and pharmacological approaches. The two therapies with maximum evidence to support them are psychodynamic psychotherapy and DBT. If patients have a high suicide risk or a high rate of self-harming behaviors, they may benefit more from a highly structured psychotherapeutic framework; DBT has shown to be particularly effective in improving suicidal and self-harming behaviors. In terms of pharmacological treatment, SSRIs and olanzapine are the medications with maximum evidence to support their use. On the other hand, mood stabilizers are frequently prescribed to target mood instability and irritability/anger.

D. PROGNOSTIC

Perpetuating factors and factors associated with relapse in BPD include the presence of alcohol-related problems or major depressive disorder as well as higher neuroticism and conscientiousness. On the other hand, protective and good prognostic factors include a high IQ, having a steady work or study status after remission, absence of narcissistic entitlement, and absence of parental divorce.

8. Risk Assessment

Risk assessment in BPD should include the risk for acute and chronic suicidality, considering important risk factors such as number and severity of previous attempts, and presence of comorbidities such as major depressive disorder and alcohol abuse. One should remember that even though many patients with BPD have nonlethal self-harm behaviors that may appear to be inconsequential, the rate of completed suicide among this population is 10%, as high as for other severe mental illnesses such as schizophrenia. When prescribing medications, one should assess the risk for overdose and be careful in prescribing medications with a low therapeutic window, such as tricyclics.

KEY POINTS (ABPN Examination)

A. When interviewing a patient with suspected Borderline Personality Disorder

1. Patients can often present with rapidly changing mood lability, which can be easily mistaken for a mood disorder.
2. Do not forget to make a thorough assessment of safety, including suicidal ideations, intent, or plans, as well as any recent self-harm behavior, such as cutting or overdosing.

B. When presenting a patient with suspected Borderline Personality Disorder

1. Acknowledge that the diagnosis of a personality disorder cannot be made during an acute crisis and that the presence of a more pervasive and long-standing behavioral pattern must be present to make the correct diagnosis.
2. If diagnosis is unclear, state that you would use a structured diagnostic interview like SCID-DSM-IV for clarification.

(continued)

KEY POINTS (ABPN Examination) (Continued)

3. Assess both chronic and acute risk of suicidality; many of these patients report chronic, if not daily, suicidal ideations, which makes it of paramount importance to be able to assess what the patient's baseline functioning is and what the current risk for suicidality is.
4. Do not forget to ask about any history of physical, sexual, or emotional abuse, which is quite common in patients with BPD.
5. Ask about comorbidities, particularly mood disorders, anxiety disorders, and substance abuse disorders, which have a high prevalence among this population.

Suggested Readings

Abraham PF, Calabrese JR. Evidence-based pharmacological treatment of borderline personality disorder: A shift from SSRIs to anticonvulsants and atypical antipsychotics? *J Affect Disord* 2008 Nov;111(1):21–30.

American Psychiatric Association. *Diagnostic and Statistical Manual of Mental Disorders: Text Revision*. Washington, DC: American Psychiatric Association, 2000.

Bohus M, Schmahl C. Psychopathology and treatment of BPD. *Nervenarzt* 2007 Sep;78(9): 1069–1080.

Bradley R, Jenei J, Westen D. Etiology of BPD. *J Nerv Ment Dis* 2005;193:24–31.

Coccaro EF, Kavoussi RJ. Fluoxetine and impulsive aggressive behavior in personality disordered subjects. *Arch Gen Psychiatry* 1997;54: 1081–1088.

Cowdry RW, Gardner DL. Pharmacotherapy of borderline personality disorder: Alprazolam, carbamazepine, trifluoperazine, and tranylcypromine. *Arch Gen Psychiatry* 1988;45: 111–119.

De la Fuente J, Lotstra F. A trial of carbamazepine in borderline personality disorder. *Eur Neuropsychopharmacol* 1994;4:479–486.

De la Fuente JM, Tugendhaft P, Mavroudakis N. Electroencephalographic abnormalities in BPD. *Psychiatr Res* 1998;77(2):131–138.

Frankenburg FR, Zanarini MC. Divalproex sodium treatment of women with borderline personality disorder and bipolar II disorder: A double-blind, placebo-controlled pilot study. *J Clin Psychiatry* 2002;63:443–446.

Gunderson JG. *BPD-A Clinical Guide*. Washington, DC: American Psychiatric Press, 2001.

Hollander E, Allen A, Lopez RP, et al. A preliminary doubleblind, placebo-controlled trial of divalproex sodium in borderline personality disorder. *J Clin Psychiatry* 2001;62:199–203.

Levy KN, Yeomans FE, Diamond D. Psychodynamic treatments of self-injury. *J Clin Psychol* 2007 Nov;639(11):1105–1120.

Lieb K, Zanarini MC, Schmal C, et al. Borderline personality disorder. *Lancet* 2004;364(9432): 453–461.

Linehan M. *Cognitive Behavioral Treatment of Borderline Personality Disorder*. New York, NY: The Guilford Press, 1993.

Linehan MM, Comtois KA, Murray AM, et al. Two-year randomized controlled trial and follow-up of dialectical behavior therapy vs. therapy by experts for suicidal behaviors and borderline personality disorder. *Arch Gen Psychiatry* 2006 Jul;63(7):757–766.

Marcus J, Ovsiew F, Hans S. Neurological dysfunction in borderline children. In: *The Borderline Child*. New York, NY: McGraw Hill, 1982:171.

Oldham JM. BPD: An overview. *Psychiatr Times* 2004;21(8).

Paris J. Chronic suicidality among patients with BPD. *Psychiatr Serv* 2002;53:738–742.

Quigley, BD. Diagnostic relapse in borderline personality disorder: Risk and protective factors. Doctoral Dissertation, Texas A&M University, August 2003.

Rinne T, van den Brink W, Wouters L, et al. SSRI treatment of borderline personality disorder: A randomized, placebo-controlled clinical trial for female patients with borderline personality disorder. *Am J Psychiatry* 2002;159:2048–2054.

Soloff PH, Cornelius J, George A, et al. Efficacy of phenelzine and haloperidol. *Arch Gen Psychiatry* 1993;50:377–385.

Tragesser SL, Solhan M, Schwarzt-Mette R, et al. The role of affective instability and impulsivity in predicting future BPD features. *J Personal Disord* 2007 Dec;21(6):603–614.

Zanarini MC, Frankenburg FR, Hennen J, et al. The longitudinal course of borderline psychopathology: 6-year prospective follow-up of the phenomenology of borderline personality disorder. *Am J Psychiatry* 2003;160: 274–283.

II. ANTISOCIAL PERSONALITY DISORDER

CASE HISTORY

PRESENT ILLNESS

Mr P is a 35-year-old white male with a long-standing history of recurrent major depressive disorder (MDD) who was admitted to a psychiatric facility following a severe suicide attempt. He stated that he had been feeling progressively more depressed during the past 3 months and had been having an increase in suicidal thoughts over the last week. He felt tired most of the time and had problems concentrating. He felt hopeless about life, found his job and his personal life unsatisfactory, and worried a lot about his critical financial situation. He was unable to think about reasons to continue living, even though he has an extensive family, who lives close to him, and several children from different partners. A few days prior to his admission, he went to a local casino for the first time in years and lost a significant proportion of his savings. He then came back home, drank a bottle of wine, and slit his wrists. He was found by a neighbor, who stopped by the patient's house to ask him to pay him back some money that he owed.

The patient was brought in to the hospital by ambulance and medically stabilized before being transferred to the psychiatric inpatient unit. At admission, he reported passive suicidal ideations but stated feeling safe in the hospital. He denied any homicidal ideations, intent, or plan, as well as any psychotic symptoms. He also denied any recent use of illicit drugs and reported drinking two beers and around two glasses of wine per day. He denied any presence of withdrawal symptoms, except for mild headache.

PSYCHIATRIC HISTORY

Patient recalls having some contact with the school counselor at his elementary school for bullying other kids, frequent lying, and cheating. The school recommended follow-up in an outpatient mental health center, but his parents never followed up with these recommendations. He was first diagnosed with MDD at age 25 and had one previous suicide attempt at age 27, which required inpatient hospitalization. He has been intermittently compliant with outpatient treatment and was on escitalopram 20 mg PO daily, for several months, which he stopped 6 months ago due to sexual side effects.

He has an extensive substance abuse history and used cocaine daily for several years starting in his teens. He stopped using cocaine 2 years ago when he was taken to the emergency department for chest pain and palpitations after inhaling this drug. He also reported drinking an average of two beers and two glasses of wine daily for the past 10 years. He tried stopping once several years ago and was admitted for an inpatient rehabilitation program, but he relapsed soon after being discharged from the program. He currently does not have any interest in reducing his alcohol intake and does not see it as a problem in his life. He denied any history of withdrawal seizures or delirium tremens.

Mr P also has had several contacts with the legal system in the past and was arrested twice in the last 2 years for possession of drugs and a Driving under the influence (DUI) and for robbing a local convenience store. He served 6 months in prison and is currently on probation. He reported getting into physical fights frequently, mostly due to altercations at bars or because of not "paying back on time." He also denies a significant history of gambling problems, except for the recent episode in which he lost a lot of money.

FAMILY HISTORY

His mother was diagnosed with bipolar disorder and somatization disorder; father had a history of alcohol dependence.

SOCIAL HISTORY

Mr P was born and raised in Connecticut; he was the third of four boys. His parents divorced when he was 5 years old, and he has had an intermittent and inconsistent contact with his father since then. He recalls his father as being frequently intoxicated and physically abusive to his mother and all children. After the divorce, his mother had to start working at the local supermarket to pay the bills and to care for her sons. He recalls his mother as "good when she wasn't having one of her episodes." She suffered from bipolar disorder and had to be hospitalized several times during the patient's childhood. Mr P was seen as the "leader" of a group of friends in school who would frequently bully younger children. He was kicked out of high school after cheating on an important final test and decided not to go back. He has held many jobs throughout his life, including driving trucks and working in Wal-Mart and in local restaurants, but he is currently not working. He was never married but had several relationships with female partners. He is the father of three children by different mothers. He does not pay child support and sees them occasionally and did not show any signs of remorse for the fact that he is not participating financially or emotionally in his children's lives. One of his main current stressors is the fact that he owes money to several of his acquaintances, has failed to pay them back, and has moved to different cities in order to avoid being found by his lenders. Even though he currently has a job, he does not see paying his debts as a priority.

PERTINENT MEDICAL HISTORY

Patient reported a history of occasional chest pain immediately after inhaling cocaine. He has had several stress tests done with negative results. He also has chronic asthma. He denied any other medical problems.

MENTAL STATUS EXAMINATION

Mr P presented as a well-developed and well-nourished white man who looked his stated age of 35 years. He was casually dressed in jeans and a T-shirt, and his general hygiene was good. He was pleasant and cooperative and showed good eye contact. His speech was normal in rhythm, volume, and speed. He reported "sad" mood with constricted, mood-appropriate affect. His thought process was goal oriented and appropriate. He reported passive suicidal ideations with the plan to cut his wrists or jump from the window, but he denied an active intent and reported feeling safe in the hospital. He denied homicidal ideations, intent, or plan as well as any delusions, auditory or visual hallucinations, or obsessions. On the Folstein Mini-Mental State Examination, he scored 30/30 indicating that he had good cognitive functioning. His insight was fair; he could identify some precipitating factors that led to the suicide attempt but did not see his intermittent compliance with treatment as a contributing factor. His judgment was also fair; he was still unsure of his willingness to comply with the treatment after his discharge.

PERTINENT PHYSICAL FINDINGS

His vital signs were a temperature of 97.1°F, heart rate 68 per minute, blood pressure 124/82 mm Hg, and respiratory rate of 14 per minute. Oxygen saturation on room air was 99.0%. His pupils were equal and reactive to light and accommodation. No jaundice, anemia, or lymphadenopathy was noted. The first and second heart sounds were heard and there was no murmur. Lungs were clear. Abdomen was soft, nontender and there was no organomegaly. Bowel sounds were heard normally. Extremities showed normal capillary perfusion. Neurological examination was normal. He weighed 200 lb. on admission.

LABORATORY DATA

The laboratory data obtained on admission revealed a BUN of 13 mg% and creatinine 1.0 mg%. HCO_3 was 23.5 mEq/L, with a chloride level of 104 mEq/L. The sodium level was 135 mEq/L, with a potassium level of 4.0 mEq/L. The white blood cells count was 7,000/cmm. Hemoglobin was 15.8 gm% with a hematocrit of 41%. The platelet count was 200,000/cmm. VDRL was nonreactive. The fasting blood glucose was 85 mg%. TSH level was normal.

HOSPITAL COURSE

Mr P was admitted to the psychiatric inpatient unit and was initially placed on constant observation due to his active suicidal ideations with a plan to jump from a window and his history of impulsive, reckless behavior. Since he had a history of sexual side effects while on an SSRI and this was a major concern for him, he was started on bupropion SR, 150 mg PO daily, which was increased over the course of one week to a final dose of 300 mg PO daily. He was placed on a detoxification protocol with lorazepam as needed, folate, vitamin B_{12}, and multivitamins. He experienced minimal alcohol withdrawal symptoms, with Clinical Institite Withdrawal Assessment of Alcohol Scale (CIWA) scores below the threshold for the need of medications. The lorazepam taper was discontinued after 3 days, and since his mood was improving and he consistently denied any more suicidal or homicidal ideations, intent, or plan, the constant observation precautions were discontinued.

During his hospital stay, he presented with calm, improving mood and was always charming with other patients and staff members. In individual therapy sessions, he would present as engaging and cooperative, but he would not provide any specific details of his interpersonal problems, his current legal situation, or about what he would like to change in order to live a happier life and would direct the conversation to topics unrelated to his treatment.

On the seventh day after his admission, he requested to be discharged from the hospital. At the time, he denied any depressive symptom, any suicidal or homicidal thoughts, as well as any side effects from bupropion. The treatment team offered to schedule an outpatient appointment for him to start cognitive behavioral therapy (CBT), but he refused, stating that he had no interest in "talk therapy." Outpatient treatment programs for his alcohol abuse were also offered, but the patient stated that he was also not interested in pursuing them. However, he agreed to follow up with an outpatient psychiatrist to continue his psychotropic medication management. No family meetings were held since the patient did not want his family to know about his psychiatric admission. However, the treatment team was able to contact the patient's current girlfriend, who felt that Mr P was now "his usual self and ready to come home." He was discharged home with the plan to follow up with an outpatient psychiatrist for medication management a week after his discharge.

DISCHARGE MEDICATIONS

Bupropion SR, 300 mg PO daily.

DSM-IV-TR MULTIAXIAL DIAGNOSIS

Axis I. Major depressive disorder; severe and recurrent, without psychotic features
Alcohol abuse
Cocaine dependence in full remission
Axis II. ASPD
Axis III. Asthma; history of cocaine—induced chest pain
Axis IV. Severity of psychosocial stressor: severe, currently on probation, severe financial difficulties, no income
Axis V. Global Assessment of Functioning:

At admission: 20; some danger of hurting self due to the presence of significant suicidal ideations with plan

At discharge: 50; unable to keep a job, persistence of some depressive symptoms

FORMULATION

A. Diagnostic

This patient meets six out of the seven clinical criteria for the diagnosis of ASPD according to the DSM-IV-TR. He is unable to conform to social norms and has been arrested in several occasions. He frequently asks friends for money and then moves to different cities to avoid paying them back. He also shows a pattern of impulsivity, as evidenced by his suicide attempts in the context of losing money. He also shows consistent irresponsibility, as evidenced by not honoring his debts and having a history of being unable to stay in jobs for prolonged periods of time. He has a history of aggressive behavior and reports frequently getting into physical fights. Finally, he was unable to show remorse when asked about his responsibilities toward his children and the fact that he is not paying any child support. He also has a history of conduct disorder as a child and is over 18 years of age, which are all required criteria for the diagnosis of this personality disorder.

Important diagnoses to rule out in this patient include bipolar disorder, which can also present with impulsivity and reckless behavior. However, this patient did not have a history of elevated mood or neurovegetative symptoms of mania, such as decreased need for sleep, increased psychomotor activity, racing thoughts, or increased energy. Schizophrenia would be highly unlikely in this patient since there is no history of either positive symptoms of schizophrenia, such as hallucinations or delusions, or negative symptoms, such as social isolation or flat affect. On the contrary, the patient was quite charming and engaging during his stay in the hospital. An important factor to rule out is antisocial behavior related to a substance use disorder. However, this patient has a history of antisocial behavior in periods where he was not consuming drugs, and his antisocial behavior does not seem to be bound to periods where he is intoxicated or experiencing withdrawal symptoms.

Important personality disorders to rule out in this patient include narcissistic personality disorder and histrionic personality disorder. Patients with narcissistic personality disorder also show lack of empathy and can be exploitative at times. However, their central preoccupation revolves around feeling "unique" and "special," needing constant admiration, and dreaming about power and success, all of which are not seen in this patient's presentation. This patient's charm could raise the suspicion of histrionic personality disorder. However, he lacks the self-dramatization, the need to be the center of attention, and easy suggestibility, which characterizes histrionic personality disorder.

Patients with ASPD often produce a negative and occasionally hostile counter transference in their treaters. Staff often feels manipulated by this type of patients; it is frequently hard to come to terms with their criminal and violent histories. However, there is the risk of missing important diagnoses that could potentially be treated in patients with ASPD. This patient presents with clear criteria for a major depressive episode that warrants pharmacological treatment and psychotherapy. Diagnoses to rule out include substance-induced mood disorder, which could be secondary to his alcohol use, and mood disorders due to a medical condition. However, recent data suggest that if a patient meets the criteria for major depressive disorder, he should be treated with pharmacological agents even in the presence of a concurrent substance use disorder. On the other hand, the laboratory results did not point to a particular medical disorder that could be contributing to his depressive episode.

Mr P meets the criteria for alcohol abuse since he has used the substance while driving and was actually arrested for it. However, he does not meet the criteria for alcohol dependence at the time since he does not need increased amounts of alcohol to achieve intoxication and he does not experience withdrawal symptoms. He does not show a persistent desire to control or reduce his alcohol use, he does not spend a great deal of time in activities necessary to obtain alcohol, and he does not think alcohol is a problem for him. His cocaine abuse is currently in sustained full remission since he has not met the criteria for cocaine abuse or dependence in over 12 months.

B. Etiologic

This patient has some important biological, psychological, and social predisposing factors for ASPD. Even though his father was not formally diagnosed with this disorder, the fact that he was physically abusive to his wife and his children and that he failed to act as a responsible father in providing financial and emotional support for his family strongly suggests the presence of antisocial traits. His father's history of alcohol dependence and his mother's history of somatization disorder have both been associated with the development of ASPD. It is unknown if he has any genetic or neuroanatomic risk factors, such as decreased prefrontal gray matter volume, that could contribute to his risk for ASPD. He was exposed to physical and emotional abuse as a child, which is the most consistent predisposing factor for ASPD. Some perpetuating factors that are present in his presentation include his continuous abuse of alcohol.

C. Therapeutic

Mr P requires therapeutic interventions for different aspects of his clinical presentation. His major depressive disorder should be treated with an antidepressant. Due to his history of SSRI-induced sexual side effects and his history of poor compliance with treatment, the treatment team should spend a significant amount of time discussing different treatment options, risks and benefits, and alternative treatments with him. Bupropion, which is not associated with sexual side effects, is a good treatment option for him.

In regard to his alcohol abuse, the most important factor is to assess how the patient feels about this and what his treatment alternatives are. This patient does not think alcohol is a problem in his life, and he has no interest in quitting at this point. Since he is in a precontemplation stage, the most beneficial intervention for him would be to use motivational interviewing, so that he can start to become aware of the problematic aspects of his alcohol intake, such as getting arrested for driving under the influence or getting into fights when he is drinking in bars, to move him to a contemplation stage. Once he reaches the action stage, one can decide if he would benefit from a 12-step program or from pharmacological interventions, such as disulfiram or acamprosate, among others.

The most difficult aspect of this patient's treatment is his ASPD. There are no randomized, controlled trials looking at the use of medications in this disorder. Scant case reports are the only current evidence for the pharmacological treatment of ASPD. On the other hand, some psychotherapeutic interventions, such as CBT or group therapy, have shown some benefit in treating ASPD and should be offered as treatment options for patients. Unfortunately, Mr P is not interested in pursuing psychotherapy, which is a frequent problem in patients with ASPD.

D. Prognostic

Mr P presents with several poor prognostic factors in ASPD. He shows a diversity of deviant behavior, such as robbing, lying, and stealing money from friends. He also has a current diagnosis of alcohol abuse, which is considered a poor prognostic factor in this personality disorder. However, he was able to stop using cocaine and has been in sustained full remission for 2 years. He is now 35 years old, which has been associated with a decline in antisocial behaviors. In terms of his suicidal behavior, he has important risk factors for another suicide attempt. He has had prior suicide attempts, which is the most important risk factor for future suicidality; he is a white male, he abuses alcohol, and he meets the criteria for a major mood disorder, which are all risk factors for a future suicide attempt.

ANTISOCIAL PERSONALITY DISORDER

1. Introduction

Patients with ASPD have difficulties conforming to social norms and obligations, difficulties respecting the rights of others, criminal tendency, and lack of remorse. These difficulties start during childhood and persist into adulthood. This personality disorder is frequently encountered in prisons and correctional facilities. Recent research has helped to further clarify the etiology and prognosis of this prevalent and particularly challenging personality disorder.

2. Epidemiology

Three percent of the male population and 1% of the female population meet the criteria for ASPD. However, approximately 75% of male inmates and 56% of female inmates in prisons meet the criteria for this disorder. The prevalence peaks between the ages of 24 and 44 years and decreases at the ages of 45 to 64 years. ASPD is five times more common among first degree relatives, and the risk seems to be higher among the offspring of females with ASPD.

This personality disorder has been associated with several psychiatric disorders, including substance use disorders, mood disorders, anxiety disorders, and impulse disorders, such as pathological gambling. Among alcoholics, approximately 49% of men and 20% of women meet the criteria for ASPD. ASPD is also comorbid among patients who abuse illicit drugs. A recent study found that 40% of pathological gamblers had ASPD in comparison to 3.2% of controls. Other studies have linked the presence of somatization disorder and ASPD among first degree relatives; interestingly, in a family with a member with ASPD, female relatives have higher rates of somatization disorder and male relatives have higher rates of ASPD.

Longitudinal studies examining the natural history of ASPD suggest that approximately one third of patients experience remission, another third experience some improvement without remission, and 40% do not experience an improvement. Mortality rates are high in this population, both from natural and unnatural causes. Patients with ASPD also have a high prevalence of traumatic injuries, accidents, and suicide attempts. Medical problems are also common in this population. ASPD has been associated with a higher frequency of past-year medical conditions, coronary heart and gastrointestinal diseases, liver diseases, arthritis, a number of inpatient hospitalizations, inpatient days, emergency department visits, and injuries.

3. Etiology

Biological, genetic, and environmental factors seem to play an important role in the development of ASPD. There has been increasing interest in recent years in identifying genetic markers involved in the development of psychiatric problems, including aggression and antisocial behaviors. Although studies trying to identify specific genes related to the development of sociopathy and ASPD have yielded mixed results, some have reported an association between the short alleles of the serotonin transporter–linked polymorphic region in conferring a higher risk for the development of aggression. On the other hand, the absence of a functional monoamine oxidase-A (MAO-A) gene has also been associated with violence and aggression. A recent study found that adults who had been maltreated as children who had the high-risk MAO-A alleles were more likely to develop conduct disorder, antisocial personality symptoms, and violence than adults maltreated as children with the low-risk MAO-A alleles, with this latter group having rates of these problems that were comparable to the nonmaltreated control subjects. This suggests that there is an interaction between environmental factors and a genetic susceptibility in increasing the risk of aggression and ASPD. However, another study found that this gene and environmental interaction was only valid when comparing children exposed to low versus moderate trauma and that children exposed to severe trauma had higher aggression levels regardless of genotype, which suggests that this particular gene ceases to exert any protection when the environment becomes extremely aversive.

Researchers have speculated that damage to the prefrontal lobe can cause sociopath-like behavior. Recent studies have shown that psychopathy levels are associated with low prefrontal gray volumes. Interestingly, when looking at psychopaths who had been unsuccessful in staying away from the legal system, these subjects had a 22% reduction in prefrontal gray volumes when compared to controls. However, there were no significant differences in prefrontal gray volume between psychopaths who had been successful in not "being caught" by the legal system and controls. Another study found that subjects with ASPD had a 11% reduction in prefrontal gray matter volume without the presence of clear brain lesions, in addition to reduced autonomic activity during the tested measure. Since the prefrontal cortex plays a role in fear conditioning and stress responsivity, the authors suggest that this reduction in gray matter and in autonomic activity could predispose patients with ASPD to be less responsive to punishments or social norms and to make choices which are more risky and less socially adaptive.

Child maltreatment, including physical and sexual abuse, as well as neglect and exposure to domestic violence have been consistently associated with the development of aggression and sociopathy. Some of the risk factors associated with the development of violence and ASPD include a history of child maltreatment, large family size, poverty, living in a high-crime neighborhood, having been in foster care and a family history of ASPD, externalizing disorders, and alcohol abuse. On the other hand, protective factors for the development of ASPD include an easy temperament and good problem-solving skills, in addition to parental cooperation, high level of family support, secure attachment, and effective discipline practices.

4. Diagnosis

In 1941, Hervey Cleckley described 16 criteria to define what was then called "psychopathy." He used the term "the mask of sanity" to describe the superficial charm and calm attitude that often characterizes these patients. Some of his other clinical criteria included the lack of anxiety, unreliability, deceitfulness, lack of remorse, inadequately motivated antisocial behavior, failure to learn from punishment, egocentricity, poverty of affect and emotional bonds, lack of insight, and failure to plan ahead. Many of his criteria are still valid when making the diagnosis of ASPD.

The DSM-IV-TR requires the presence of a pervasive pattern of disregard for and violation of other people's rights since the age of 15 years, in addition to at least three of the core features of ASPD (Table 3F.3).

Clinicians often describe being shocked while listening to the complicated and disordered personal stories of patients who at first sight seem quite charming and "in control." Patients can describe having been involved in violent crimes, participating in illegal activities, or having deceived people in their lives without expressing much anxiety or discomfort. They frequently find excuses to exonerate them from their hurtful behavior, or in more severe cases, they simply acknowledge that they are not remorseful of their actions. They are usually manipulative and tend to be particularly abusive toward people they see as "weaker" (e.g., wives, children). They show lack of impulse control and often engage in reckless behaviors; they frequently don't plan ahead and are unable to think about the

TABLE 3F.3 Diagnostic Criteria for Antisocial Personality Disorder

A. *A pervasive pattern of instability of disregard for and violation of the rights of others occurring since the age of 15 years, as indicated by three (or more) of the following:* 1. Failure to conform to social norms with respect to lawful behaviors as indicated by repeatedly performing acts that are grounds for arrest 2. Deceitfulness, as indicated by repeated lying, use of aliases, or conning others for personal profit or pleasure 3. Impulsivity or failure to plan ahead 4. Irritability and aggressiveness, as indicated by repeated physical fights or assaults 5. Reckless disregard for the safety of self or others 6. Consistent irresponsibility, as indicated by repeated failure to sustain consistent work behavior or honor financial obligations 7. Lack of remorse, as indicated by being indifferent to or rationalizing having hurt, mistreated, or stolen from another
B. The individual is at least 18 years of age
C. There is evidence of conduct disorder with onset before the age of 15 years
D. The occurrence of antisocial behavior is not exclusive during the course of schizophrenia or a manic episode

Adapted from American Psychiatric Association. *Diagnostic and Statistical Manual of Mental Disorders: Text Revision*. American Psychiatric Association, 2000.

consequences of their actions. They may abandon their job, without thinking about how they will pay their bills or find a new job, and they may also change relationships in an abrupt manner. They are also frequently arrogant (they may think that working or a specific romantic partner is beneath them) and show a consistent lack of empathy.

On the other hand, even though it could appear as if patients with ASPD are self-entitled and oblivious to the outside world, these individuals suffer from elevated rates of mood disorders, particularly major depressive disorder and suicidal tendency. The presence of high negative emotionality, impulsivity, and low constraint seem to be strongly associated with suicidal behavior in this population. ASPD is associated with many psychiatric and medical comorbid illnesses, which should always be ruled out when examining a patient with this disorder (Table 3F.4).

5. Treatment

A. NONPHARMACOLOGICAL TREATMENTS

Patients with ASPD rarely come to treatment voluntarily and instead are usually referred by the legal system or other sources. The lack of motivation for change, poor insight, and fear of intimacy make the psychotherapeutic treatment of ASPD particularly challenging. It is unclear if intensive psychoanalytic treatment of this condition is helpful, and there are limited data that point to the contrary. Group therapy has shown to be helpful in some patients with ASPD, since individuals with this disorder tend to feel more comfortable in discussing their symptoms and problems with other peers.

CBT has shown some positive results in the treatment of ASPD, especially in the residential setting. Many of these structured programs integrate specific modalities for ASPD, such as training manuals for the development of social skills and moral thinking and aggression management.

Multisystemic Therapy was developed to treat children and adolescents with antisocial behaviors. This treatment modality believes that antisocial behavior is caused by several factors in a child's multisystemic social network and that an effective treatment strategy should intervene in all the affected systems. Multisystemic Therapy has shown to significantly reduce the number of violent crimes, drug abuse, school

TABLE 3F.4 Disorders Comorbid with Antisocial Personality Disorder

A. Psychiatric Disorders	B. Medical Disorders
Mood disorders	Traumatic brain injuries
Substance use disorders	Coronary heart disease
Anxiety disorders, posttraumatic stress disorder	Liver disease
Impulse disorders	Arthritis
Narcissistic personality disorder	
BPD	
Histrionic personality disorder	
Somatization disorder	

problems, mental health problems, and family functioning.

B. PHARMACOLOGICAL TREATMENTS

There are very limited data to show that pharmacotherapy is beneficial in the treatment of ASPD. A few case reports have documented the efficacy of quetiapine in treating impulsivity, hostility, aggressiveness, irritability, and rage reactions in patients with ASPD. Another case report described risperidone as being effective in treating aggression and impulsivity in one patient with ASPD. One study found valproic acid to be somewhat helpful in treating aggression in small number of patients with ASPD. In summary, there is currently not enough evidence to suggest that pharmacotherapy is helpful in the treatment of ASPD. Pharmacotherapy in this population should only be used when necessary and in the presence of comorbid conditions, such as mood or anxiety disorders.

6. Prognosis

Few studies have followed patients with ASPD over long periods of time. However, this disorder seems to have a chronic course and can become less marked or even reach remission as the individuals reach the fourth decade of life. The prevalence of ASPD peaks in persons aged 24 to 44 years and drops off in persons aged 45 to 64 years. One study followed subjects with ASPD over an average of 29 years and found that 27% of subjects had remitted, 31% had improved, and 42% did not show an improvement. Persons with ASPD also have less legal problems as they age. However, one study showed that even though convictions decline with age in ASPD, many of these individuals continue to be criminally active.

7. General Formulation for ASPD

A. DIAGNOSTIC

ASPD is a cluster B personality disorder that can only be diagnosed if a patient has a history of symptoms of conduct disorder. Substance use disorders can obscure and complicate the accurate diagnosis of ASPD. Antisocial behaviors, aggression, and violence are commonly encountered among subjects who are acutely intoxicated. Furthermore, individuals may engage in criminal behavior to obtain the drug of choice when they are undergoing withdrawal symptoms. Therefore, in order to accurately diagnose ASPD, one must elucidate if the antisocial symptoms were present during childhood and in periods of time where the patient was not using substances. Bipolar disorder should also be included in the differential diagnosis of ASPD. During the course of a manic episode, patients can engage in reckless, impulsive behavior that may resemble some of the characteristics of ASPD. However, a manic episode is time limited and is not characterized by a chronic and long-standing pattern of reckless, impulsive behavior in addition to criminality and aggression. Patients with schizophrenia can also show erratic and impulsive behaviors, as well as problems with conforming to social norms, but this is usually in relation to a specific delusion, and it is accompanied by perceptual alterations and negative symptoms of schizophrenia, which are not part of ASPD.

Narcissistic personality disorder, histrionic personality disorder, and BPD should be included in the differential diagnosis of ASPD. Patients with narcissistic personality disorder also show a similar superficial pattern in their relationships, a grandiose sense of self, and a lack of empathy for others.

However, patients with narcissistic personality disorder are not characterized by showing a disregard for the rights of others and for social norms. They also do not engage in criminal or irresponsible acts and are more preoccupied with feelings of envy and admiration than patients with ASPD. Patients with histrionic personality disorder can be reckless and impulsive and also are superficial in their relationships. However, they do not usually engage in antisocial acts and frequently show exaggerated and inflated emotions, which are not commonly seen in patients with ASPD. Patients with BPD are often described as manipulative and impulsive. However, their main goal is to receive attention, or validation, whereas patients with ASPD manipulate for secondary purposes, such as money or power.

B. ETIOLOGIC

Important predisposing biological factors for ASPD include the family history of sociopathy, somatization disorder, and substance abuse. Ongoing research suggests that some candidate genes, such as the MAO-A gene or the serotonin transporter gene, could play a role in the development of antisocial symptoms, particularly in the presence of exposure to childhood abuse and significant trauma. Low prefrontal gray matter volumes have also recently been shown to be associated with ASPD. The most consistent predisposing factor for the development of aggression and ASPD is child maltreatment. This risk factor seems to act in an additive and perpetuating manner; the risk of ASPD seems to correlate with the severity and chronicity of the exposure to abuse and trauma during childhood and adolescence. Other psychological and social predisposing factors include poverty and urban settings, living in a high-crime neighborhood, and having been in foster care.

C. THERAPEUTIC

The treatment of ASPD is challenging since patients rarely come for treatment on a voluntary basis. There is some evidence to suggest that CBT can be helpful in adults with ASPD and children with conduct disorder. Multisystemic Therapy has also been found to be beneficial for children and adolescents with antisocial behaviors. The evidence for the utility of psychodynamic approaches in the treatment of ASPD is conflicting. Patients may also benefit from group therapy, since they usually find it easier to disclose their complicated histories among peers.

Evidence for the pharmacological treatment of ASPD is scarce, if not nonexistent. Case studies have reported beneficial effects of risperidone, quetiapine, and valproic acid in decreasing aggression and impulsivity in patients with ASPD. However, more research is needed to be able to make any evidence-based recommendations for the pharmacological treatment of this disorder. However, due to the high prevalence of comorbidities in ASPD, pharmacological treatment should be offered if patients meet criteria for other psychiatric illnesses, such as mood disorders, anxiety disorders, or substance use disorders.

D. PROGNOSTIC

Most of the research looking at prognostic factors in ASPD focuses on the progression from conduct disorder to ASPD. Risk factors for this progression include deviant behavior before the age of 10 years, a greater diversity of deviant behavior, and history of substance use. On the other hand, factors associated with remission include lower symptom severity during initial evaluation and current sobriety. Reaching the fourth decade of life seems to be a good prognostic factor for ASPD since symptoms and involvement with the legal system tend to decrease after this age in patients with ASPD.

8. Risk Assessment

Patients with ASPD have several important risk factors for suicide. ASPD in itself has been associated with a higher risk of suicide attempts. On the other hand, frequent comorbidities, such as major depressive disorder, history of child abuse, or substance use disorders, significantly increase the risk for future suicide attempts.

Another important risk to assess in patients with ASPD is their increased risk for accidents, important medical problems such as coronary artery disease, and unnatural causes of death, usually related to their criminal activity. It is not uncommon for patients with ASPD to come to the hospital with the secondary gain of hiding from someone who wants to hurt them.

Finally, these patients also have a history of violent and criminal behavior that should be taken seriously. One should pay particular attention when assessing homicidal ideations, intent, or plans in patients with this disorder. This assessment should also include an assessment of the presence of domestic violence, or any ongoing child abuse or neglect, which the patient could be perpetrating.

KEY POINTS (ABPN Examination)

A. When interviewing a patient with antisocial personality disorder

1. Patients can present as being very calm and charming and most often tend to minimize their symptoms and lie about their criminal and legal history.
2. Contrary to prior beliefs, mood and anxiety disorders are frequently encountered in this population and should be assessed thoroughly.
3. Assess for the presence of exposure to childhood trauma and chronic and acute domestic and community violence. Patients with ASPD have frequently been exposed to significant trauma and may experience PTSD symptoms.
4. Enquire about substance abuse as it is highly prevalent in this population and has been associated with increased risk for violence.

B. When presenting a patient with antisocial personality disorder

1. Acknowledge that the diagnosis of a personality disorder cannot be made during an acute crisis and that a more pervasive and long-standing behavioral pattern must be present to make the correct diagnosis.
2. If diagnosis is unclear, state that you would use a structured diagnostic interview like SCID-DSM-IV for clarification.
3. As patients can present in a calm and charming manner and tend to minimize their symptoms and lie about their criminal and legal history, it is critical to state that obtaining collateral information is a priority.

Suggested Readings

American Psychiatric Association. *Diagnostic and Statistical Manual of Mental Disorders: Text Revision*. Washington, DC: American Psychiatric Association, 2000.

Armelius BA, Andreassen TH. Cognitive-behavioral treatment for antisocial behavior in youth residential treatment. *Cochrane Database Syst Rev* 2007 Oct 17;(4):CD005650.

Beitchman JH, Baldassarra L, Mik H, et al. Serotonin transporter polymorphisms and persistent, pervasive childhood aggression. *Am J Psychiatry*. 2006 Jun;163:1103–1105.

Black DW, Baumgard CH, Bell SE. A 16-to-45 year follow-up of 71 men with antisocial personality disorder. *Compr Psychiatry* 1995 Mar;36(2):130–140.

Cale EM, Lilienfeld SO. Sex differences in psychopathy and antisocial personality disorder. A review and integration. *Clin Psychol Rev* 2002 Nov;22(8):1179–1207.

Carr A. Contributions to the study of violence and trauma: Multisystemic therapy, exposure therapy, attachment styles, and therapy process research. *J Interpers Violence* 2005 Apr;20(4):426–435.

Caspi A, McClay J, Moffitt TE, et al. Role of Genotype in the cycle of violence in maltreated children. *Science* 2002;297(5582):851–854.

Douglas KS, Lilienfeld SO, Skeem JL, et al. Relation of antisocial and psychopathic traits to suicide-related behavior among offenders. *Law Hum Behav.* 2008 Dec;32(6):511–525.

Farrington DP, Loeber R. Epidemiology of juvenile violence. *Child Adolesc Psychiatr Clin N Am* 2000 Oct;9(4):733–748.

Goldstein RB, Dawson DA, Chou SP, et al. Antisocial behavioral syndromes and past-year physical health among adults in the United States: Results from the National Epidemiologic Survey on Alcohol and Related conditions. *J Clin Psychiatry* 2008 Mar;69(3):368–380.

Hirose S. Letter to the Editor: Effective treatment of aggression and impulsivity in antisocial personality disorder with risperidone. *Psychiatry Clin Neurosci* 2001;55:161–162.

Myers M, Stewart DG, Brown S. Progression from conduct disorder to antisocial personality disorder following treatment for adolescent substance abuse. *Am J Psychiatry* 1998 Apr;155:479–485.

Pietrzak RH, Petry NM. Antisocial personality disorder is associated with increased severity of ganbling, medical, drug and psychiatric problems among treatment-seeking pathological gamblers. *Addiction* 2005 Aug;100(8):1183–1193.

Raine A, Lencz T, Bihrle S, et al. Reduced prefrontal gray matter volume and reduced autonomic activity in antisocial personality disorder. *Arch Gen Psychiatr*, 2000 Feb;57(2):119–127.

Raine A, Lencz T, Bihrle S, et al. Reduced prefrontal gray matter volume and reduced autonomic activity in antisocial personality disorder. *Arch Gen Psychiatry* 2000;57:119–127.

Reeves RR, Struve FA, Patrick G. Auditory and visual P300 evoked potentials do not predict response to valproate treatment of aggression in patients with borderline and antisocial personality disorders. *Clin EEG Neurosci* 2005 Jan;36(1):49–51.

Sadock BJ, Sadock VA. Kaplan & Sadock's Synopsis of Psychiatry. 9th Ed. New York, NY: Lippincott Williams & Wilkins, 2003.

Walker C, Thomas J, Allen TS. Treating impulsivity, irritability and aggression of antisocial personality disorder with quetiapine. *Int J Offender Ther Comp Criminol*. 2003 Oct;47(5):556–567.

Yang Y, Raine A, Lencz T, et al. Volume reduction in prefrontal gray matter in unsuccessful criminal psychopaths. *Biol Psychiatry*. 2005 May 15;57(10):1103–1108.

G. Somatoform disorders and sleep disorders

Vikrant Mittal, MD, MHS

I. SOMATOFORM DISORDERS

CASE HISTORY

PRESENT ILLNESS

Ms X is a 44-year-old single white woman who was admitted to the medicine unit for the fifth time in last 3 months. She complained about abdominal pain which required opioid analgesics for relief. Tylenol with codeine helps somewhat but does not completely alleviate the pain. According to the patient, she has had this pain even before her husband passed away but "it was not this bad." She reports vomiting and diarrhea, associated with the abdominal pain, though she reports that at times she gets diarrhea without the abdominal pain. She quotes one of the surgeons, "It is because of my ischemic bowel syndrome." She complains that recently she has noticed initial tingling followed by complete numbness in her upper extremities after a bout of vomiting. Ms X also mentions the headache, a bandlike phenomenon associated with awakening in the morning. She has seen many neurologists, gastroenterologists, and internists, but nobody has been able to help her with the problems.

She has been unable to work for the past 5 years because of her symptoms and claims that they have "destroyed her life." The patient also goes on to report that recently she has also been having some knee and lower back pain. She mentions that her mother had similar pain associated with her arthritis. Ms X reported that she is not able to enjoy anything in life and has not met with her friends in weeks.

She reported weight fluctuation associated with her gastrointestinal symptoms and their flare-ups, though her appetite is not affected. She reports anergia and anhedonia secondary to her pain problems. She denies any thoughts to harm herself or anybody else. She denies any auditory or visual hallucinations.

PSYCHIATRIC HISTORY

Over the last 6 years, Ms X has been seen by the psychiatric consult service on multiple occasions during her many admissions to the medical floor due to the medical team's concern that Ms X has an underlying psychopathology contributing to her physical symptoms in the absence of clear medical etiology. She was reported to have hysteria in one of the past emergency room evaluations 7 years ago. She has been noted to be given a diagnosis of depressive disorder not otherwise specified (NOS), with somatization disorder ruled out in the past. She denied a history of psychiatric admissions or illicit substance abuse. She had seen a psychologist for the first time, after her last hospitalization, 2 weeks ago. The patient reports that she has had psychotropic medication trials with selective serotonin reuptake inhibitors (SSRIs) which have not been effective. It is noted that her medical admissions have increased in frequency over the course of the year, since the death of her husband and ensuing financial stressors.

FAMILY HISTORY

The patient's father had a diagnosis of alcohol dependence and antisocial personality disorder.

SOCIAL HISTORY

Ms X is an only child who was raised by a single mother in New York City. Her father left the family when the patient was 1 year of age. Her mother worked two jobs to support the family. Ms X finished high school and completed college in arts from Columbia University. A history of physical or sexual abuse was unclear. The patient was married for 7 years until her husband passed away 6 years ago. They have one son who is 12 years of age. She is currently self-employed at a family-owned restaurant. The business was doing poorly even prior to her husband's death and the financial strain has been worrisome for the patient. She has reported that she has been unable to have any intimate relationships since her husband died.

PERTINENT MEDICAL HISTORY

The patient has history of cholecystectomy at age 28. She has multiple colonoscopies, which revealed a mild form of ischemic bowel disease.

MENTAL STATUS EXAMINATION

Ms X is a white woman who appeared to be older than her stated age. She was casually dressed and her general hygiene was good. She was pleasant and cooperative but avoided eye contact. Her speech fluctuated in tone and volume. It was normal for the most part but became of soft tone and low volume when she talked about her pain. Her psychomotor activity was normal to retarded. She had a full range of affect and cried when talking about the pain. Her thought process was goal oriented. She denied any suicidal or homicidal ideations, intent or plan, as well as any delusions, auditory or visual hallucinations, or obsessions. On the Folstein Mini-Mental State Examination, she scored 30/30 indicating intact cognitive functioning. Her insight was fair; she was agreeable to continue seeing her therapist. Her judgment was fair; she agreed to let her primary care physician be aware of the present admission and psychiatric evaluation.

PERTINENT PHYSICAL FINDINGS

Her vital signs were within normal limits. Neurological examination was normal.

LABORATORY DATA

CBC, electrolytes, liver function tests, and cholesterol and thyroid function tests were within normal limits. Nerve conduction studies were within normal limits. Folate and other vitamin levels were all at the higher limits of normal.

HOSPITAL COURSE

Ms X was continued on the pain medications as per the pain management consult. A letter was sent to the primary care physician updating him about the recent multiple admissions, pain consult, and psychiatry consult.

DISCHARGE MEDICATIONS

No psychotropic medications prescribed at discharge.

DSM-IV-TR MULTIAXIAL DIAGNOSIS

Axis I. Somatization disorder
Axis II. None
Axis III. Ischemic bowel disease
Axis IV. Financial stressor, single mother
Axis V. Global assessment of functioning: 55

FORMULATION

A. Diagnostic

This patient meets most of the DSM- IV-TR criteria for somatization disorder. She has a history of complaints that started before age 30, leading to severe social and functional impairment which are in excess of what is to be expected of her symptoms and concluded from the tests and the laboratory work. The patient's symptoms include four separate areas with pain, two gastrointestinal symptoms, one sexual symptom, and one pseudo neurological symptom. These occur together and at different point of times, without any association.

In somatization disorder, symptoms are not generated for a secondary gain as in malingering or factitious disorder. Other common differential diagnosis is hypochondriasis. The patient here shows multiple vague, multiorgan symptoms, and complaints of neglect by physicians with need to legitimize the sick role. She also endorses depressive symptoms. In hypochondriasis, patients show an exaggeration of normal bodily sensations, focus on body vulnerability, fear of serious illness, and obsessive personality traits. Presence of an organic medical cause should be ruled out by thorough testing and laboratory work. Differential diagnosis should also include anorexia nervosa, depressive disorder, and anxiety disorders.

B. Etiologic

Biologically, she is at risk given a family history of antisocial personality disorder and alcohol dependence in her father. She was raised in a lower socioeconomic environment which is another risk factor. Psychologically, being abandoned by her father at an early age can predispose her to major mental illness, particularly depression. The patient being raised by a single parent, with two jobs, points to emotional loneliness. It is made worse as she did not have any sibling. Little is known about her socialization during childhood. She has multiple financial and social stressors like the death of her husband, her business in huge debt that puts her at risk of symptom relapse. The events of admission can be linked to these stressors. She has some reduced risk given that she is educated and is of the white race.

C. Therapeutic

The first line of treatment is psychotherapy. The patient should be encouraged to continue with her psychotherapist who can help the patient with cognitive behavioral therapy (CBT). The therapy should focus on having regular appointments, establishing a shared agenda, limiting the diagnostic tests and visits to the hospital. The treatment plan should also include managing the family issues that can precipitate an event. There should be constant contact between the primary care physician, psychotherapist, and the psychiatrist.

For pharmacotherapy, there is some evidence of benefit from a fluvoxamine trial. One uncontrolled study showed that tricyclic antidepressants might be better than SSRI. The role of antidepressants in these patients is not clearly understood, it is thought to help in controlling the mood issues.

D. Prognostic

Short-term prognosis depends on the presence of various psychosocial stressors that she is facing and is rather grim. Another important prognostic factor from both short-term and long-term perspective is the establishment of a working relationship with her psychotherapist and her participation in CBT. Ms X has some important positive prognostic factors, such as the absence of substance abuse disorder and higher education level.

SOMATIZATION DISORDER

1. Introduction

Somatization disorder is also known as Briquet syndrome or hysteria and is one of the most common types of somatoform disorders. It involves a patient complaint list from multiple organ systems which cannot be medically explained. The patient normally presents with a history of seeing multiple physicians, having multiple surgeries, receiving multiple prescriptions, and repeated investigations. Patients with somatization disorder incur huge costs related to their health care. Other types of somatoform disorders are undifferentiated somatoform disorder, conversion disorder, hypochondriasis, body dysmorphic disorder, pain disorder, and somatoform disorder NOS.

Of the other somatoform disorder, in conversion disorder, the patient has functional loss of a body part or has abnormal movements. In hypochondriasis, there is unusual conviction about having a particular disease. Body dysmorphic disorder is a disorder of preoccupation with imaginary or false perceptions of defects in the physical appearance. Pain disorder involves having pain with a high intensity or simulation which is not explainable by normal physiological mechanisms or tests. Somatoform disorder NOS is used when the patient does not meet the criteria for any of the above disorders. Undifferentiated somatoform disorder is diagnosed when somatoform disorder NOS has been present for more than 6 months.

2. Epidemiology

The lifetime prevalence of somatization disorder is 0.2% to 2% in women and 0.2% in men. The onset of illness is mostly noted in the teen years. Other risk factors include older age, less education, lower socioeconomic status, nonwhite race, and immigrant status. The common association within the family is of somatization disorder in women and antisocial personality in men. No clear association has been established between somatization disorder and substance abuse disorders.

3. Etiology

There is no clear etiology established for somatization disorder. The main theory that is suggested is the interplay of the various cognitive-perceptual, behavioral, psychobiological, and affective processes. It has also been suggested that the endocrine system, the immune system, and various neurotransmitters play an important role. A state of physiological hyperactivity even when there is no stressor is considered to be a risk factor. One of the studies showed decreased levels of CD9 T lymphocytes and interleukin-6. Levels of branched chain amino acids have been noted to be low in patients with somatization disorder. There is no clear association of cortisol levels with the somatoform disorders.

It is hypothesized that low levels of 5-HIAA and tryptophan in patients with fibromyalgia may be relevant from an etiologic point of view in somatization disorder. EEG evoked potentials have been used to study attention and perception processes; these indicate increased N1-components and decreased mismatch negativity in somatization disorder. In a positron emission tomography (PET) study, it has been shown that patients with somatization disorder have lower glucose metabolism rates in each caudate nuclei, left putamen, and right precentral gyrus. There was significant enlargement of caudate nuclei volumes, bilaterally. Genetically, there is a high association of antisocial personality, borderline personality, and histrionic personality with the somatization disorder.

4. Diagnosis

The DSM-IV-TR criteria for somatization disorder are shown in Table 3G.1.

5. Treatments

A. NONPHARMACOLOGICAL TREATMENTS

The nonpharmacological treatment can be divided into the following two groups as defined by Mai F in Somatization disorder: A practical review. *Can J Psychiatry* 2004; 49(10):652–662.

1. General Principles

(a) Comprehensive clinical assessment (history, mental state, and physical examination).
(b) Interview key family member.
(c) Minimize number of clinicians involved. Ensure a consistent, coordinated management plan.
(d) Minimize invasive diagnostic and therapeutic procedures.
(e) Ensure regular, structured sessions. Avoid as-needed visits to doctors and emergency departments.
(f) Recognize reality of symptoms and provide diagnostic feedback to both the patient and the family member. When appropriate, try to link symptoms to stressful life events.
(g) Identify and minimize secondary reinforcers.
(h) Treat associated medical and psychiatric conditions appropriately.

2. Cognitive Behavioral Therapy

(a) Develop treatment contract (listing agreed approximate frequency, duration, and number of sessions).
(b) Set realistic short- and long-term goals. Review these regularly.
(c) Focus on practical ways of coping with symptoms and limitations.
(d) Encourage the patient to keep a daily log of thoughts, feelings, and coping behaviors. Review these regularly.
(e) Promote daily physical, social, recreational, and occupational activities.
(f) Promote daily relaxation activities and exercises.
(g) Promote patient control and autonomy.

CBT is the treatment of choice that helps in alleviating a wide range of physical symptoms, associated mood disturbances, and thus, overall physical and social functioning of the patient.

B. PHARMACOLOGICAL TREATMENTS

The importance of even a single consultation has been highlighted in the literature, especially for the

TABLE 3G.1 Diagnostic Criteria for Somatization Disorder

A. A history of many physical complaints beginning before age 30 years that occur over a period of several years and result in treatment being sought, or significant impairment in social, occupational, or other important areas of functioning.

B. Each of the following criteria must have been met, with individual symptoms occurring at any time during the course of the disturbance:
1. Four pain symptoms: a history of pain related to at least four different sites or functions (e.g., head, abdomen, back, joints, extremities, chest, rectum, during menstruation, during sexual intercourse, or during urination).
2. Two gastrointestinal symptoms: a history of at least two gastrointestinal symptoms other than pain (e.g., nausea, bloating, vomiting other than during pregnancy, diarrhea, or intolerance of several different foods).
3. One sexual symptom: a history of at least one sexual or reproductive symptom other than pain (e.g., sexual indifference, erectile or ejaculatory dysfunction, irregular menses, excessive menstrual bleeding, vomiting throughout pregnancy).
4. One pseudoneurological symptom: a history of at least one symptom or deficit suggesting a neurological condition not limited to pain (conversion symptoms such as impaired coordination or balance, paralysis or localized weakness, difficulty swallowing or lump in throat, aphonia, urinary retention, hallucinations, loss of touch or pain sensation, double vision, blindness, deafness, seizures; dissociative symptoms such as amnesia; or loss of consciousness other than fainting).

C. Either (1) or (2):
1. After appropriate investigation, each of the symptoms in Criterion B cannot be fully explained by a known general medical condition or the direct effects of a substance (e.g., a drug of abuse, a medication).
2. When there is a related general medical condition, the physical complaints, or resulting social or occupational impairment are in excess of what would be expected from the history, physical examination, or laboratory findings.

D. The symptoms are not intentionally produced or feigned (as in factitious disorder or malingering).

Adapted from American Psychiatric Association. *Diagnostic and Statistical Manual of Mental Disorders*. Washington, DC: American Psychiatric Association, 2000.

patients managed by the primary care physician. The psychiatrist should evaluate the patient for any potential need for antidepressant treatment. The drug of choice is fluvoxamine even though any other SSRI medication can be used. The use of medication helps in reducing disability and improving the outcome.

6. Prognosis

The prognosis of the illness depends on the early recognition of the problem by the primary care provider and establishment of a working relationship between the patient and the primary care provider. Following this, an early initiation of the CBT can lead to improvement in the functionality of the person. The course of illness is often a chronic, relapsing, and remitting one.

7. General Formulation for Somatization Disorder

A. DIAGNOSTIC

Somatization disorder is a type of somatoform disorder and it should meet the DSM-IV-TR criteria as outlined above. It is important to differentiate it from factitious disorder and malingering which involve a secondary gain. In somatization disorder, the patient seeks to establish a diagnosis in order establish a sick role. The other differentiation to be made is from hypochondriasis in which the patient exaggerates normal body sensations and believes them to be a serious illness.

A family history of antisocial personality, borderline personality, or histrionic personality is an important risk factor in the development of somatization disorder. The most commonly associated mood disorders—depression and anxiety—should also be identified.

B. ETIOLOGIC

There is no clear etiology for the disorder although genetic correlation has been established with certain personality disorders. Current theory hypothesizes an interplay of the various cognitive-perceptual, behavioral, psychobiological, and affective processes along with important modifiers coming from the endocrine system, immune system, and various neurotransmitters.

C. THERAPEUTIC

The treatment of choice for somatization disorder is CBT. A moderate amount of improvement has been documented with this form of therapy. The role of antidepressants—tricyclics and SSRIs—is limited to treating mood symptoms.

D. PROGNOSTIC

Early recognition of illness and the presence a stable primary care provider are prime positive prognostic indicators for maintenance of functionality in a patient. Female sex, lower educational levels, lower socioeconomic strata, nonwhite race, and immigrant status are all negative risk factors.

8. Risk Assessment

Somatization disorder patients are at increased risk of attempting suicide. There is an unconfirmed association of somatization disorder with the anxiety and depressive disorders. Somatization patients have at least twice the utilization of outpatient and inpatient medical care and double the total medical care costs irrespective of comorbid psychiatric and medical issues.

Patients with somatization disorder also have medical comorbidities but they are at increased risk of developing iatrogenic medical and surgical problems due to "doctor shopping". They may have high rates of use of alcohol and other recreational drugs.

KEY POINTS (ABPN Examination)

A. When interviewing a patient with somatization disorder

1. Remember to inquire about all the symptoms and the timeline.
   - Onset of unexplained medical symptoms at age earlier than 30 years.
   - Multiple chronic multisystem complains along with four pain symptoms involving multiple sites, such as the head, neck, back, stomach, and limbs.
   - Presence of two or more unexplained gastrointestinal symptoms, such as nausea and indigestion.
   - Presence of at least one sexual complaint and/or menstrual complaint
   - And at least one pseudoneurological symptom, such as blindness or inability to walk, talk, or lift an extremity.
2. Ask about suicidality, as it is an important risk factor.
3. Ask about comorbidities, particularly mood disorders, anxiety disorders, and substance abuse disorders, which have a high prevalence in this population.

B. When presenting a patient with somatization disorder

1. Enumerate the various symptoms that the patient listed in the presenting symptoms.
2. Describe the presence or absence of "secondary gain" in the patient.
3. Indicate the presence or absence of "sick role" in the patient.
4. Discuss the stresses in the patient's life and try to link them to the current presentation.
5. Do not forget to discuss the importance of having only a few stable medical providers, i.e., avoid "Doctor shopping."
6. Elaborate on the importance of psychotherapy and management of psychiatric and medical comorbidities.

Susggested Readings

American Psychiatric Association. *Diagnostic and Statistical Manual of Mental Disorders*. 3rd Ed. Washington, DC: American Psychiatric Association, 1987.

American Psychiatric Association. *Diagnostic and Statistical Manual of Mental Disorders*. Washington, DC: American Psychiatric Association, 2000.

Barsky AJ, Orav EJ, Bates DW. Somatization increases medical utilization and costs independent of psychiatric and medical comorbidity. *Arch Gen Psychiatry* 2005;62:903–910.

Brown TM. Somatization. *Medicine* Aug 2004;32(8): 34–35.

Cloninger CR, Bayon C, Przybeck TR. Epidemiology and Axis I comorbidity of antisocial personality. In: Stoff DM, Breiling J, Maser JD, eds. *Handbook of Antisocial Behavior*. New York, NY: Wiley, 1997:12–21.

Escobar J, Swartz M, Rubio-Stipec M, et al. Medically unexplained symptoms: Distribution, risk-factors, and co-morbidity. In: Kirmayer LJ, Robbins JM, eds. *Current Concepts of Somatization: Research and Clinical Perspectives*. Washington, DC: American Psychiatric Press, 1991: 63–78.

Fallon BA. Pharmacotherapy of somatoform disorders. *J Psychosom Res* 2004; 56:455–460.

Garralda E. Somatization and somatoform disorders. *Psychiatry* 2005;4(8):97–100.

Hakala M, Karlsson H, Kurki T, et al. Volumes of the caudate nuclei in women with somatization disorder and healthy women. *Psychiatry Res Neuroimaging* 2004;131:71–78.

Hakala M, Karlsson H, Ruotsalainen U, et al. Severe somatization in women is associated with altered brain metabolism. *Psychol Med* 2002;32: 1379–1385.

Hasin D, Katz H. Somatoform and substance use disorders. *Psychosom Med* 2004;69:870–875.

James L, Gordon E, Kraiuhin C, et al. Augmentation of auditory evoked potentials in somatization disorder. *J Psychiatr Res* 1990;24:155–163.

Kroenke K. Efficacy of treatment for somatoform disorders: A review of randomized controlled trials. *Psychosom Med* 2007;69:881–888.

Kroenke K, Swindle R. Cognitive–behavioral therapy for somatization and symptom syndromes: A critical review of controlled clinical trials. *Psychother Psychosom* 2000;69(4): 205–215.

Mai F. Somatization disorder: A practical review. *Can J Psychiatry* 2004; 49(10):652–662.

Noyes R, Happel R, Muller B, et al. Fluvoxamine for somatoform disorders: An open trial. *Gen Hosp Psychiatry* 1998;20:339–344.

Noyes R, Stuart S, Watson DB, et al. Distinguishing between hypochondriasis and somatization disorder: A review of the existing literature. *Psychother Psychosom* 2006;75:270–281. DOI: 10.1159/000093948.

O'Malley PG, Jackson JL, Santoro J, et al. Antidepressant therapy for unexplained symptoms and symptom syndromes. *J Fam Pract* 1999;48(12): 980–990.

Rief W, Barsky AJ. Psychobiological perspectives on somatoform disorders. *Psychoneuroendocrinology* 2005;30(10):996–1002.

Rief W, Sharpe M. Somatoform disorders—new approaches to classification, conceptualization, and treatment (Editorial). *J Psychosom Res* 2004;56:387–390.

Sadock BJ, Sadock VA. *Kaplan & Sadock's Synopsis of Psychiatry*. 9th Ed. New York, NY: Lippincott Williams & Wilkins, 2003.

Salmon P, Peters S, Stanley I. Patients' perceptions of medical explanation for somatization disorders: Qualitative analysis. *BMJ* 1999;318:372–376.

Sumathipala A. What is the evidence for the efficacy of treatments for somatoform disorders? a critical review of previous intervention studies. *Psychosom Med* 2007;69:889–900.

II. INSOMNIA

CASE HISTORY

PRESENT ILLNESS

Mr Y, a 34-year-old, African American man comes to an outpatient psychiatrist's office, accompanied by his wife with a complaint of not being able to sleep. He reports that this is taking a toll on his work life. According to the patient, he has difficulty falling asleep and maintaining sleep during the night. He reports that even if he sleeps, he wakes up within a couple of hours and then has difficulty going back to sleep. He states that he used to be able to sleep for 8 hours a day, but now he is able to sleep only for about 5 to 6 hours. The patient does not recall exactly when the problem started but was able to say that it was after his wife came to the United States from Africa 7 months ago.

He reports having many problems at work because of his sleep issues. He reports decreased energy at work and feeling tired during the day. He reports some problem at home with his wife as he feels he does not have enough energy to do things at home. His wife, who came with him for the appointment, is supportive and does not report any marital problems. She denies that her husband snores while sleeping. She also reports that she has never seen him sleep during the daytime. If he is able to sleep, he reports that he has no problems with concentration. There were no identifiable stressors or relievers for the insomnia. No history of weight change or appetite change was reported. He denied any self-injurious behavior or any suicidal ideation, thoughts or plan. He denied any thoughts of harming anybody else. He denied any signs or symptoms of mania or hypomania. He denied any history of delusions. He denied any history or current use of illicit substances.

PSYCHIATRIC HISTORY

He reports that he had similar problems more than 10 years ago, when he was a senior in college. He reports that he was prescribed a medication by his primary care physician, but does not recall the name of that medication at this time.

FAMILY HISTORY

Mr Y denies any history of psychiatric illness, substance abuse or suicides in the family.

SOCIAL HISTORY

Mr Y was born in Farmington, CT. He is the sixth of nine children in his family. His parents were both school teachers. Mr Y completed his PhD in chemistry and works as a senior chemist in a private company. He has been married for the past 2 years and does not have any children.

PERTINENT MEDICAL HISTORY

He has no active medical problems. He has no history of seizures or head injury.

MENTAL STATUS EXAMINATION

Mr Y is noted to be well built, African American male, who looked his stated age. He was casually dressed and had good general hygiene. He was pleasant and cooperative with fairly good eye contact. His speech was normal in rate, with appropriate volume and rhythm. No psychomotor agitation or retardation was noted. He reported his mood as anxious and displayed a full range of affect. His thought process was linear and goal directed. He denied any suicidal or homicidal ideations, intent or plan, as well as any delusions, auditory or visual hallucinations, or obsessions. His insight was fair; he was able to understand the negative aspects of insomnia on his life. His judgment was fair, in that he seeks treatment for his illness. On the Folstein Mini-Mental State Examination, he scored 30/30 indicating that he had good cognitive functioning.

PERTINENT PHYSICAL FINDINGS

His vital signs were a temperature of 96.7°F, heart rate 84 per minute, blood pressure 120/86 mm Hg, and respiratory rate of 17 per minute. Oxygen saturation on room air was 97.0%. His pupils were equal and reactive to light and accommodation. No jaundice, anemia, or lymphadenopathy was noted. The first and second heart sounds were heard and there was no murmur. The lungs were clear. The abdomen was soft, nontender and there was no organomegaly. Bowel sounds were heard normally. The extremities showed normal capillary perfusion. The neurological examination was normal. He weighed 210 lb.

LABORATORY DATA

The laboratory data obtained were as follows: sodium level: 140 mEq/L, potassium: 3.9 mEq/L, bicarbonate: 21.7 mEq/L, chloride: 110 mEq/L, Blood Urea Nitrogen (BUN): 17 mg%, creatinine: 0.5 mg%, white blood cell count: 6,500/cmm, hemoglobin: 14.8 gm%, hematocrit: 40%, platelet count: 300,000/cmm, and fasting blood glucose: 90 mg%. The TSH level was within range at 2.0 mIU/L. Venereal Disease Research Laboratory test (VDRL) was nonreactive. His lipid panel and liver function tests were within the normal range.

OUTPATIENT COURSE

The patient is started on temazepam 15 mg oral once at bedtime. The patient is given information on sleep hygiene. He was to follow up in 1 week with the outpatient clinic.

DSM-IV-TR MULTIAXIAL DIAGNOSIS

Axis I. Primary insomnia
Axis II. Deferred
Axis III. None acute
Axis IV. Problems at work
Axis V. Global assessment of functioning: 60

FORMULATION

A. Diagnostic

This patient meets the criteria for primary insomnia as evidenced by his inability to initiate or maintain sleep for the last 7 months in the absence of any other medical problems. These symptoms are not associated with any depressive or other mood symptoms. His symptoms are producing significant dysfunction in both his social and occupational activities. There is no associated psychotic symptomatology. All his laboratory tests were within normal range, ruling out other common causes of insomnia like thyroid problems, vitamin deficiencies, infections, or tumors.

Differentiating between primary insomnia and insomnia secondary to mental disorders is most often the challenging question. In this case, there are no associated mental disorders which greatly aids in the diagnosis. Patients with insomnia are more prone to develop mood disorders, and it is important to look at the timeline of development of the disorder versus the insomnia to find out what came first. One should also look for other causes like restless leg syndrome. The patient mentioned the arrival of his wife as the point of initiation of his insomnia, but no stressor were identified secondary to the relationship issues or finances.

A fact mentioned by his wife rules out circadian rhythm disorder. She mentioned that he does not sleep during the day time, suggesting that he does not have circadian abnormalities which include advanced and delayed sleep phase disorders. The patient did not meet the criteria for any other Axis I disorders—major depressive disorder, anxiety disorders, substance abuse disorder, or other mood disorders. Of the above, major depressive disorder is the most commonly associated psychiatric disorder with insomnia. This patient also did not meet the criteria for a psychotic or cognitive disorder. Further confirmation would be established on the patient's response to the benzodiazepines, the first line of treatment for insomnia.

B. Etiologic

There is no genetic predisposition for the patient to have this illness, and there is no genetic correlation known for the primary insomnia. No other primary causative factor for the insomnia was noted in this patient.

C. Therapeutic

The patient was started on first-line treatment—temazepam for the treatment of primary insomnia. Temazepam is one of the eight benzodiazepines that are called benzodiazepine receptor agonists. It is an FDA-approved sedative-hypnotic drug for the treatment of insomnia. It would benefit the patient in allaying the anxiety symptoms and early morning awakening that he has reported. He was informed that the medication is to be used as a treatment option for only 2 to 4 weeks given the potential for physical dependence, withdrawal, and tolerance. The other side effects to take note of temazepam are orthostatic hypotension and anticholinergic side effects. He has been advised not to drive or operate heavy machinery after taking the medication.

For nonpharmacological treatments, he was made aware of maintaining good sleep hygiene and trained in the guided imagery and deep muscle relaxation techniques. For long-term management of his insomnia, CBT was recommended.

D. Prognostic

Mr Y has no known mood disorder at the present time, which is a good prognostic sign. As the patient has good social support provided by his wife with no accompanying significant socioeconomic stressor, he has a better chance of achieving symptom remission. A negative prognostic sign is the history of a similar episode in the past. Achievement of full remission would also depend on his participation in the treatment, both pharmacological and nonpharmacological.

INSOMNIA

1. Introduction

Insomnia is defined as difficulty with sleep initiation, maintenance or inability to have a quality, refreshing sleep resulting in the impairment of daytime functioning. DSM-IV-TR recognizes primary insomnia as a diagnosis when it is present for at least 1 month leading to significant social, functional, or occupational disturbance. In addition, sleep disturbance should not be associated only with a mental disorder, substance abuse or dependence, circadian rhythm disorders or active psychosocial stressor. Insomnia can be acute or chronic. Acute insomnia is considered when the patient has less than 4 weeks of sleep difficulties. When insomnia lasts for more than 4 weeks, it becomes chronic insomnia. Persistence of chronic insomnia is greatly associated with development of mental illness, most commonly major depressive disorder.

2. Epidemiology

Prevalence of primary insomnia varies from 5% to 35% in different studies. When including all the criteria, insomnia occurs in 5% to 10% of the population. The female: male sex ratio is approximately 1.4:1. There are a number of known risk factors for insomnia that have been identified, the most common of which is the presence of concurrent depressive symptoms. There is increasing evidence which suggests a strong correlation with people who are separated or divorced, of low income, low socioeconomic status, have high chronic life stress, and of African American race and insomnia. Additionally, increasing age, comorbid medical illness, and comorbid psychiatric illness are other consistent risk factors.

3. Etiology

There is no known causative basis for primary insomnia. The current theory that is widely accepted is that it is a state of hyperarousability. There is increasing evidence of cognitive and affective hyperarousal in insomnia in the recent studies. Physiological states of increased arousal are indicated by elevated cortisol or adrenocorticotropic hormone (ACTH) in the evening time, increased heart rate, variations in heart rate, and increase in the whole body metabolic rate.

In primary insomnia, EEG has been shown to have an increased Non-Rapid Eye Movement (NREM) activity in the frequency ranges from 14 to 45 Hz. In individuals with primary insomnia, PET studies also support the hyperarousal theory, as there is an elevated whole brain metabolism during both sleep and wakefulness. They are also noted to have localized activation in the affective and arousal centers during non-REM sleep.

4. Diagnosis

The DSM-IV-TR criteria for primary insomnia are shown in Table 3G.2.

5. Treatments

A. NONPHARMACOLOGICAL TREATMENTS

There are various of therapies available for the treatment of insomnia. The recommended therapies are

a. Stimulus control therapy: This therapy focuses on reassociating bed with sleepiness to promote rapid onset of sleep. Patients are asked not to go to bed until they are feeling sleepy and not to associate any other activity with the bed.
b. Paradoxical intention: This theory conceptualizes that anxiety to perform (sleep) prevents the patient from sleeping. The patient is asked to stay awake as long as possible and not to sleep. In doing this, anxiety would be reduced and the patient would be able to sleep.
c. Relaxation technique: It is based on the theory that deep muscle relaxation would reduce muscular tension and in turn, cognitive arousal, as they are related, thus helping in achieving better sleep.
d. Cognitive behavioral therapy: It focuses on altering the maladaptive beliefs and attitudes about sleep and sleep loss.
e. Sleep restriction therapy: This is used to increase the efficiency of sleep by reducing the amount of awake time and poor quality sleep time in the bed.
f. Sleep hygiene education: In this technique, the person is taught to improve his or her behaviors that interfere with sleep, for example, regular exercise, avoiding naps, and limiting alcohol and caffeine intake.

If these treatments reduce sleep onset latency or increase the total sleep time by 30 minutes, they are considered effective.

TABLE 3G.2 Diagnostic Criteria for Primary Insomnia

1. The predominant complaint is difficulty initiating or maintaining sleep, or nonrestorative sleep, for at least 1 month.
2. The sleep disturbance (or associated daytime fatigue) causes clinically significant distress or impairment in social, occupational, or other important areas of functioning.
3. The sleep disturbance does not occur exclusively during the course of Narcolepsy, breathing-related sleep disorder, circadian rhythm sleep disorder, or parasomnia.
4. The disturbance does not occur exclusively during the course of another mental disorder (e.g., major depressive disorder, generalized anxiety disorder, or delirium).
5. The disturbance is not due to the direct physiological effects of a substance (e.g., a drug of abuse, a medication) or a general medical condition.

Adapted from American Psychiatric Association. *Diagnostic and Statistical Manual of Mental Disorders (DSM-IV-TR)*. Washington, DC: American Psychiatric Association, 2000.

B. PHARMACOLOGICAL TREATMENTS

The pharmacological treatments include benzodiazepine receptor agonists, melatonin receptor agonist, some sedating antidepressants and antihistaminic drugs.

1. FDA approved benzodiazepine receptor agonists can be differentiated into short-acting and long-acting drugs. The short-acting ones include zolpidem, zaleplon, eszopiclone, triazolam, and temazepam. The long-acting ones are flurazepam, quazepam, and estazolam.
2. Melatonin receptor agonist includes ramelteon, which acts on the MT1 and MT2 receptors, thus aiding in the sleep.
3. Other treatments for insomnia include antidepressants such as trazodone, doxepin, amytriptyline and antihistaminic such as diphenhydramine. Some herbal supplements such as valerian root and melatonin are also used to treat insomnia.

6. Prognosis

For early remission, short-term pharmacological treatment is the best option. Long-term, continued remission of insomnia can be greatly aided by the nonpharmacological treatment. In some insomnia studies, CBT has been shown to be as effective as the pharmacological treatment or better. Numerous studies suggest that after 1 year, the rate of remission of the symptoms is around 50%. Patients with untreated insomnia are at higher risk for developing mood disorder, especially major depressive disorder.

7. General Formulation for Insomnia

A. DIAGNOSTIC

Primary insomnia is established when the patient meets all the criteria of DSM-IV-TR. The important point to note is the absence of any predisposing factor before the development of insomnia. This is important in the presence of a mood disorder, the timeline for which needs to be established in relation to insomnia with a good history. The duration of insomnia needs to be at least 1 month to establish the diagnosis. There should not be any kind of substance abuse or circadian rhythm disorder history present.

B. ETIOLOGIC

The exact mechanism is not known but the generally accepted hypothesis is that of hyperarousal in patients with insomnia. This is substantiated by increased activity in the range of 15 to 45 Hz seen on EEG, physiological markers like cortisol/ACTH ratio in the evening, and studies done with PET scans showing increased metabolism in the brain during sleep and wakefulness. Polysomnography is rarely used.

C. THERAPEUTIC

The first line of treatment for short duration are the benzodiazepine receptor agonists or the melatonin receptor agonist. Medications like the sedating antidepressants can be used if the aforementioned medications fail. Some authors consider psychotherapy to be as effective in treating primary insomnia as the pharmacological interventions.

D. PROGNOSTIC

The prognosis of primary insomnia is fair with nearly 50% of the patients achieving remission. The chances of maintaining remission after short-term medication trial are greatly enhanced by continuing with one of the forms of psychotherapy. Participation and follow-up of the patient are paramount in achieving and maintaining the remission.

8. Risk Assessment

There are various risk factors associated with primary insomnia which should be addressed during the course of evaluation to establish the diagnosis and followed during the course of treatment. The important risk factors are higher rates of accidents, absenteeism at work, poor quality of life, and impaired memory function. Patients should be progressively evaluated for the development of a mood disorder. Development of drug dependence is a major concern, as patients can become dependent on the medications used to treat insomnia, especially the benzodiazepines.

KEY POINTS (ABPN Examination)

A. When interviewing a patient with primary insomnia

1. Insomnia needs to be differentiated as primary insomnia or insomnia secondary to other causes.
2. History taking is vital; one should try to get clear time lines for the development of insomnia in relation to other psychiatric disorders, if present.
3. Presence or continuation of any inciting stressor/s—substance use, emotional, etc.—needs to be established through history.

B. When presenting a patient with primary insomnia

1. Describe if the symptoms of insomnia are primary or secondary to mood disorder.
2. Discuss medical and psychiatric co-morbidities in the patient.
3. Highlight the consequences of insomnia; social, educational, occupational and medical in the patient.

SUGGESTED READINGS

American Psychiatric Association. *Diagnostic and Statistical Manual of Mental Disorders: Text Revision*. 4th Ed. Washington, DC: American Psychiatric Association, 2000.

Becker PM. Insomnia: Prevalence, impact, pathogenesis, differential diagnosis, and evaluation. *Psychiatr Clin N Am* 2006;29:855–870.

Benka R. Diagnosis and treatment of insomnia: A Review. *Psychiatr Serv* 2005;56(3):332–343.

Buysse DJ, Germain A, Moul DE. Diagnosis, epidemiology, and consequences of insomnia. *Prim Psychiatry* 2005;12:37–44.

Daniel J. Buysse Chronic insomnia. *Am J Psychiatry* Jun 2008;165(6):678–686.

Jacobs GD, Pace-Schott EF, Stickgold R, et al. Cognitive behavioral therapy and pharmacotherapy for insomnia. A randomized controlled trial and direct comparison. *Arch Intern Med* 2004;164:1888–1896.

Kuppermann M, Lubeck DP, Mazonson PD, et al. Sleep problems and their correlates in a working population. *J Gen Intern Med* 1995;10:25–32.

Morin CM, Culbert JP, Schwartz SM. Nonpharmacological interventions for insomnia: A meta-analysis of treatment efficacy. *Am J Psychiatry* 1994;151:1172–1180.

Morin CM. Psychological and behavioral treatments for primary insomnia. In: Kryger MH, Roth T, Dement WC, eds. *Principles and Practice of Sleep Medicine*. Philadelphia, PA: Elsevier Saunders, 2005:726–737.

Nofzinger EA, Buysse DJ, Germain A, et al. Functional neuroimaging evidence for hyperarousal in insomnia. *Am J Psychiatry* 2004;161:2126–2129.

Nowell PD, Buysse DJ, Reynolds CF, et al. Clinical factors contributing to the differential diagnosis of primary insomnia and insomnia related to mental disorders. *Am J Psychiatry* 1997;154: 1412–1416.

Ohayon MM. Epidemiology of insomnia: What we know and what we still need to learn. *Sleep Med Rev* 2002;6:97–111.

Perlis ML, Smith MT, Andrews PJ, et al. Beta/gamma EEG activity in patients with primary and secondary insomnia and good sleeper controls. *Sleep* 2001;24(1):110–117.

Perlis ML, Smith MT, Pigeon WR. Etiology and pathophysiology of insomnia. In: Kryger MH, Roth T, Dement WC, eds. *Principles and Practice of Sleep Medicine*. Philadelphia, PA: Elsevier Saunders, 2005:714–725.

Perlis ML, Youngstedt SD. The diagnosis of primary insomnia and treatment alternatives. *Comp Ther* 2000;26(4):298–306.

Ringdahl EN, Pereira SL, Delzell JE. Treatment of primary insomnia. *JABFP* Apr 2004;7(3):212–219.

Roth T, Ancoli-Israel S. Daytime consequences and correlates of insomnia in the United States: Results of the 1991 National Sleep Foundation Survey II. *Sleep* 1999;22(suppl): S354–S358.

Roth T, Roehrs T. Insomnia: Epidemiology, characteristics, and consequences. *Clin Cornerstone* 2003;5(3):5–12.

Sateia MJ, Nowell PD. Insomnia. *Lancet* 2004;364:1959–1973.

Silber MH. Chronic insomnia. *N Engl J Med* Aug 2005;353:803–810.

Simon GE, VonKorff M. Prevalence, burden, and treatment of insomnia in primary care. *Am J Psychiatry* 1997;154:1417–1423.

H.1. Psychodynamic psychotherapy

Sunanda Muralee, MD, Rajesh R. Tampi, MD, MS

INTRODUCTION

Psychodynamic psychotherapy is a form of psychotherapy where the primary focus is to reveal the unconscious content of a patient's psyche in an effort to alleviate psychic tension. Psychodynamic psychotherapy is similar to psychoanalysis as it attributes emotional problems to the patient's unconscious motives and conflicts. However, it differs from classical psychoanalysis in that the psychodynamic psychotherapists do not necessarily accept Freud's view that these unconscious motives and conflicts are ultimately sexual in nature. Psychodynamic psychotherapy views the patient's developmental experiences as critical in forming his or her adult personality. This type of therapy relies heavily on the interpersonal relationship between patient and therapist. It takes into account both transference, in which the patient experiences the therapist as a significant figure from the past, and countertransference, in which the therapist experiences the patient as a significant figure from the past. While these concepts are present in any patient-therapist relationship, psychodynamic psychotherapy sees these concepts (particularly transference) as therapeutic material to be understood. Similarly, resistance, which is seen as a frustrating nuisance to other treaters, is explored and examined for its underlying meaning in psychodynamic therapy.

INDICATIONS

Psychodynamic psychotherapy can be used in individual therapy, group therapy, and family therapy and to understand and work within institutional and organizational contexts. It has also been shown to be helpful in treating patients with depressive disorders, anxiety disorders, sexual disorders, somatoform disorders, and personality disorders. Therapy sessions may be scheduled from 1 to 3 days per week, with greater frequency for more in-depth treatment. Each session typically lasts for 45 to 50 minutes. It is not usually possible at the outset of treatment to estimate the number of sessions that will be necessary to achieve the person's goals.

THEORIES

A. Freud's Theories

1. TOPOGRAPHIC THEORY

This theory divides the mental apparatus into the systems of *conscious, preconscious, and unconscious*. These systems are not anatomical structures of the brain but mental processes.

2. STRUCTURAL THEORY

This theory divides the mental apparatus into *the id, the ego, and the superego*. The id consists of sexual and aggressive wishes, which Freud defined as "drives." The ego is comprised of those forces that oppose the drives, i.e., defenses. Defenses are an example of synthetic functions and serve the purpose of protecting the conscious mind from awareness of forbidden impulses and thoughts. The superego represents the conscience, i.e., values, ideals, shame, and guilt. The "drives" may be either conscious or unconscious processes. The conscious versus unconscious conflict is the quality of any mental operation.

DEFENSE MECHANISMS

These mental processes are used to lessen distress and anxiety provoked by threatening or uncomfortable people or situations. These can be divided into the following types:

1. **Level 1 defense mechanisms (Psychotic):** When present, they are almost always pathological. These defenses distort the external experiences to eliminate the need to cope with reality. They are often seen in patients with psychosis.

Defense	Explanation
Denial	Refusal to accept external reality because it is too threatening.
Distortion	A gross distortion of external reality to meet internal needs.
Delusional projection	Delusional and persecutory views of external reality.

2. **Level 2 defense mechanisms (Immature):** These mechanisms lessen distress and anxiety provoked by threatening people or by uncomfortable reality. These defenses are often seen in patients with personality disorders and in adolescents.

Defense	Explanation
Projection	Attributing one's own unacknowledged, unacceptable/unwanted thoughts and emotions to another in order to allow the expression of the unacceptable impulses or desires without becoming consciously aware of them.
Projective identification	It is considered a self-fulfilling prophecy, whereby a person, believing something false about another, relates to that other person in such a way that the other person alters his or her behavior to make the belief true. The second person is influenced by the projection and begins to behave as though he or she is actually characterized by the projected thoughts or beliefs.
Acting out	The expression of one's unconscious wishes/impulses as inappropriate or aggressive behaviors.

(continued)

Idealization	Perceiving another individual as having more positive qualities than what he or she may actually have.
Hypochondriasis	Conversion of negative feelings toward others into negative feelings toward self and the expression of these feelings as somatic symptoms.
Passive aggression	Expression of feelings of aggression toward others in an indirect or in a passive way.
Fantasy	Retreating into a fantasy state in order to resolve inner and outer conflicts.

3. **Level 3 defense mechanisms (Neurotic)**: These defenses are seen in patients with personality disorders and anxiety disorders. They help in the short-term coping of stressful situations but cause long-term problems in relationships.

Defense	Explanation
Regression	Transient reversion of the ego to an earlier stage of development to handle unacceptable impulses.
Repression	Pulling thoughts into the unconscious and preventing painful or dangerous thoughts from entering consciousness.
Displacement	Shifting of unacceptable impulses to a more acceptable or less threatening object or person.
Dissociation	Transient alteration of one's personal identity or character to avoid feeling emotionally distressed.
Reaction formation	Conversion of unconscious wishes or impulses that are perceived to be dangerous or threatening into their opposites. Behaving or feeling completely opposite of how one really wants to behave or feel.
Isolation	The separation of feelings from ideas and events.
Intellectualization	Focusing on the intellectual aspects of a situation so as to distance oneself from the associated anxiety-provoking emotions.

4. **Level 4 defense mechanisms (Mature)**: These defense mechanisms are usually found among emotionally healthy adults and are considered the most mature of defenses. They help the person integrate conflicting emotions and thoughts, while still remaining effective.

Defense	Explanation
Altruism	Constructive service to others that brings joy and personal satisfaction.
Humor	Expression of ideas and feelings, especially those that are unpleasant, in a humorous way so as to give pleasure to others.
Sublimation	Transformation of negative emotions or thoughts into positive actions, behaviors, or emotions.
Suppression	The conscious decision to delay paying attention to an emotion or need in order to cope with reality.
Identification	The unconscious modeling of another person's character and behaviors.
Introjection	Identifying with some idea or object so deeply that it then becomes a part of that person.

3. DREAM ANALYSIS

Freud described dream interpretation as "the royal road to unconscious." In his book *The Interpretation of Dreams,* Freud opined that the foundation of all dream content is wish fulfillment. He argued that the reasons for dreams are found in the events of the day preceding the dream. Freud viewed dreams as a disguised fulfillment of repressed wishes. He stated that distorting operations were applied to the repressed wishes in forming the dream as recollected. These distortions make the manifest content of the dream differ from the latent-dream content. The operations that distort the dream content include four processes. They are condensation, displacement, representation, and symbolism. Freud also described secondary elaboration as the dreamer's natural tendency to make "sense" or "story" out of the various elements of the manifest content as recollected.

Process	Explanation
Condensation	Several associations and ideas are condensed into one theme.
Displacement	To prevent the censor's suspicion, the dream object's emotional significance is separated from the real object or content and attached to an entirely different object.
Representation	Thoughts are represented as visual images.
Symbolism	A person, action, or idea is replaced by a symbol.

4. PSYCHOSEXUAL STAGES

Freud opined that personality development also centered on the effects of the sexual pleasure drive on the individual psyche. He felt that at particular points in the developmental process, body parts are particularly sensitive to sexual or erotic stimulation. These erogenous zones include the mouth, anus, and the genital region.

Freud stated that the child cannot focus on the primary erogenous zone of the next stage without resolving the developmental conflicts of the previous stage. Each child at a given stage of development has certain needs and demands. The child gets frustrated when these needs are not met. On the other hand, overindulgence on the part of the caregivers also makes the child reluctant to progress beyond the particular stage. Both frustration and overindulgence tend to lock the child's libido permanently into the stage in which they occur, resulting in fixation. For normal development, a child has to progress through the stages, resolving each conflict and then moving on. If the child fixates at a particular stage, then the methods of obtaining satisfaction characterized by the stage will dominate his adult personality.

Stage	Age (years)	Pleasure Source	Conflict	Personality Development
Oral	0–2	Mouth: sucking, biting, and swallowing	Weaning away from mother's breast	The frustrated oral character is characterized by pessimism, envy, suspicion, and sarcasm. The overindulged oral character, often excessively satisfied, is optimistic, gullible, and full of admiration for others around him.
Anal	2–4	Anus: defecating or retaining feces	Toilet training	If the parents are too lenient, it will result in the formation of an anal expulsive character, who is messy, disorganized, reckless, and careless. If the parents are very strict, the child develops into an anal retentive character, who is neat, precise, orderly, careful, stingy, withholding, obstinate, meticulous, and passively aggressive.

(continued)

Phallic	4–6	Genitals	Oedipus complex (boys), Electra complex (girls). Castration anxiety	Fixation at the phallic stage develops a phallic character, who is self-assured, narcissistic, and proud. The failure to resolve the conflict causes a person to be afraid or incapable of close love. Freud postulated that fixation could be the root cause of homosexuality.
Latency	6 to puberty	Sports, hobbies, and same-sex friends	Sexual drive lies dormant	Children channel their repressed libidinal energy into pursuits such as school, athletics, and same-sex friendships.
Genital	Puberty onward	Physical and sexual changes reawaken the repressed needs and these sexual feelings toward others lead to sexual gratification	Social rules and norms	The less psychosexual conflict the person has, the greater his or her capacity to form normal relationships with the opposite sex. However, if the person remains fixated on the genital stage, he or she will struggle with repression and defenses.

B. Jung's Theories

Jung divided the psyche into three parts. The first part is the "ego," which Jung identified with the conscious mind. The "personal unconscious" includes memories that are brought to mind and those that have been suppressed. The third part is the "collective unconscious," which is the reservoir of our experiences as a species and includes the knowledge we are all born with. It influences all of our experiences and behaviors.

The contents of the collective unconscious are called "archetypes." An archetype is an unlearned tendency to experience things in a certain way. The archetypes have no form but act as an "organizing principle" on the things that we perceive or do. Different archetypes include the mother, father, child, hero, maiden, wise old man, trickster, hermaphrodite, self, and shadow. Jung stated that there is no fixed number of archetypes and they overlap and easily blend into each other as needed.

"Anima and animus" include the male or female roles we play. For most, that role is determined by the person's physical gender. In most societies, the expectations placed on men and women differ based on their different roles within the society. The anima is the female aspect present in the collective unconscious of men, and the animus is the male aspect present in the collective unconscious of women. The anima or animus is the archetype through which you communicate with the collective unconscious.

Jung also described three principles for the operation of the psyche. In the "Principle of Opposites," every wish immediately suggests its opposite type. It is this opposition that creates the power (or libido) of the psyche. The "Principle of Equivalence" states that the energy created from the opposition is divided between both sides equally. The "Principle of Entropy" describes the tendency for oppositions to come together and for the energy to decrease over a person's lifetime. Jung called the process of rising above our opposites and seeing both sides of who we are as "Transcendence." "Synchronicity" is the term he used to describe the occurrence of two events that are casually linked but are meaningfully related.

Jung developed a personality typology that described the distinction between "Introversion" and "Extroversion." Introverts prefer their internal world of thoughts, feelings, fantasies, and dreams, while extroverts prefer the external world of things and people and activities. Jung suggests there are four basic ways or functions that we use to deal with our inner and outer worlds. The first is "Sensing," in which the person gathers information by means of the senses. "Thinking" is the means of evaluating information or ideas rationally or logically. "Intuiting" is the perception that works outside of the usual conscious processes. "Feeling" is the evaluation of all the information available by weighing one's overall emotional response.

Jung stated that the goal of life is to realize the self. The self is an archetype that represents the transcendence of all opposites, so that every aspect of your personality is expressed equally. You are then neither and both male and female, neither and both ego and shadow, neither and both good and bad, neither and both conscious and unconscious, and neither and both an individual and the whole of creation.

C. Erikson's Theory

Erik Erikson believed that the ego exists from birth and the course of development is determined by the interaction of the body, mind, and cultural influences. He organized life into eight stages that extend from birth to death.

Age	Ego Developmental Outcome	Basic Strength	Additional Information
Birth to 18 months (infancy)	Trust vs. mistrust	Drive and Hope	This stage is also called the Oral Sensory Stage. If the child passes successfully through this stage, it will learn to trust that life is basically okay and will have basic confidence in the future. If it fails to experience trust and is constantly frustrated as its needs are not met, it may end up with a deep-seated feeling of worthlessness and a mistrust of the world in general.
18 months –3 years (early childhood)	Autonomy vs. shame	Self-control, courage, and will	In this stage, the child masters the skills for survival. It learns to walk, talk, and feed itself and become toilet trained. It develops autonomy as it gains more control over its body and acquires new skills. It also learns right from wrong. If it develops shame during the process of toilet training or in learning other skills, it may feel great shame and doubt of its capabilities and may suffer from low self-esteem.
3–5 years (play age)	Initiative vs. guilt	Purpose	During this period, the child experiences a desire to copy the adults around it. It also takes the initiative in creating play situations. It also begins to explore the world around it and uses the word "Why?" to get answers. At this stage, the child becomes involved in the Oedipal struggle and resolves this struggle through "social role identification." If frustration develops over the natural desires and goals, the child will experience guilt.
6–12 years (school age)	Industry vs. inferiority	Method and competence	This phase is also called latency. During this stage, the child learns, creates, and accomplishes numerous new skills. He develops a sense of industry. If the child experiences unresolved feelings of inadequacy and inferiority among peers, he can develop serious problems in terms of competence and self-esteem.

(Continued)

12–18 years (adolescence)	Identity vs. role confusion	Devotion and fidelity	Development during this stage depends primarily upon what we do for ourselves. During this stage, when we are neither a child nor an adult, we attempt to define our own self. We also struggle with social interactions and grapple with moral issues. During this process, some may withdraw from responsibilities, a phase Erikson called a "moratorium." If unsuccessful in navigating this stage, we will experience role confusion and upheavals.
18–35 years (young adulthood)	Intimacy and solidarity vs. isolation	Affiliation and love	Young adults seek companionship and development of one's family. If negotiating this stage is successful, then the adult can experience intimacy on a deeper level. If not successful, isolation and distance from others may develop. Without satisfying relationships, the world of the person begins to shrink.
35–65 years (middle adulthood)	Generativity vs. self-absorption or stagnation	Production and care	During this stage, the person becomes occupied with creative and meaningful work and with issues surrounding his or her family. The primary task of the person is to perpetuate culture and transmit values of the culture through the family. Strength comes through the care of others and production of something that contributes to the betterment of society, which is called generativity. In this stage, the main fear is inactivity and meaninglessness. As the children leave home, relationships or goals change. The person may be faced with major life changes—the midlife crisis—and struggle with finding new meanings and purposes. If the person does not get through this stage successfully, he or she can become self-absorbed and stagnate.
65 years to death (late adulthood)	Integrity vs. despair	Wisdom	Erikson stated that much of life is spent on preparing for the middle adulthood stage and the last stage is for recovering from it. Older adults often look back on their lives with happiness and are content, feeling fulfilled with a deep sense that life has meaning and the contributions made to life, a feeling Erikson called "Integrity." The strength in this stage comes from wisdom. There is a detachment from concerns for the whole of life and acceptance of death as the completion of life. Some adults may reach this stage and despair at their experiences and perceived failures. They may fear death as they struggle to find a purpose to their lives. They may also end up with a strong dogmatic view that only their view has been correct.

D. Piaget's Theory

Piaget proposed the theory of cognitive development called genetic epistemology. He described "four levels of development": infancy, preschool, childhood, and adolescence. Each stage is characterized by a cognitive structure that affects all of the child's thinking and actions. Each stage also represents the child's understanding of reality during that period. Progress from one stage to the next is due to the accumulation of errors in the child's understanding of his or her environment. This process causes cognitive disequilibrium that then restructures the entire thought process.

Concept	**Description**
Stage	The period in a child's development in which he is capable of understanding some things but not others.
Schema	The representation in the mind of perceptions, ideas, and actions that go together.
Adaptation	Process of becoming a part of the world.
Assimilation	The process of taking information from the environment to the mind and changing the evidence of his senses to make it fit.
Accommodation	The difference made to one's concepts by the process of assimilation.
Operation	The cognitive process of working through a concept.
Stage	
Sensorimotor (birth–2 years)	During this stage, the child learns about himself and his environment through motor and reflex actions. Thoughts are derived from sensation and movement. The child is able to differentiate self from objects. He is able to recognize self as an agent of action and begins to act intentionally. The child achieves *object permanence.*
Preoperational (2–7 years)	During this stage, the child learns to use language and to represent objects by images and words. The thinking is still *egocentric*. He has difficulty taking the viewpoint of others. The child begins to use symbols to represent objects. He also classifies objects by a single feature, i.e., single-colored blocks regardless of shape or all the blocks regardless of color. The child has difficulty conceptualizing time. His thinking is influenced by fantasy. The child takes in information and then changes it in his mind to fit his ideas.
Concrete operational (7–11 years)	During this stage, the child can think logically about objects and events. He achieves *conservation* of number (age 6), mass (age 7), and weight (age 9). He can classify objects according to several features and can order them in series along a single dimension such as size. During this stage, accommodation increases. The child develops an ability to think abstractly and to make rational judgment about concrete or observable phenomena.
Formal operational (11 years and up)	The child thinks logically about abstract propositions and test hypotheses systematically. At this stage, the child is capable of hypothetical and deductive reasoning. He becomes concerned with the hypothetical, the future, and the ideological problems.

E. Kernberg's Theory of Personality Development

Kernberg was a major proponent of Ego Psychology and Object Relations. He opined that the self is an intrapsychic structure that consists of multiple self representations. Realistic self integrates both good and bad self-images. It combines both the libidinal and aggressive components. Normal narcissism is seen as the libidinal investment of the self. This libidinal investment stems from the several relationships between the self and other intrapsychic structures including the ego, the superego, and the id. Narcissistic personality disorder develops due to the process of pathological differentiation and integration of ego and superego structures from pathological object relationships. Pathological narcissism constitutes the libidinal investment in the self in a primitive and pathological way. This pathological structure develops defense mechanisms against early self and object images that are either libidinal or aggressive.

Kernberg also opined that the defensive structure of a person with narcissistic personality disorder is similar to someone with borderline personality disorder as they both use the defenses of splitting and projective identification in their relationships.

Type of Narcissism	**Description**
Normal infantile narcissism	The regulation of self-esteem occurs through gratifications related to the age. These include infantile system of values, demands, and prohibitions.
Normal adult narcissism	The self-esteem is based on normal structures of the self. The whole representations of objects, stable object relationships, and solid moral systems have been introjected and the superego is fully developed and individualized.
Pathological narcissism	The three subtypes include: • Regression to the regulation of infantile self-esteem: In this subtype, the ego is dominated by infantile pursuits, values, and prohibitions. The regulation of self-esteem is mainly dependent on defense against infantile pleasures. These defenses are then discarded in adult life. • Narcissistic choice of object: The representation of the infantile self is projected on an object and then identified through that object. In this subtype, the functions of the self and the object have been exchanged. • Narcissistic personality disorder: This is the most severe subtype.

F. Kohut's Theory of Self-psychology

Kohut described the self as an adaptable structure with a static core which is defined early in life. Central to his theory was the concept of self and "defects" within the self. He opined that the failure of the parents to empathize with their children and the responses of their children to these failures were the causes of almost all psychopathology. Kohut also proposed human empathy as a therapeutic skill.

Kohut also described self-objects that are external objects which function as part of the self-machinery. These self-objects include people, objects, or activities that complete the self and are essential for the normal functioning of that person. He opined that when the self-object is not accessible, it will lead to frustration. This frustration is resolved by imagining the object's presence and creating a surrogate self-object until the real self-object becomes available. Kohut also described the need to establish a self-object that can be idealized. He also described ego-twinship, which is the need to feel a likeness to another human being.

Kohut's concept of personality differed from that of Kernberg. He opined that narcissistic and borderline personality disorders are separate in their development. He felt that narcissistic personality results from the pathological development in which aggressive drives play a central role. They are also more appropriate for psychological treatment as they are characterized by a more resilient self. Kohut and Kernberg also differed in their treatment approaches as Kohut encouraged the patient's narcissistic desires to be opened up during the process of transference while Kernberg encouraged the use of confrontation to help the patient integrate his or her internal fragmented world.

G. Klein's Theory of Object Relations

Melanie Klein was an important proponent of Object Relations theory. She was the first person to use traditional psychoanalytic techniques with children. She opined that parental figures played a significant role in the child's fantasy life. She also described the paranoid-schizoid position and the depressive positions. These are a set of psychic functions that correspond to a given phase of development and that usually appear during the first year of life. These can reactivate at any time in one's life. The earlier and more primitive position is the paranoid-schizoid position and if the individual's environment and upbringing are satisfactory, he or she will progress through to the depressive position.

The *paranoid-schizoid position* is thought to occur in the first 6 months of age. Central to the paranoid-schizoid position is the concept of paranoid anxiety. This is the anxiety of imminent annihilation. In this position, the immature ego deals with its anxiety by splitting off bad feelings and projecting them outward, resulting in paranoia. The schizoid describes the defense mechanism of splitting the good object from the bad object. Klein opined that a healthy development indicates that the infant has to split its external world into two categories: the good and the bad. The good symbolizes love and gratification and the bad the feelings of frustration and hatred. This split makes it possible for the infant to introject and identify with the good object. It is a means of identifying what is good and what is bad for survival. When the ego develops sufficiently, the bad can be integrated and the ambivalence and conflict can be tolerated. With maturity and the resolution of the depressive position, the ego is able to bring together the good and bad objects, thereby leading to whole object relations. In achieving this position, there is the process of mourning the loss of the idealized object and this is usually associated with depressive anxiety.

H. Kohlberg's Theory of Moral Reasoning

Kohlberg's theory proposes that moral reasoning is the basis for ethical behaviors. He opined that the process of moral development was principally concerned with justice and that it continues throughout the individual's lifetime. He proposed six identifiable developmental stages occurring sequentially, with each more adequate at responding to moral dilemmas than its predecessor. These six stages can be generally grouped into three levels of two stages each: preconventional, conventional, and postconventional.

Levels	Stages
Level I: Preconventional This type of moral reasoning is especially common in children	**Stage One: Obedience and punishment orientation.** Individual focuses on the direct consequence of his action on himself. An action is perceived to be morally wrong if the perpetrator is punished. The worse the punishment for the act, the worse the act. It gives an inference that even innocent victims are guilty in proportion to their suffering. Thinking is egocentric. There is no recognition of others' points of view. There is deference to superior power or to prestige. **Stage Two: Self-interest orientation.** In this stage, right behavior is defined by whatever is in the individual's best interest. There is only a limited interest in the needs of others if it furthers the individual's own interests. Concern for others is not based on loyalty or respect but rather on a self-serving mentality.

(continued)

Level II: Conventional This is the moral reasoning typical of adolescents and adults	**Stage Three: Interpersonal accord and conformity.** Individuals are receptive to approval or disapproval from others based on societal roles. They try to be a "good boy" or "good girl" to live up to these expectations. They judge the morality of an action by evaluating its consequences in terms of a person's relationships. The desire to maintain rules and authority exists in order to support and maintain these social roles. **Stage Four: Authority and social order maintaining orientation.** Moral reasoning at this stage indicates that society must learn to transcend individual needs. Ideals are often prescribed. Judgment is provided on what is right or wrong. There is a duty to uphold laws and rules. When someone does violate a law, it is morally wrong. Culpability is important at this stage.
Level III: Postconventional No individual consistently operates at this level	**Stage Five: Social contract orientation.** Each individual is viewed as holding different opinions and values. Laws are regarded as social contracts rather than rigid dictums. Those societal rules that do not promote the general welfare need to be changed when necessary for the greater good of the society. Majority decision making, compromises, and democratic process are all given due consideration. **Stage Six: Universal ethical principles.** Moral reasoning is based on ethical principles. Laws are only valid if they are just. Commitment to justice carries with it an obligation to disobey unjust laws. Decisions are reached categorically and not hypothetically.

IMPORTANT POINTS TO REMEMBER

- In psychodynamic psychotherapy, the therapist's job is to listen and to help identify patterns of thinking, feeling, and interactions that may be contributing to the patient's current struggles.
- During the sessions, the patient becomes more aware of his or her thoughts and feelings and learns effective ways of dealing with problems.
- Awareness and insights are thought to stimulate psychological growth and change in the patient.
- This therapy places great importance on the relationship between the therapist and the patient, i.e., the therapeutic dyad.
- The relationship between the therapist and the patient is unique because the therapist maintains a uniform, neutral, and accepting stance.
- There are mainly theoretical frameworks that the therapists can use to help their patients but the decision to use a particular framework depends entirely on the therapists.
- Treatment continues until the troubling symptoms have been reduced or alleviated and the patient is consistently making use of more adaptive methods of coping with greater insight.
- Following the completion of therapy, the patient should ideally be able to handle difficulties in a more adaptive manner, have improved interpersonal relationships, be productive at work, and continue to develop new insights into his or her thoughts, feelings, and behaviors.

SUGGESTED READINGS

Gabbard GO. *Psychodynamic Psychiatry in Clinical Practice*. 4th Ed. Arlington, VA: American Psychiatric Publishing, Inc., 2008:3–127.

Kaplan HI, Sadock BJ. *Kaplan and Sadock's Synopsis of Psychiatry*. 8th Ed. Philadelphia, PA: Lippincott Williams & Wilkins, 1998:206–239, 885–893.

Tyson P, Tyson RL. *Psychoanalytic Theories of Development. An Integration*. New Haven: Yale University Press, 1990:7–322.

H.2. Cognitive behavioral therapy

Gauri Khatkhate, MD, Kirsten M. Wilkins, MD

INTRODUCTION

Cognitive behavioral therapy (CBT), formulated by Aaron T. Beck in the early 1960s, is based on the theory that one's affect and behavior are determined by cognitions which are based on underlying assumptions. For example, the cognitive theory of depression postulates that cognitive dysfunctions comprise the core of depression and that symptoms of depression (i.e., feelings of worthlessness, guilt, and hopelessness) are consequences of faulty thinking patterns. The goal of therapy is to help patients recognize, challenge, and change these distorted constructs in order to alleviate depression.

CBT is a structured, time-limited therapy, typically carried out weekly. Therapy is usually conducted on an individual basis, although CBT groups have been utilized as well. CBT is oriented toward resolution of current problems, and the therapist and patient actively collaborate toward this goal. This therapy is comprised of three core components: didactic aspects, cognitive techniques, and behavioral techniques. CBT has been shown to be one of the most useful psychotherapeutic modalities for the treatment of depression, and has shown efficacy in the treatment of other disorders as well.

INDICATIONS

CBT has a substantial evidence base supporting its use as monotherapy for the treatment of mild to moderate major depressive disorder and as adjunct therapy along with medications for severe major depressive disorders. It has also been shown to have a therapeutic effect in the treatment of panic disorder, generalized anxiety disorder, bulimia nervosa, substance use disorders, and schizophrenia. Other indications for which it has been explored include personality disorders, somatoform disorders, obsessive-compulsive dis order, posttraumatic stress disorder, and smoking cessation. Patients who are ideal for CBT are psychologically minded and are able to recognize their emotions and become aware of distorted thought patterns.

According to Aaron T. Beck, the criteria that justify the use of CBT alone include failure to respond to two more antidepressants; partial response to adequate doses of antidepressants; failure to respond to or partial response to other psychotherapies; variable mood that correlates with negative cognitions; adequate reality testing; inability to tolerate medication side effects or evidence of substantial risk with pharmacotherapy. Factors that suggest CBT alone is *not* indicated include evidence of coexisting schizophrenia, dementia, or substance-related disorders; medical illness or medication likely causing depression; poor reality resting; history of manic episode or family member with bipolar I disorder; little evidence of cognitive distortions; and absence of precipitating environmental stresses.

CBT can be used in both inpatient and outpatient psychiatric treatment settings. Gender, educational level, socioeconomic status, and ethnic background do not appear to influence the outcome of CBT. Though initially developed for individual therapy, CBT has been modified for group therapy, couples' problems, and family therapy.

BASIC TERMS

Theoretical Framework

The *cognitive model* theorizes that disturbances in one's mood and behavior arise from dysfunctional thinking. Therefore, it is not the particular situation, but rather how the patient perceives the situation, that leads to a change in the patient's mood. These situation-specific words and images that enter one's mind are called *automatic thoughts*. CBT aims to help patients identify, challenge, and then modify these automatic thoughts in order to improve mood and behavior.

Underlying automatic thoughts are more global, generalized ideas about oneself, called *core beliefs*. These beliefs develop in childhood, and can be positive (e.g., "I am likeable") or negative (e.g., "I am unworthy"). These beliefs may extend to other people and the world. Core beliefs generally belong to one of two categories: helpless core beliefs and unlovable core beliefs. Between automatic thoughts and core beliefs are intermediate beliefs, a set of rules, attitudes, and assumptions that influence the patient's thinking, but which may not be explicitly discussed in treatment. Typically, therapy begins with a focus on identifying and modifying automatic thoughts; later, the same is done for the underlying core beliefs.

Treatment Structure

CBT is a problem-oriented, short-term treatment that typically lasts between 5 and 20 sessions for uncomplicated cases, though more complex or treatment-resistant cases may take longer. The focus is on the here and now, but a longitudinal perspective is used to develop a more complete understanding of the patient and his difficulties. As in all forms of therapy, the therapeutic relationship is considered key to successful treatment. In CBT this relationship is highly collaborative, with the patient and therapist working together to identify current dysfunctional patterns of thought and behavior and to replace them with more adaptive ones. The first step in CBT is a comprehensive history and mental status examination leading to a multiaxial diagnosis. The diagnosis is used to develop a case conceptualization that also takes into account formative experiences, interpersonal and situational concerns, biological factors, patient strengths, patterns of automatic thoughts, and underlying core beliefs. The patient and therapist then come up with a set of goals for treatment that helps the therapist to develop a treatment plan. In addition to developing the case conceptualization, treatment goals, and treatment plan, the therapist works to establish trust and rapport, to normalize the patient's problems, and to instill hope. The patient is educated about his illness and about the cognitive model. Because this treatment may be new or different for the patient, it is important to understand his expectations about therapy and to socialize him into cognitive therapy.

CBT is highly structured, and sessions often begin with a brief update and check on mood symptoms (and medications, if prescribed). This is typically followed by "bridging" from the previous session; that is, reviewing the patient's understanding and any pertinent issues. Then, an agenda is set, in which both patient and therapist identify important issues to address in the session. Homework is a key element of CBT and allows the patient to practice the techniques that have been learned in session throughout the week. If completed, homework is reviewed in session. If not completed, reasons for not completing it are explored and homework may be completed in session. Finally, sessions end with feedback/summary, wherein the patient has a chance to provide the therapist with input on how they felt about the session and raise any concerns or questions. Early CBT sessions tend to be more structured than later sessions. As therapy progresses, patients are less symptomatic and have acquired the skills needed to be more responsible for managing their own treatment. Focus then shifts more toward anticipating difficulties that may occur after termination and developing strategies for relapse prevention. In chronic or recurrent illness, an intermittent booster session may be scheduled after the main treatment is complete.

Therapeutic Strategies

CBT, as previously noted, has three components: didactic aspects, cognitive techniques, and behavioral techniques. Didactic strategies are used to educate the patient about his illness and the treatment process. The ultimate goal in CBT is for the patient to become his own therapist. One of the principles of CBT is that when patients suffer from illnesses such as depression or anxiety, they are more likely to commit *cognitive errors* that lead to changes in mood and behavior. A list of common errors is included in Table 3H.2.1. Patients can be taught to observe their thoughts, to recognize errors, and to replace dysfunctional thoughts with more realistic appraisals. This process is known as *cognitive restructuring*. Commonly used methods include Socratic questioning, the keeping of thought records, examining the evidence, and cognitive rehearsal. Behavioral strategies are also used in CBT. One example is behavioral activation, in which patients are helped to choose one or two manageable activities that

TABLE 3H.2.1 Cognitive Errors

1. *All-or-nothing thinking*: viewing a situation in black-and-white terms
2. *Catastrophizing*: predicting negative outcomes without considering other, more likely, possibilities
3. *Discounting the positive*: telling oneself that positive experiences or qualities do not count
4. *Emotional reasoning*: assuming something is true because it "feels" true, despite evidence to the contrary
5. *Labeling*: using fixed, global labels for self or others without considering more reasonable alternatives
6. *Magnification/minimization*: magnifying the negative and minimizing the positive when examining self, others, or a situation
7. *Mental filter*: focusing excessively on one negative detail instead of on the whole picture
8. *Mind reading*: assuming you know what others are thinking without considering other possibilities
9. *Overgeneralization*: making sweeping conclusions that go beyond the current situation
10. *Personalization*: believing other people's behavior is a direct reflection on you without considering other explanations
11. *"Should" and "must" statements*: you have fixed expectations of how you and others should behave and overestimate how bad it is if these are not met
12. *Tunnel vision*: you only see the negative aspects in a situation

Adapted from Beck JS. *Cognitive Therapy: Basics and Beyond*. New York: The Guilford Press, 1995.

might change the way they feel and to develop a plan for carrying them out. Patients rate activities on the sense of mastery and pleasure that they provide. Other techniques include graded exposure to feared situations, breaking down large tasks into smaller, more achievable ones, the scheduling of pleasant activities, and relaxation training.

IMPORTANT POINTS TO REMEMBER

- CBT was developed by Aaron T. Beck to treat patients with depression and anxiety disorders. It has also been shown to be useful in the treatment of bulimia nervosa, substance abuse, and schizophrenia, among others.
- CBT may be used as monotherapy in mild to moderate major depression, when antidepressants have not been effective due to poor response or side effects, or when other psychotherapies have failed.
- The cognitive model, on which CBT is based, theorizes that problems with mood and behavior arise from dysfunctional automatic thoughts, which in turn are based on negative core beliefs about the self, others, and the world.
- CBT uses a set of didactic, cognitive, and behavioral strategies to help patients examine their thoughts, detect distortions, and replace them with more adaptive and realistic ones.
- The treatment is problem oriented and time limited with structured sessions and emphasis on the here and now.
- Homework is a key element of CBT that allows patients to practice skills in real world situations.
- An ultimate goal of CBT is for patients to gain the tools they need to act as their own therapists once treatment is complete.

SUGGESTED READINGS

Beck JS. *Cognitive Therapy: Basics and Beyond*. New York, NY: The Guilford Press, 1995.

Deckersbach T, Gershuny BS, Otto MW. Cognitive-behavioral therapy for depression: Applications and outcomes. *Psychiatr Clin N Am* 2000;23: 795–809.

Dobson KS. A meta-analysis of the efficacy of cognitive therapy for depression. *J Consult Clin Psychol* 1989;57:414–419.

Hoffman SG, Smits JAJ. Cognitive-behavioral therapy for adult anxiety disorders: A meta-analysis of randomized, placebo-controlled trials. *J Clin Psychiatry* 2008;69:621–632.

Rush JA, Beck AT. Cognitive therapy. In: Sadock BJ, Sadock VA, eds. *Comprehensive Textbook of Psychiatry*. 7th Ed. Philadelphia, PA: Lippincott Williams & Wilkins, 2000:2167–2178.

Wright JH, Basco MR, Thase ME. *Learning Cognitive Behavioral Therapy: An Illustrated Guide*. Arlington, VA: American Psychiatric Publishing, Inc., 2006.

H.3. Dialectical behavioral therapy

Natalie Weder, MD

INTRODUCTION

Dialectical behavioral therapy (DBT) was developed by Marsha Linehan in the 1990s to treat people with borderline personality disorder (BPD) and who presented with suicidality and repeated self-harming behaviors. Since then, DBT has evolved to become a treatment for different multidiagnostic psychiatric illnesses.

DBT is based on a biosocial theory of BPD, in which a child with high emotional vulnerability is placed in an "invalidating environment." It is thought that in this invalidating environment, there is a mismatch between the child's emotional expression and vulnerability, and the caretaker's ability to process and tolerate it. The child's expressions of emotions are then met with erratic and inappropriate responses from the caretaker, which contribute and reinforce the development of emotional dysregulation and distress. DBT follows both cognitive and behavioral principles, but the unique feature of this therapy is that validation and acceptance of clients are core therapeutic components.

DBT is based on the concept of "dialectics"; both the patient and the therapist accept the existence of opposing views and perspectives, and try to find a synthesis to a particular problem. Clients are accepted as they are, but within the dialectic, are also encouraged to change and to develop skills and coping mechanisms to have a "life worth living." The treatment includes weekly individual sessions with a skilled therapist, a skills training group, a therapist consultation team, and individual coaching for clients. It is a highly structured form of therapy, is evidence-based, and has solid scientific data proving its effectiveness in treating this particular population.

INDICATIONS

DBT was initially designed for women with BPD, especially if they were presenting with recurrent suicidal and self-harming behaviors. Several randomized controlled trials comparing DBT with treatment as usual and other standardized treatment like client-centered therapy and psychodynamic psychotherapy modalities have consistently found that this therapy significantly reduces the rate of intentional self-injury, a reduction in total psychiatric hospitalization days, self-rated anger, global mental health functioning, and treatment dropout rates in clients with BPD, when compared to these other treatment modalities.

Since substance abuse is a common and important problem faced by many clients who suffer from BPD, Marsha Linehan's group created a modified version of standard DBT specifically targeted for clients with BPD and substance abuse. In this modification, more attachment strategies were developed to prevent clients from dropping out of treatment, clients were encouraged to receive replacement pharmacotherapy for their substance abuse, and clinicians undertook a more active role as case managers, to address important issues common to clients with substance abuse, such as legal and housing difficulties. Although studies showed that DBT remains effective in reducing self-harming behaviors and core problems of BPD in patients who have comorbid substance abuse, more studies are needed to determine if DBT can also be helpful in treating substance abuse per se.

DBT has also shown to be helpful in treating adults over the age of 60 years with major depressive disorder when compared to pharmacotherapy. Two studies have examined the efficacy of DBT to treat clients with eating disorders. One study found that DBT significantly reduced the number of binge and purge episodes when compared to controls on a waiting list, while the other study reported that in addition to reducing binge and purge episodes, DBT significantly reduced the patient's weight, shape, and eating concerns. However, both studies had small sample sizes and controls were not receiving any standard intervention.

BASIC TERMS

Theoretical Framework

DBT integrates concepts from different theoretical frameworks, such as cognitive and behavioral therapies, as well as Zen practice and mindfulness. Following the biosocial theory in which clients with BDP have a biological predisposition to high emotional vulnerability and were frequently raised in an invalidating environment, this therapy tries to create a more validating framework for clients, which is accepting but also encourages change and the development of adaptive behaviors.

Assumptions

DBT has several assumptions about clients. One of these assumptions is that clients are doing the best they can and want to improve, but at the same time, they need to do better and try harder to lead a better life. It also believes that although clients may not have caused all of their own problems, they have to solve them anyway, and need to learn new behaviors in order to be able to lead a better life.

Following these assumptions, the therapists pay close attention to specific behaviors that may be reinforcing unwanted outcomes, such as episodes of self-harm or anger outbursts. While keeping awareness of both sides of each dialectic, both the therapist and client try to find a synthesis that will then lead to a more adaptive behavior. Mindfulness, which is taught as a skill during treatment, helps clients to be more aware and nonjudgmental of their environment and their behaviors, and at the same time it provides a means to cope with intense emotions, without having to act out on them.

Treatment Structure

DBT is divided into individual sessions with a therapist and weekly group sessions which focus on building skills and individual consultation to the client, which are usually done via telephone consultations. Clients commit to a contract at the start of treatment, and are required to attend a minimum number of sessions to be able to continue the treatment.

DBT also acknowledges that the therapist's well-being is a critical part of the treatment, and it requires therapists to attend a weekly consultation session, to prevent them from feeling burnt-out and to make therapists and skills-group leaders work as a team and obtain knowledge and support from each other.

Treatment Hierarchy

Another important aspect of DBT is its treatment target hierarchy. Individual therapists follow this hierarchy during sessions, to keep track of the client's progress and treatment goals, and to make sure that important problem behaviors are not missed during sessions. The following are the four components of DBT's target hierarchy:

1. Reducing life-threatening, self-harm, or suicidal behaviors
2. Reducing therapy interfering behaviors
3. Reducing quality of life–interfering behaviors
4. Improving the use of adaptive skills

Stages of Treatment

DBT has four different stages of treatment which are addressed in a hierarchical order. Clients in the first stage present with behaviors that are life threatening. Once a client has control of these types of behavior, the treatment moves to the next stage. The second stage focuses on emotional experiencing and working on issues related to trauma and posttraumatic stress. The third stage deals with achieving individual goals and improving one's self-respect. Finally, clients in the fourth stage focus on increasing one's joy and dealing with feelings of loneliness or emptiness. Most of the research examining DBT's efficacy has focused on the first stage of treatment, and particularly in reducing self-harming and suicidal behaviors.

IMPORTANT POINTS TO REMEMBER

- DBT was developed by Marsha Linehan to treat clients with BPD and suicidal behaviors.
- Several randomized controlled studies have shown its efficacy in reducing suicidal behavior and other core problems of clients with BPD.
- Some studies have shown that it is also beneficial in treating clients with BDP and substance abuse, depression in the elderly, and eating disorders.
- The treatment is highly structured, and involves weekly individual sessions, skills-training groups, and individual coaching.
- The treatment follows a dialectical framework, in which both therapist and client accept a situation the way it is, acknowledge the opposing aspects of it, and come to a synthesis which then leads to more adaptive behaviors.

SUGGESTED READINGS

Koons CR, Robins CJ, Tweed J, et al. Efficacy of dialectical therapy in women veterans with borderline personality disorder. *Behav Ther* 2001;32:371–390.

Linehan MM. *Cognitive-Behavioral Treatment of Borderline Personality Disorder*. New York, NY: Guilford, 1993a.

Linehan MM, Comtois KA, Murray AM, et al. Two year randomized controlled trial and follow-up of dialectical behavior therapy vs therapy by experts for suicidal behaviors and borderline personality disorder. *Arch Gen Psychiatry* 2006b;62:1–10.

Lynch TR, Morse JQ, Mendelson T, et al. Dialectical behavior therapy for depressed older adults: A randomized pilot study. *Am J Geriatr Psychiatry* 2003;11:33–45.

Lynch TR, Trost WT, Salsman N, et al. Dialectical behavior therapy for borderline personality disorder. *Annu Rev Clin Psychol* 2007;3: 181–205.

Turner RM. Naturalistic evaluation of dialectical behavior therapy-oriented treatment for borderline personality disorder. *Cogn Behav Pract* 2000a;7:413–419.

van den Bosch LMC, Verheul R, Schippers GM, et al. Dialectical behavior therapy of borderline patients with and without substance use problems: Implementation and long-term effects. *Addict Behav* 2002;27:911–923.

H.4. Interpersonal therapy

Nicole A. Foubister, MD, Clarence Watson, MD, JD

INTRODUCTION

Interpersonal therapy (IPT) is a time-limited treatment directed at improving interpersonal skills that may have contributed to the development of depression. Treatment is focused on developing these skills in 12 to 16 sessions.

INDICATIONS

IPT, initially developed to treat adult depression, has since been applied to the treatment of depression in adolescents, the elderly, and people with human immunodeficiency virus (HIV) infection. In addition, it has been used with dysthymic disorder, bipolar disorder, and depressed patients with marital difficulties. IPT has also been modified for the treatment of substance abuse, bulimia, and anorexia nervosa.

BASIC TERMS

There are seven types of interventions that are commonly used in IPT, many of which reflect the influence of psychodynamic psychotherapy. These include a focus on a patient's emotions, an exploration of resistance to treatment, discussion of patterns in relationships, taking a detailed past history, an emphasis on current interpersonal experiences, exploration of the therapist/patient relationship, and the identification of patient's wishes and fantasies. IPT emphasizes the ways in which a person's current relationships and social context cause or maintain symptoms rather than exploring the deep-seated sources of the symptoms. IPT is distinctive for its brevity and its treatment focus. Goals of treatment are the improvement in current interpersonal skills with subsequent rapid symptom reduction, amelioration of depressive symptoms, and improved social adjustment.

The IPT framework considers clinical depression as having three components: the development of symptoms, which arise from biological, genetic, and/or psychodynamic processes; social interactions with other people, which are learned over the course of one's life; and personality, made up of the more enduring traits and behaviors that may predispose a person to depressive symptoms. IPT intervenes at the levels of symptom formation and social functioning, and does not attempt to alter aspects of the patient's personality.

Treatment with IPT is based on the premise that depression occurs in a social and interpersonal context which must be understood for improvement to occur. Interpersonal psychotherapy utilizes reassurance, clarification of feeling states, improvement in interpersonal communications, testing perceptions, development of interpersonal skills, and medication as indicated. Treatment occurs in three phases, the first of which is gathering a history, formulating a diagnosis, and introducing the framework for treatment. Data obtained from this review assist in identifying one of four problem areas that will guide therapy: unresolved grief, social role disputes (often marital), social role transitions, and interpersonal deficits. Use of medications is determined based on symptom severity, previous response, and patient preference. The patient is placed in the sick role, and the depressive syndrome is related to the patient's main interpersonal theme.

In the first session, the psychiatric history includes a review of the client's current social functioning and their patterns and mutual expectations in current close relationships. Changes in relationships prior to the onset of symptoms are clarified, such as the death of a loved one, a child leaving home, or worsening marital conflict.

IPT is psychoeducational and involves teaching the client about the nature of depression and the ways that it manifests itself in his or her life and relationships. In the initial sessions, depressive symptoms are reviewed in detail, and the accurate naming of the problem is essential. The therapist explains depression, its treatment, and how the patient has adopted the "sick role." The concept of the "sick role" based on the notion that illness is not merely a condition but a social role that affects the attitudes and behaviors of the patient and those around him or her. The patient learns how the sick role has increasingly come to govern his or her social interactions.

The middle phase of treatment is directed toward resolving the identified problem area with specific goals and strategies used for each problem area.

In **unresolved grief**, the goals of treatment are to facilitate the mourning process and assist the patient in finding new activities and relationships to offset the loss. In normal bereavement, a person experiences symptoms such as sadness, disturbed sleep, and difficulty functioning which usually resolve in 2 to 4 months. Unresolved grief in depressed patients is usually either delayed grief, which has been postponed and then experienced long after the loss; or distorted grief, in which there is no felt emotion of sadness but there may be nonemotional symptoms, which are often somatic in nature.

Interpersonal role disputes occur when the patient and at least one other significant person have differing expectations of their relationship. The dispute is identified, a plan of action is chosen, and a resolution is sought through modified expression or improved communication. The therapist does not direct the patient to one particular resolution strategy, and patients are encouraged to terminate an unsuccessful plan of action in exchange for another. The therapist does not attempt to preserve unworkable relationships.

Depression associated with **role transitions** occurs when a person has difficulty coping with life changes that require new roles. These may be such transitions as retirement, a career change, moving, or leaving home. The patient is assisted in mourning and accepting the loss of the old role. Therapy is terminated when a client has given up the old role; expressed the accompanying feelings of guilt, anger, and loss; acquired new skills; and developed a social network around the new role.

Interpersonal deficits are the focus of treatment when the patient has a history of inadequate or unsupportive interpersonal relationships. The patient may never have established lasting or intimate relationships as an adult, and may experience a sense of inadequacy, lack of self-assertion, and guilt about expressing anger. Generally, patients with a history of extreme social isolation come to therapy with more severe emotional disturbances. Rather than focusing on current relationships, IPT therapy in this area focuses on the patient's past relationships; the present relationship with the therapist; and ways to form new relationships. In the treatment of interpersonal role deficits, the therapist encourages the patient to establish relationships and diminish social isolation.

The expected outcomes of IPT are a reduction or elimination of symptoms, improved interpersonal functioning, and a greater understanding of the presenting symptoms and ways to prevent their recurrence. The efficacy of IPT for the treatment of acute depression has been demonstrated in several randomized controlled trials.

IMPORTANT POINTS TO REMEMBER

- IPT is directed at improving interpersonal relationships that may have contributed to the development of depression.
- IPT identifies "here and now" concerns such as grief, loss of an important relationship, or new transitions such as motherhood.
- One of four main problem areas (unresolved grief, interpersonal role disputes, role transitions, or interpersonal deficits) is identified as the main focus of treatment.
- Specific goals and strategies are used for each individual problem area.
- Treatment in limited in duration, usually 12 to 16 sessions.

SUGGESTED READINGS

American Psychiatric Association. *Diagnostic and Statistical Manual of Mental Disorders: Text Revised*. 4th Ed. Washington, DC: American Psychiatric Association, 2000.

Apple R. Interpersonal therapy for bulimia nervosa. *J Clin Psychol* 1999;55(6):715–725.

Barkham M, Hardy G. Counseling and interpersonal therapies for depression: Towards securing an evidence-base. *Br Med Bull* 2001;57:115–132.

Frank E, Thase M. Natural history and preventative treatment of recurrent mood disorders. *Annu Rev Med* 1999;50:453–468.

Klerman G, Weissman M, Rounseville B, et al. *Interpersonal Psychotherapy of Depression*. New York, NY: Basic Books, 1984.

Klerman G, Weissman M. *New Applications of Interpersonal Psychotherapy*. Washington, DC: American Psychiatric Press, Inc., 1993.

McIntosh V. Interpersonal psychotherapy for anorexia nervosa. *Int J Eat Disord* 2000;27:125–139.

Mufson L. *Interpersonal Psychotherapy for Depressed Adolescents*. New York, NY: Guilford Press, 1993.

Mufson L, Weissman M, Moreau D, et al. Efficacy of interpersonal psychotherapy for depressed adolescents. *Arch Gen Psychiatry* 1999;56(6):573–579.

Weissman M, Markowitz J. An overview of interpersonal psychotherapy. In: Markowitz, J, ed. *Interpersonal Psychotherapy*. Washington, DC: American Psychiatric Press, 1998:1–33.

Weissman M, Markowitz J. Interpersonal psychotherapy: Current status. *Arch Gen Psychiatry* 1994;51(8):599–606.

Weissman M, Markowitz J, Klerman G. *Clinician's Quick Guide to Interpersonal Psychotherapy*. New York, NY: Oxford University Press, 2007.

H.5. Group therapy

Sunanda Muralee, MD, Rajesh R. Tampi, MD, MS

INTRODUCTION

Group therapy is a form of psychotherapy in which one or more therapists treat a small group of clients together as a group. This term can refer to any form of psychotherapy when delivered in a group format but is most commonly used to denote psychodynamic therapy where the group context and group process are explicitly utilized as a mechanism of change by developing, exploring, and examining interpersonal relationships within the group. The concept of group therapy can include any process that takes place in a group setting, including support groups, skills training groups (such as anger management, mindfulness, relaxation training, or social skills training), and psychoeducation groups.

INDICATIONS

Group therapy can be practiced in inpatient and outpatient settings, partial hospitalization programs, halfway houses, community settings, and in private practice. Group therapy has been effective in the treatment of depression, posttraumatic stress disorder, borderline personality disorder, and inpatient substance abuse. The efficacy of group therapy has also been demonstrated in patients with alexithymia and in patients with cancer in helping them with coping with their illness. It is also widely used by nonmental health professionals in the adjuvant treatment of physical disorders.

BASIC TERMS

A. Common Therapeutic Assumptions

1. **Attachment:** Human beings are social animals and there is a universal and primary need for attachment.
2. **Cohesion:** Cohesive relationships help in new interpersonal learning.
3. **Amplification:** Relationships within a group help make the individual aware of his or her own true feelings and impulses and help him or her manage these feelings and impulses.

Relationships within the group help reduce isolation and shame while providing empathy and support to the individual. They also help members expand their emotional and behavioral repertoire.

B. Theories in Group Therapy

1. **General Systems Theory.** This theory integrates the intrapsychic, interpersonal, and social perspectives within the group. It focuses on growth and change, rather than on conflicts and deficits. It also maintains that groups possess common properties and these exist to carry out defined functions and goals. The relationship within the group is constantly impacted by factors from within the group and from the outside of the group that affects its members. It stresses the importance of understanding and maintaining boundaries; boundaries are seen as being permeable, allowing for the sufficient exchange of information, but being impermeable by providing protection and separation to the group. The group leaders ensure the appropriate functioning of the group by monitoring boundaries, the group process to support desired behaviors, providing information, feedback, and guiding member interactions in a positive direction. The structure of the group evolves from such ongoing interaction within the group.
2. **Cognitive Behavioral Theory.** It uses behavioral principles and techniques such as social skills training, cognitive restructuring, stress inoculation, and problem solving as curative factors of group therapy. The group setting provides opportunities for patients to eliminate maladaptive patterns of thinking and behavior and to learn and practice adaptive skills,

behaviors, and cognitions. The emphasis within the group is the present and the future and not the past. The individual members of the group and the group contract for mutually agreeable goals and the therapist then functions as consultant to the group. The members of the group support each other with constructive feedback, altruistic behavior, and peer reinforcement. They learn to interact with authority by dealing with the group therapist.

3. **Transactional Analysis.** It was developed by Eric Berne in the mid-1950s and borrows extensively from psychoanalytic concepts including structural theory and the concept of regression. The focus is on the individual within the group while other members function as supportive audience. It focuses primarily on ego states; the parent, adult, and child. The ego states are further subdivided into Critical and Nurturing subcategories. It uses labels like scripts, decision, and redecisions to maintain contracts.
4. **Existentialism.** This theory divides the world into two basic forms: being-in-itself which consists of nonhuman forms and animals and being-for-itself, which consists of humans and transcendent consciousness. This theory places emphasis on the concept of conscious choice and includes the ideas of human consciousness and intentionality, freedom, responsibility, authenticity, and engagement. The state of consciousness is in relation to the external world. Within the group setting, an individual's personal myth, intentionality in the world, and authentic self, as they are seen by the group, can be presented, verified, and accepted.

C. Bion's Subgroups

Based on his observation of the group process, Bion described two subgroups within every group. They are the work group and the basic assumption group.

1. **Work group:** This group is involved with actual work task in the group and is geared toward the completion of the task.
2. **Basic assumptions group:** This refers to the unconscious thoughts and fantasies that lead the group away from its primary goal. The groups then begins to act in an "as-if manner." The group behaves on an assumption that is different from the main task at hand. There are three types of basic assumption.

1. **Dependency:** Group members behave as if they are weak and totally dependant on the therapist for functioning.
2. **Fight or flight:** Group members become nonreflective and regress to the point where they see only two ways to proceed forward with the group, i.e., fight the therapist or give up control completely.
3. **Pairing:** Group members try to pair up and produce a solution to rescue the entire group.

The group therapist has to be vigilant for the development of these basic assumptions within the group, so it can be interpreted and used in a constructive manner. If unchecked, these assumptions can destroy the framework of the group and prevent the group from undertaking its primary task.

D. Curative Factors

The 12 important curative factors within a group described by Yalom are as follows:

1. **Universality:** These shared experiences and feelings among group members that include universal human concerns, serve to remove a group member's sense of isolation, validate his or her experiences and raise his or her self-esteem.
2. **Cohesiveness:** This is the primary therapeutic factor in the group. Humans have the instinctive need to belong to groups, and personal development can only take place in an interpersonal context. A cohesive group is one in which all members feel a sense of belonging, acceptance, and validation.
3. **Altruism:** The group is a place where members help each other, and the experience of being able to give something to another person helps lift a member's self-esteem and help develop more adaptive coping styles and interpersonal skills.
4. **Instillation of hope:** Members at various stages of development or recovery can be inspired by or encouraged by another member who has overcome similar problems in his or her life.
5. **Imparting information:** Members find it very helpful to learn factual information from other members in the group.
6. **Corrective recapitulation of the primary family experience:** Members often unconsciously identify the group therapist and other

group members with their own parents and siblings. They then develop a form of transference specific to the group process. The therapist's interpretations of the process can help the group members gain understanding of the impact of childhood experiences on their personality. By this experience, they may learn to avoid unconsciously repeating unhelpful past interactive patterns in current relationships.

7. **Development of socializing techniques:** The group setting provides a safe and supportive environment for members to take risks by extending their repertoire of interpersonal behaviors and improving their social skills.
8. **Imitative behavior:** Members can develop social skills through a process of observing, imitating, and modeling the therapist and other group members.
9. **Existential factors:** Learning that one has to take responsibility for one's own life and the consequences of one's decisions.
10. **Interpersonal learning:** Group members achieve a greater level of self-awareness through the process of interacting with others in the group, who give feedback on a member's behavior and impact on others.
11. **Self-understanding:** It refers to the achievement of greater levels of insight into the genesis of problems and the unconscious motivations which underlie behaviors.
12. **Catharsis:** It describes the experience of relief from emotional distress through the free and uninhibited expression of emotion.

E. Differences Between Groups

Guides	Psychodynamic Group	Cognitive Behavioral Group	Supportive Group
Indications	• Depressive disorders • Anxiety disorders • Personality disorders • Trauma	• Anxiety disorders • Depressive disorders • Substance abuse disorders • Personality disorders	• Trauma • Bereavement • Life crises
Content	• Current and past relationships • Group dynamics	• Cognitive distortions • Specific symptoms	• Current crisis
Goals	• Resolution of conflict within self and with others	• Specific symptom relief	• Resolution of crisis
Therapists role	• Reduction of shame and guilt • Challenging defenses • Interpreting intrapsychic conflicts	• Challenging thoughts/ assumptions • Improving responses/ behaviors	• Giving support and advise • Strengthening existing defenses

F. Legal and Ethical Considerations

- Except where disclosure is required by law, the therapist can only legally and ethically give information about a group member to others only after obtaining an appropriate consent from that member.
- The therapist is responsible to the society as well as to the group members, when the group members pose a danger to themselves or to others.
- Although the group members should protect the identity of other members and maintain confidentiality, the group members are not legally bound to do so. During the preparation of members for group therapy, the therapist should routinely instruct prospective members to keep all materials discussed within the group as being confidential. Theoretically, in legal cases, one member of a group can be asked to testify against another.

- Patients with a demonstrated history of assaultive behavior and psychotic patients who pose a potential for violence should not be placed in a group. Sexual intercourse by a therapist with a patient or a former patient is unethical; in many states, such behaviors are considered a criminal act.
- The therapist should advise prospective group members that each patient is responsible for reporting any sexual contact between members. The therapist should identify sexual, vulnerable, or exploitive patients in the selection and preparation of patients for the group. Patients who sexually exploit others should be informed that such behavior is not acceptable in the group.

IMPORTANT POINTS TO REMEMBER

- Group therapy refers to any form of psychotherapy delivered in a group format.
- It can be organized in inpatient, partial hospital, outpatient programs, and in private clinics.
- Group therapy has been successfully used to treat depression, anxiety disorders, substance abuse, personality disorders, and eating disorders.
- The four basic theories of group therapy are general systems theory, cognitive behavioral theory, transactional analysis, and existentialism.
- There are 12 curative factors described by Yalom in group therapy.
- The group therapist is responsible for maintaining the confidentiality of the group and ensuring safety of group members.
- The success of a group depends upon the appropriate selection of its members and the motivation of the therapist and its members.

SUGGESTED READINGS

Gabbard GO. *Psychodynamic Psychiatry in Clinical Practice.* 4th Ed. Washington, DC: American Psychiatric Publishing, Inc., 2008:129–155.

Hales RE, Yudofsky SC, Gabbard GO. *The American Psychiatric Publishing Textbook of Psychiatry.* 5th Ed. Washington, DC: American Psychiatric Publishing, Inc., 2008, http://www.psychiatryonline.com/content.aspx?aid=334425, last accessed on January 11, 2009.

Kaplan HI, Sadock BJ. *Kaplan and Sadock's Synopsis of Psychiatry.* 8th Ed. Philadelphia, PA: Lippincott Williams & Wilkins, 1998:897–910.

Yalom I, Leszcz M. *The Theory and Practice of Group Psychotherapy.* 5th Ed. New York, NY: Basic Books, 2005:19, 272.

H.6. Family therapy

Nicole A. Foubister, MD, Clarence Watson MD, JD

INTRODUCTION

Family therapy is a form of psychotherapy that involves all the members of a family. It is based on the belief that the family is a unique social system with its own structure and patterns of communication and that these patterns are determined by many factors, including the parents' beliefs and values, the personalities of all family members, and the influence of the extended family. Family therapists posit that as a result of these variables, each family develops its own unique personality, which affects all of its members. According to family systems theory, as a result of these variables, family units develop a homeostasis which must be maintained at any cost and which affects each of the family members.

The family therapist's goal is to facilitate an understanding that the "labeled patient's" symptoms serve the function of maintaining the family's homeostasis. Although some types of family therapy are based on behavioral or psychodynamic principles, the most widespread form is based on family systems theory. This approach regards the entire family as the unit of treatment, and emphasizes such factors as relationships and communication patterns, rather than traits or symptoms in individual members.

INDICATIONS

Family therapy can be utilized for the following: marital problems; divorce; eating disorders; substance abuse; affective disorders, such as depression or bipolar disorder; chronic health problems, such as asthma or cancer; grief; loss and trauma; parenting skills; emotional abuse or violence; sibling or parental conflict; and dealing with chronic mental illness. Although family therapy can be used for all of the aforementioned issues, it is most commonly utilized when a child has behavioral or school problems.

Family therapy aims to understand and treat emotional problems and personal crises by working with the entire family. For example, if a child is acting out, systemic family therapy will examine the whole family and relationships between family members and try to determine how these relationships are contributing to and maintaining the problem. In this example, a child may act out (without its conscious knowledge) because it senses that its parents are not getting along well. Thus, by acting out, the child is indicating that the problem lies within him or her. The child's parents may then use this identified problem to focus their attention on the child rather than their own relationship difficulties. These behaviors may serve the function of keeping the whole family together, instead of risking the breakup of the parents' relationship and hence the family. Therefore, the therapist explores what function the problem may serve for the family unit.

BASIC TERMS

Supportive family therapy is often used as a method for allowing family members to express how they feel about a problem in a safe, caring setting. The problem may be difficult to manage at home (e.g., caring for a sick parent), and the therapeutic environment provides an opportunity for families to talk openly about how the problem affects them. The therapist may also offer practical advice and information about further sources of help.

Family therapy using *cognitive behavioral therapy* techniques attempts to change the ways people think or behave in order to treat the problem. Homework tasks may be set, or specific behavioral programs may be drawn up.

Family therapy using *psychodynamic techniques* examines the individuals' own subconscious minds. It attempts to reduce the problem(s) by uncovering what is occurring under the surface. It is hoped that by providing the individuals in the family with the reasons underlying the problems, members will be able to deal with their difficulties more successfully.

Systemic family therapy attempts to identify the problems, relationships, ideas, and attitudes of all the family members. This strategy includes identifying dyads, triangles, and boundaries. Dyads are subsystems between two family members (e.g., the executive subsystem usually contains the two parents). Boundaries are barriers between subsystems (e.g., between the parents and the children). Boundaries may be too rigid or too permeable. Triangles are dysfunctional alliances between two family members against a third member. Once these relationships become clear, the therapist will attempt to shift the problem(s), attitudes, and relationships to a position that is more beneficial, less damaging, or more realistic. Interventions may include education, homework, experimentation (e.g., suggesting that the family try behaving or relating in a different way), or attempting to provide insight to family members. The emphasis is on the whole family, with avoidance of blame on one or more individuals.

The *Bowen model*, also known as the family system model, focuses on a person's differentiation from his family of origin and his ability to be his true self in the face of pressures that threaten the loss of love or social position. This style of therapy assesses the family's level of enmeshment and ability to differentiate, and analyzes emotional triangles. The therapist's role is to act as a coach to stabilize or shift the triangles that are producing the presenting symptoms. The therapist works with family members to achieve adequate personal differentiation so that the triangle does not reoccur. Bowen family therapy aims to resolve emotional cutoffs, foster creativity, increase family cohesion, and increase the family's tolerance for conflict. The Bowen model uses the genogram, which is a survey of the family going back for several generations, with education provided about multigenerational family processes. Finally, the Bowen model encourages use of self and aims to achieve family reconstruction.

Techniques Used in Family Therapy

Family therapy encourages mutual accommodation, a process in which family members identify each other's needs and work toward meeting them. In addition, family therapy works toward normalizing boundaries between subsystems and reducing the likelihood of triangles. The therapist works with family members toward redefining blame and encouraging family members to reconsider their own responsibility for problems.

IMPORTANT POINTS TO REMEMBER

- Family therapy is a form of psychotherapy that involves all members of a family.
- Each family has a unique personality and homeostasis that family members strive to maintain.
- Family therapy shifts the focus from the "identified patient" and presents the problem in the context of the family unit and maintenance of homeostasis.
- Presenting complaints are assessed based on their purpose and significance within the family unit.
- Family therapy utilizes mutual accommodation and aims to normalize boundaries and reduce triangles.
- Family therapy is most commonly used for behavioral problems in children and adolescents.

Suggested Readings

Bowen M. *Family Theory in Clinical Practice*. New York, NY: Aronson, 1978.

Diamond G, Liddle HA. Resolving a therapeutic impasse between parents and adolescents in multidimensional family therapy. *J Consult Clin Psychol* 1996;64:481–488.

Diamond GS, Serrano AC, Dickey M, et al. Current status of family-based outcome and process research. *J Am Acad Child Adolesc Psychiatry* 1996;35(1):6–16.

Glick ID. Family therapies: Efficacy, indications, and treatment outcomes. In: Janowksy DS, ed. *Psychotherapy Indications and Outomes*. Washington, DC: American Pyschiatric Press, 1993:303.

Kim EY, Miklowitz DJ. Expressed emotion as a predictor of outcome among bipolar patients undergoing family therapy. *Affect Disord* 2004;82(3):343–352.

Miklowitz DJ, Richards JA, George EL, et al. Integrated family and individual therapy for bipolar disorder: Results of a treatment development study. *J Clin Psychiatry* 2003;64(2): 182–191.

Miller IW, Keitner GI, Ryan CE, et al. Family treatment for bipolar disorder: Family impairment by treatment interactions. *J Clin Psychiatry* 2008;69(5):732–740.

I. Cross cultural psychiatry

Sunanda Muralee, MD, Rajesh R. Tampi, MD, MS

CASE HISTORY

PRESENT ILLNESS

Mr K is a 60-year-old, married, Indian man who was admitted to a tertiary care psychiatric hospital as an involuntary patient. He had become severely depressed over the past few months and was complaining of lack of energy, endorsing delusions (i.e., "I have not had a bowel movement for two months"; "If I take the medications, my stomach will explode."), cognitive difficulties (i.e., "I am forgetting everything at work; I am a stupid person"), eating less and had lost approximately 15 lb in this time. He was also not compliant with his psychotropic medications for 1 month (i.e., "I stopped taking them because they were not working and I didn't tell my wife about this"). He also reported worsening of his performance at work. His family reported that he was very anxious at home, was pacing constantly, and was unable to sleep. He denied any suicidal or homicidal thoughts at the time of admission to the hospital.

PSYCHIATRIC HISTORY

The patient's first psychiatric admission was to a local hospital in the fall of 2004 for a 2-week period. Ever since that time, he has had outpatient psychiatric follow-up near his home. He had several trials of medications including venlafaxine, mirtazapine, bupropion, olanzapine, methylphenidate, aripiprazole, risperidone (did not tolerate the side effects), and lorazepam at different points in time. In 2006, he was admitted to the local teaching hospital where he received Electroconvulsive Therapy (ECT) followed by maintenance treatments for approximately 1 year. He discontinued maintenance ECT even though it was helpful as he felt that it was causing him to have memory loss. His family reported that when he was receiving maintenance ECT, he was functioning very well at home and at work.

FAMILY HISTORY

There is no known family history of psychological or psychiatric problems.

SOCIAL HISTORY

Mr K was born in Delhi, India. He majored in physics and mathematics at college. He came to the United States in 1980. He is married and has four children (two boys and two girls). He works in the area of quality control at a local manufacturing unit where he is employed as an inspector. According to his family, he has always been a loner and a "workaholic." He is described as not having any friends outside of his home or having any specific hobbies. Other than going to work regularly, he spends most of his time at home.

PERTINENT MEDICAL HISTORY

He has a history of hypothyroidism and is currently treated with levothyroxine at 50 mcg PO once a day. He is status post prostate surgery and bilateral inguinal hernia repair.

MENTAL STATUS EXAMINATION

Mr K presented as a slightly built Asian Indian man who looked older than his stated age of 60 years. He was casually but cleanly dressed, and his general hygiene was good. He was pleasant and cooperative. His speech lacked spontaneity, but he replied appropriately when asked. His psychomotor activity was slow. He had a restricted range of affect, and his mood appeared depressed. His thought process was slowed. He reported somatic delusions, such as "I haven't had a bowel movement in two months." He was not responding to any internal stimuli. He did not endorse any suicidal thoughts or plans at admission. He denied any homicidal ideations. On the Folstein Mini-Mental State Examination (MMSE), he scored 27/30 indicating that he had good general cognitive function. He scored 4/15 on the Executive Interview (EXIT) indicating that his executive functioning was good. He scored a 13/15 on the Geriatric Depression Scale (GDS) indicating that he was severely depressed. His insight was limited, he did not believe that he was depressed, and attributed all his problems to his inability to move his bowels and the fact that he was "losing my memory."

PERTINENT PHYSICAL FINDINGS

His vital signs were a temperature of 97.6°F, heart rate 69 bmp, blood pressure 112/72 mm Hg, and respiratory rate of 18 per minute. Oxygen saturation on room air was 93.7%. His pupils were equal and reactive to light and accommodation. No jaundice, anemia, or lymphadenopathy was noted. The first and second heart sounds were heard and there was no murmur. His lungs were clear. The abdomen was soft, nontender, and there was no organmegaly. Bowel sounds were heard normally. The extremities showed normal capillary perfusion. The neurological examination was normal. He weighed 94 lb at admission.

LABORATORY DATA

Data obtained at admission revealed a Blood Urea Nitrogen (BUN) of 6 mg% and a creatinine of 1.0 mg%. The HCO_3 (Bicarbonate) was 23.7 mEq/L, with a chloride level of 107 mEq/L. The sodium level was 138 mEq/L, with a potassium level of 3.7 mEq/L. The white blood cells count was 5,500/cmm. The hemoglobin was 13.9 gm% with a hematocrit of 41%. The platelet count was 187,000/cmm. Venereal Diease Research Laboratory (VDRL) was nonreactive. The prelbumin level was normal at 15.8 mg%. The fasting blood glucose was 102 mg%. The chest x-ray was normal. The CT scan of the head was normal.

HOSPITAL COURSE

The patient was restarted on his outpatient medications including aripiprazole at 10 mg PO q.h.s, venlafaxine XR at 75 mg PO q.h.s., and lorazepam at 0.5 mg PO twice a day. We also restarted him on levothyroxine at 100 mcg PO once a day, senokot two pills PO twice a day along with docusate 100 mg PO twice a day for constipation.

As he had an inadequate response to pharmacotherapy, it was decided to restart him on ECT treatment. Although he believed that he was not depressed and all his ailments were due to physical problems, he agreed to the treatments as he did not want to disappoint his family. He received eight ECT treatments while in the hospital. He tolerated these treatments reasonably well except for some postictal confusion that cleared in a few hours after the treatment.

During his hospital stay, he was always been pleasant and cooperative. He, however, remained focused on somatic complaints: saying that he was unable to eat because his stomach was going to explode and that he had not had a bowel movement. He had some reluctance to drink nutritional supplements such as Ensure or Glucerna because of his irrational fear that he would acquire diabetes as a result of taking these supplements.

During the course of his hospital stay, the dose of aripiprazole was increased to 20 mg PO q.h.s. The venlafaxine XR dose was titrated to 150 mg PO q.h.s. The lorazepam was continued at 0.5 mg PO twice a day. He was continued on levothyroxine at 100 mcg PO per day and senakot two pills twice a day along with docusate 100 mg PO twice a day for constipation.

Information obtained from the patient's family indicated that Mr K had never really adjusted to his life in the United States. He has remained here for economic reasons and for the welfare of his family. He was a loner and had no friends or hobbies. He is a passive man and leaves all the care of the home to his younger and more capable wife. He was described by his wife as "good but lifeless man." His kids described him as a "good but uninvolved provider." At work, he was considered a hard and honest worker, but had no friends. He had worked his way up to the supervisor's position. He was well liked by his subordinates who considered him a "kind man." Further discussions with him about his life in the United States indicated that he had not transcultured to the life here. He always longed to go back to his home in Delhi, but could not do so because his family was well adapted to the life here and it was not financially viable for them.

The patient never believed that he was depressed. He attributed all his symptoms to his thyroid disease and to the fact that he was constipated. He saw symptoms affecting his "mind and brain" as a sign of weakness and he did not want to be considered weak. He never believed that any of the medications that were prescribed to him had helped or would help. He took the medications reluctantly and did so only to please his family. He was afraid that he would lose his memory because of the ECT and would not be able to work.

After eight ECT treatments, he was doing better. His mood was much improved. He was less anxious and he was eating better. Repeat MMSE and EXIT testing showed that the scores were unchanged from admission but it still did not convince him of the fact that his memory had not worsened during the hospital stay. He remained fearful of losing his memory as he would then not be able to go to work and provide for his family. He remained skeptical about ever feeling better and was doing well at work. Given his response to ECT, he was discharged home on maintenance ECT and pharmacotherapy.

DISCHARGE MEDICATIONS

Aripiprazole 20 mg PO q.h.s., venlafaxine XR 150 mg PO q.h.s., lorazepam 0.5 mg PO b.i.d, levothyroxine at 100 mcg PO once a day, senakot two pills PO b.i.d, and docusate 100 mg PO b.i.d.

DSM-IV-TR MULTIAXIAL DIAGNOSIS

Axis I. Major depressive disorder, recurrent, current episode severe with psychotic features.

Dysthymia. Anxiety disorder, Not Otherwise Specified (NOS)

Axis II. Dependent personality traits

Axis III. Hypothyroidism, constipation
Axis IV. Severity of psychosocial stressor: moderate, relationship issues, and financial concerns
Axis V. Global assessment of functioning:

At admission: 25, psychotic depression, severe anxiety, unable to function at home or at work.

At discharge: 45, depression and anxiety are resolving, the patient is able to start functioning in the community.

CULTURAL THEMES

1. Somatic presentation of depression and anxiety
2. Lack of understanding of mental illness
3. Lack of belief in treatments and hence reluctance with compliance/noncompliance
4. Lack of transculturation/acculturation
5. Gender roles in cultures

CULTURAL FORMULATION

Mr K is a 60-year-old, married, Indian man with a history of major depressive disorder and anxiety who was admitted to the hospital for worsening symptoms of depression and anxiety. He does not believe that he is depressed or anxious, and blames his symptoms on his constipation and other somatic complaints. He also believes that the treatments that he is getting are of no help and are making his memory worse. He is well supported by his family, but has no other peer supports outside his home. He has never transcultured to the United States, leaving him very isolated. On the other hand, his family has adapted very well to life in the United States and they have made their own world without including him. He remains stuck in the role of wanting to be the chief provider for his family when he has not been able to do so effectively in the recent past. His social isolation and continued lack of insight into his illness along with his mistrust of the treatments provided to him put him at a very high risk for treatment noncompliance. This will lead to a recurrence of his psychiatric symptoms and the need for possible psychiatric hospitalizations. Given his risk of noncompliance with treatments, aftercare plans should include psychoeducation for the patient and his family along with closer involvement of his family in his care. Close monitoring of symptoms, including cognitive performance, and side effects should be done. Involvement of peer support with his own cultural group and at work may be helpful to improve his functioning in the community. Provision of mental health providers from the same cultural group or a similar group should help with developing trust in the system of care.

1. Introduction

A. DEFINITIONS

The United Nations charter states that culture is the "set of distinctive spiritual, material, intellectual, and emotional features of society or a social group and that it encompasses, in addition to art and literature, lifestyles, ways of living together, value systems, traditions and beliefs."

Culture	Race	Ethnicity
It is a pattern of beliefs, customs, and behaviors that are acquired socially and transmitted from one generation to another. It can also be defined as a tool by which people adapt to their environment	A concept under which human beings traditionally and historically chose to group themselves. This is based on their common physiognomy. Physical, biological, and genetic connotations are fully integrated in the definition	It is a subjective sense of belonging to a given group of people who share a common origin as well as a common matrix of cultural beliefs and practices. It is an integral part of one's sense of identity, self image, and intrapsychic life

B. LEVELS OF CULTURE

Physical aspects of culture include art, literature, architecture, food, clothing, and transportation. They are directly observed and are more likely to yield to change and adaptation.

Ideological aspects of culture include beliefs and value systems of people including religion, psychology, and philosophy. These are observed indirectly through behaviors of people and are less likely to yield to change and adaptation.

C. UNDERSTANDING CULTURE

Culture has three elements:

- **Values**
- **Norms**
- **Artifacts**

Values comprise ideas about what in life seems important and they guide the rest of the culture. Norms consist of expectations of how people will behave in different situations. Each culture has different methods, called sanctions, of enforcing its norms. Sanctions vary with the importance of the norm; norms that a society enforces formally have the status of law. Artifacts are things or material culture and are derived from the culture's values and norms.

D. ADAPTATION OF CULTURES

Culture comprises symbolical codes and can thus pass via teaching from one person to another meaning that cultures, although bounded, would change. Cultural change could result from invention and innovation, but it could also result from contact between two cultures. Under peaceful conditions, contact between two cultures can lead to people "borrowing" (learning) from one another diffusion anthropology or transculturation. Under conditions of violence or political inequality, people of one society can "steal" cultural artifacts from another, or impose cultural artifacts on another acculturation. All human societies participate in these processes of diffusion, transculturation, and acculturation, and few anthropologists today see cultures as bounded. Remember that neither culture nor ethnicity is a fixed trait.

2. Epidemiology (Why Is It Important?)

A. DEMOGRAPHICS

Between 1990 and 2000 within the United States, the Hispanic Americans sustained a 58% growth rate, while Asian Americans and Pacific Islanders had a 17% growth rate. The African Americans had a 16% growth rate, whereas the white had a growth rate of 3%. In other words, the United States is a pluralistic and multiethnic society, which has permeated all aspects of life and society, including medicine and psychiatry.

B. HEALTH DISPARITIES

U.S. Surgeon General's Supplemental Report (Mental Health: Cultures, Race, and Ethnicity) states that:

1. Minorities have less access to, and availability of, mental health services.
2. Minorities are less likely to receive needed mental health services.
3. Minorities in treatment often receive poorer quality of mental health care.
4. Minorities are underrepresented in mental health research.
5. Disparities impose a greater disability burden on minorities.
6. Racism and discrimination are stressful events that adversely affect health.
7. Mistrust of mental health services is an important reason deterring minorities from seeking treatment.

C. DIFFERENCES IN PRESENTATION OF ILLNESS

Patients may present with somatic complaints when they have underlying depression or anxiety. Nonpsychotic patients may report hearing voices of the ancestors. Spirits and interactions with the dead may be acceptable in some cultures. Delusions and their presentation may have a cultural bias.

D. MISDIAGNOSIS

African Americans and Hispanics are more likely to be misdiagnosed with psychotic illness rather than an affective illness. They are also more likely to receive higher doses of antipsychotics and are more likely to have involuntary hospitalization, seclusions, and restraints.

3. Etiology (Culture-Bound Syndromes)

The term denotes recurrent, locality-specific patterns of aberrant behavior and troubling experience that may or may not be linked to a particular DSM-IV-TR diagnostic category. They are indigenously considered afflictions or illnesses and have local names. There is seldom a one-to-one equivalence of any culture-bound syndrome with a DSM-IV-TR diagnostic entity. Central to the idioms of distress is the understanding of the unique manifestation of symptoms or cluster of symptoms among different cultural, racial, and ethnic groups. Table 31.1 lists a few important culture-bound syndromes.

TABLE 31.1 Examples of Culture-Bound Syndromes

Name	Location	Presentation
Amok	South East Asia, and Polynesian Islands	• Violent, aggressive or homicidal behaviors caused by stress • More common in males • They may have some psychotic symptoms
Ataque De Nervios May resemble mood, anxiety, dissociative and or somatoform disorders	Latin Americans	• Severe anxiety attacks or feeling of out of control • Due to stress in the family • They may have amnesia for the episode • Similar to panic disorder but has precipitants and no apprehension
Brain Fag May resemble anxiety, depressive or somatoform disorders	West Africa	• Affects High School or University students • This is in response to challenges in school • Patient is usually fatigued and with poor concentration • Head and neck pain, chest tightness, blurred vision are also seen
Bouf'ee Delirante Resembles brief psychotic disorder	West Africa and Haiti	• It is a French term • There is sudden outburst of agitation, aggression, hallucinations, delusions and confusion
Falling Out Resembles conversion or a dissociative disorder	Southern United States and Caribbean Islands	• Sudden collapse with or without dizziness is seen • Eyes are open but the patient is unable to see • The patient can hear, but is powerless to move
Ghost sickness	American Indians	• It is a preoccupation with death and the deceased • Bad dreams, weakness, feelings of danger, loss of appetite, fainting, anxiety, hallucinations, loss of consciousness may also be seen
Hwa-Byung	Korea	• It is due to a suppression of anger • Insomnia, fatigue, dysphoria, anxiety attacks, pains, and mass in the epigastrium may be seen
Koro	Malaysia and South East Asia	• It is a sudden and intense anxiety attack that the penis in males and nipples and vulva in females will recede into the body and cause death

(continued)

TABLE 31.1 Examples of Culture-Bound Syndromes (Continued)

Name	Location	Presentation
Latah	Malaysia/Indonesia	• Sudden fright with, echolalia, echopraxia, command obedience, and dissociative or trance like behaviors are seen • It is more common in women
Nervios May resemble anxiety/ depression/adjustment disorder/somatoform disorder or a dissociative disorder	Latin Americas	• It is a vulnerability to stressful life experiences • Headache, irritability, stomach disturbance, sleep problems are also seen
Shin-Byung	Korea	• Anxiety and somatic complaints along with weakness, dizziness, fear, anorexia, insomnia, and gastrointestinal problems are seen • Dissociation and thought of being possessed by ancestral spirits is also seen
Susto(Soul Loss)	Latin Americas	• It is attributed to a frightening event that results the soul leaving the body and causing unhappiness or sickness • It is due to a strains in social roles • Neurovegetative and somatic symptoms may occur

4. Diagnosis (Cultural Formulation Based on DSM-IV-TR, Appendix I)

This outline should be used to supplement the multiaxial diagnostic assessment and to address difficulties that may be encountered in applying DSM-IV-TR criteria in a multicultural environment. This formulation uses a systematic review of various cultural themes that may affect the care of the individual. The clinician may provide a narrative summary for each of the categories discussed. A cultural formulation includes all of the following.

A. CULTURAL IDENTITY

It includes ethnic or cultural references and the degree to which an individual is involved with their original culture and the host culture. It pays attention to language abilities and preferences of that individual.

B. CULTURAL EXPLANATION

This indicates the individuals understanding of distress and the need for support. It is often communicated by symptoms or beliefs. It is helpful in developing an interpretation, diagnosis, and a treatment plan.

C. CULTURAL FACTORS RELATED TO PSYCHOSOCIAL ENVIRONMENTS AND LEVELS OF FUNCTIONING

This includes cultural manifestations or interpretations of stressors, as well as available network systems of supports.

D. CULTURAL ELEMENTS OF THE RELATIONSHIP BETWEEN THE PATIENT AND THE PSYCHIATRIC PRACTITIONER

It notes the cultural and social status difference between the patient and clinician. Differences in language and in patterns of communication

TABLE 31.2 Pharmacological Agents Metabolized Through the CYP P450 System

CYP1A2	CYP2C19	CYP2D6	CYP3A4
Atypical antipsychotics	Benzodiazepines	Opiates	Benzodiazepines
Typical antipsychotics	Tricyclic antidepressant	β-blockers	Mood stabilizers
Coumadin	SSRIs	Amphetamines	Codeine
Theophylline	Propranolol	Selective serotonin reuptake inhibitors	Typical antipsychotics
		Tricyclic antidepressants	Atypical antipsychotics
		Venlafaxine	
		Typical antipsychotics	
		Atypical antipsychotics	

are also kept in mind. Attention to the existence of cultural stereotypes and overidentification or rejection of the patient on the part of the clinician is also carefully considered.

E. OVERALL CULTURAL ASSESSMENT FOR DIAGNOSIS AND CARE

A cultural formulation requires a thoughtful discussion as to how the different cultural, racial, and ethnic considerations will specifically influence the diagnoses and treatment plan of the individual, e.g., transference and countertransference. The cultural competence of the practitioner must be considered and if there are problems, it must be addressed.

5. TREATMENTS (ETHNICITY AND PSYCHOPHARMACOLOGY)

A. Nonbiological Issues Affecting Pharmacology

1. **Cultural beliefs:** It plays an important role in determining whether an explanation and treatment plan makes sense to a patient.
2. **Traditional and/or alternative methods:** Many herbal medicines that can interact with psychotropic drugs, e.g., *datura candida* and swertia japonica have anticholinergic properties; ephedra sinica (Ma-Huang), a weight loss supplement, causes mania and psychosis; and St John's wort (hypericum perforatum) can interact with drugs such as indinavir and cyclosporine.
3. **Patient compliance:** Compliance with medications may be affected by:
   a. Incorrect dosing
   b. Medication side effect
   c. Polypharmacy
   d. Poor therapeutic alliance
   e. Lack of community support
   f. Financial issues
   g. Substance abuse
   h. Concerns about toxic effects and addiction potential of the medications
4. **Social network:** The way a family interacts and functions has significant impact on psychiatric treatments. Some patients may need a lot of social support to get well and the family usually provides that support.
5. **Other factors that affect medication compliance include**
   a. Language barriers
   b. Misdiagnosis
   c. Placebo response
   d. Mistrust in the system
   e. Beliefs and expectation

B. Biological Aspects of Pharmacology

Culture, race, and ethnicity may effect the psychopharmacological agents in three major ways. The three ways are

1. Pharmacogenetics
2. Pharmacokinetics
3. Pharmacodynamics

TABLE 31.3 Ethnic Variations in Cytochrome Metabolizations

Ethnic Group CYP 2C19	Poor Metabolizers (%)	Ethnic Group CYP2D6	Poor Metabolizers (%)
Whites	3.5	Whites	7.5
Hispanic Americans	4.8	Hispanic Americans	4.5
African Americans	18.5	African Americans	1.9
Asian Americans (Chinese)	17.4	Asian Americans (Chinese)	2.0

1. **Pharmacogenetics:** It focuses on the genetic and environmental factors that control and influence the functions of drug metabolizing enzymes. Some individuals are poor metabolizers of drugs, while others are extensive metabolizers, indicating genetic polymorphism of the cytochrome P450 (CYP) enzyme system, e.g., East Asians and Native Americans lack the enzyme aldehyde dehydrogenase, causing accumulation of acetaldehyde in the body, thus leading to facial flushing when drinking alcohol.
2. **Pharmacokinetics:** The focus here is on the fate and distribution of medications in the body. These processes have direct effect on the absorption, distribution, metabolism, biotransformation, and excretion of medications, e.g., he ethnic variations are seen in the CYP metabolization of medications. Tables 31.2 and 31.3 outline some of the CYP substrates and the ethnic variations in the CYP metabolizations.
3. **Pharmacodynamics:** Pharmacodynamic research focuses on how medications affect the body, by interacting with the receptors that bind with endogenous and exogenous substances. Table 31.4 outlines some of the common pharmacodynamics interactions based on ethnic differences.

TABLE 31.4 Pharmacodynamics Based on Ethnicity

Medication	African American	Hispanic American	Asian American
1. Tricyclic antidepressants			
Dose	Lower	Lower	Lower
Side effects		Higher	
2. SSRIs			
Dose	Lower		
3. Typical antipsychotics			
Dose	Same	Lower	Lower
Side Effects			Higher
Tardive dyskinesia	Higher		
Prolactin response			Higher
4. Atypical antipsychotics			
Dose	Higher		Lower
5. Lithium			
Dose			Lower
6. Benzodiazepines			
Dose			Lower

KEY POINTS (ABPN Examination)

A. When interviewing a patient of a different culture

1. First ask the patient how he/she would like to be addressed, before addressing him or her.
2. Clarify issues regarding confidentiality.
3. Acknowledge language barriers, if any.
4. Speak clearly and clarify statements, issues, and concerns.
5. Pay attention to communication, i.e., nonverbal, expressive styles, and meaning of words.
6. Ask about the use of traditional forms of healing and medicines, especially herbs.
7. Do not forget to ask about the stigma of mental illness in that particular culture.

B. When presenting the case

1. Acknowledge barriers in communication and state that the use of an interpreter would be helpful.
2. If diagnosis is unclear, state that you would use a structured diagnostic interview like SCID-DSM-IV for clarification.
3. Acknowledge the need to spend more time with the patient and that the relationship will be more complex and it will take longer to build trust and alliance.
4. Anticipate that the patient may have frustrations from previous experiences in health care systems.
5. Discuss the stigma of mental illness and explain that you would obtain a **Cultural Consultation**, if possible.
6. Discuss the role of families, use of traditional healers/medicines, and social support structures in the treatment and prognosis of mental illness.

SUGGESTED READINGS

American Psychiatric Association. *Diagnostic and Statistical Manual of Mental Disorders (DSM-IV-TR): Text Revision*. 4th Ed. Washington, DC: American Psychiatric Association, 2000. http://www.psychiatryonline.com/content.aspx?aID=14119, last accessed on April 25, 2008.

Carter JH. Culture, Race, and ethnicity. *Psychiatr Ann* 2004 Jul;34(7):500–560.

Gaw AC. *Concise Guide to Cross-cultural Psychiatry*. 4th Ed. Washington, DC: American Psychiatric Publishing, Inc., 2004:1–203.

Sadock BJ, Sadock VA. *Kaplan and Sadock's Comprehensive Textbook of Psychiatry*. 8th Ed. Philadelphia, PA: Lippincott Williams & Wilkins, 2005. http://ovidsp.tx.ovid.com/spb/ovidweb.cgi?QS2=434, last accessed on April 25, 2008.

APPENDIX

Lekshminarayan R. Kurup, MD, Sunanda Muralee, MD, Rajesh R. Tampi, MD, MS

1. INTERVIEW TEMPLATE (30 MINUTES)

1. **Boundaries: First 1 minute**
   - My name is Dr ....
   - This is Dr ......, my examiner today.
   - Purpose of the interview is ....
   - What is your name? How would you like me to address you?
   - This interview is confidential and voluntary.
   - The duration of the interview is 30 minutes.
   - I may need to interrupt you; it is not meant to be disrespectful but due to time constraints.
   - Acknowledge language barriers if any.
   - Notes taken during this interview will be destroyed at the end of the session.
   - Is it okay to start?
2. **Demographics/Identification: Next 1 minute**
   - How old are you?
   - Where do you live?
   - What is your marital status?
   - How do you support yourself?
   - Where do you receive your mental health treatment and for what reason?
   - Are you currently receiving inpatient or outpatient psychiatric treatment?
   - If inpatient, voluntary versus involuntary?
3. **History of Present Illness: Check for here and now and in the past: Next 8 to 10 minutes**
   A. **Mood:** Depression, hypomania/mania, neurovegetative symptoms, and DSM-IV-TR criteria.

   B. **Anxiety:** Generalized anxiety, social anxiety, panic attacks, agoraphobia, obsessions, compulsions, and trauma: reexperiencing, hyperarousal, and avoidance.

   C. **Psychosis:** Look for abnormality of thought content (delusions) or form of thought (tangential, circumstantial, overinclusive, and loosening of associations), perception (illusions/hallucinations), or motor activity (catatonia).
   - Delusions: paranoia, thought insertion/broadcasting, control, grandiosity, hyperreligiosity, etc.
   - Hallucinations: auditory (voices or noises that others do not hear) and visual (strange things that others do not see) and other forms of hallucinations like tactile (touch) and gustatory (taste) or olfactory (smell).

   D. **Substance Use:** Alcohol (when last consumed; ever had withdrawal seizures, DTs, liver/pancreatitis problems, etc.), sleeping pills, phencyclidine (PCP) (illy), marijuana, heroin, intravenous (IV), human immunodeficiency virus (HIV), hepatic C virus (HCV), pain pills, cocaine, stimulants (speed), and hallucinogens (acid).
   - Abuse—CAGE (>2): substances ever controlled your life (e.g., legal, occupational/educational, and social problems), felt the need to cut down (C), felt annoyed with comments about your use (A), felt guilty for using (G), needed an eye-opener or a fix to avoid withdrawal symptoms (E).
   - Dependence-withdrawal, tolerance, etc.

   E. **Safety:** Suicide, homicide (intent, plan, reasons not to, and previous attempts), etc.

   F. **Cognition:** Memory (short-term and long-term), executive functioning (problem-solving skills), and activities of daily living (ADLs).

Basic ADLS: Dressing, eating, ambulation, toileting, and hygiene (DEATH).

Instrumental ADLS: Shopping, housework, accounting, food preparation, and transportation (SHAFT).

4. **Past Psychiatric History: Next 2 to 3 minutes**
   - 1st contact with psychiatrist and for what reason?
   - How many hospitalizations, if any?
   - What kind of psychiatric medications have you been on?
   - Ask about ECT.
5. **Past Medical History: Next 2 to 3 minutes**
   - Neurological disorders: Stroke, seizures, head trauma (TBI), loss of consciousness, etc.
   - Endocrine/Metabolic problems: Diabetes, thyroid dysfunction, etc.
   - Cardiac: Hypertension, coronary artery disease (CAD), myocardial infarction (MI), atrial fibrillation, and congestive heart failure (CHF).
   - Oncological: Lung, breast, brain, and other cancers.
6. **Medications: Next 1 to 2 minutes: Medical and psychiatric**
7. **Allergies: Next 1 minute**
8. **Social and Developmental History: Next 1 to 2 minutes**
   - Birth place
   - Developmental milestones (walked, talked, etc.)
   - Parents
   - Physical, sexual, and verbal abuse
   - Education
   - Employment
   - Intimate relationships
   - Children
   - Friends
   - Religious affiliation
   - Legal problems
9. **Family History: Next 1 to 2 minutes**
   - Depression
   - Bipolar disorder
   - Schizophrenia
   - Substance abuse
   - Anxiety disorders
   - Personality disorders
10. **Mental Status Examination: Next 3 to 4 minutes**

A. **Observe these while conducting the interview and present it during the 10-minute presentation**
   - Pt appeared X (age, grooming, dress, distinguishing features, etc.).
   - Pt behaved Y (cooperation, eye contact, psychomotor functioning, etc.).
   - Pt spoke Z (clarity, spontaneity, volume, etc.).
   - Affect (emotional state observed by the interviewer): Flat, restricted or constricted, normal or expansive, etc.
   - Mood (sustained emotional state as reported by the patient): Normal, depressed, anxious, angry, happy, euphoric, or labile.
   - Thought process: Retardation, overinclusiveness, tangentiality, flight of ideas, or loosening of association.
   - Thought content: Preoccupations (worries), obsessions (recurrent intrusive, distressing thoughts, images that patient reports as being distressing/abnormal), overvalued ideas (normal, but unshakable thoughts), and delusions (false, fixed ideas/thoughts which are not in keeping with the patient's social, educational, and cultural norms).
   - Perceptual disturbances: Illusions (false perception in the presence of stimuli) or hallucinations (false perception in the absence of stimuli).

B. **Cognition (Do this during your interview!!!)**
   - Orientation: Year, month, day, and date; state, city, and name of this place.
   - Memory (registration, retention, and recall): Three objects; recalled in 2 minutes.
   - Attention (ability to focus): Spell WORLD or EARTH; forward and then backwards.
   - Concentration (ability to maintain focus): Serial 7's or serial 3's.
   - Executive functioning (Abstraction): Similarity and differences between objects, proverb interpretation, and simple mathematics: quarters in $1…$4…$6.75.
   - Apraxia (learned motor movements): Waving good bye, blowing a kiss,

showing how to shave, and three-step command.
- Agnosia (recognition and naming of objects): Name a pen and watch.
- Aphasia/Dysphasia: Receptive or expressive or conductive.

C. Insight/Judgment
- What is the problem?
- What are you doing about it?
- Will you continue the treatment?
- What will happen if you stop the treatment?

11. Closing the Interview: Last 1 minute

Thank the patient for his or her time and cooperation. Then recap briefly the problems and the plan of treatment that was discussed and then finish off the interview.

Then present the case....

12. Presentation
- Ask for 5 minutes to organize your thoughts.
- Comment on reliability of information.
- Present in a narrative format in about 10 minutes.
- The presentation should include items 2 through 8 in an organized manner.
- Make good eye contact with the examiners and try to minimize reading from your notes.

Then summarize....

13. Summarize (1 to 2 minutes)
1. Demographics: Patient's age, marital status, gender, living arrangements, religious affiliation, and mental health history.
2. Presenting problems: Symptoms and stressors—past to present (mood, anxiety, psychosis, substance use, cognition, and safety).
3. Treatments (current and past).
4. Pertinent medical, medication, social, and family history.
5. Pertinent positives and negatives on today's mental status examination including cognition.
6. Insight and judgment.

Then give the multiaxial diagnoses....

14. DSM-IV-TR Multiaxial Diagnoses

Axis I: Primary psychiatric disorder: Mood, anxiety, psychosis, cognition, or substance use
Rule out secondary disorders (due to general medical condition, substances, or another primary psychiatric disorder)

Axis II: Personality problems/mental retardation (MR)

Axis III: Pertinent medical problems

Axis IV: Psychosocial stressors (nine categories): Problems with primary support group, social environment, educational problems, occupational problems, housing problems, economic problems, problems related to access to health care, problems related to interactions with the legal system/crime, and other psychosocial or environmental problems.

Axis V: Global assessment functioning: 91 to 100: No problems; 81 to 90: Good psychosocial functioning; 71 to 80: Mild, but transient impairment; 61 to 70: Mild, but persistent impairment; 51 to 60: Moderate, but transient impairment; 41 to 50: Moderate, but persistent impairment; 31 to 40: Severe, but transient impairment; 21 to 30: Severe, but persistent impairment; 11 to 20: Danger to self or others or self-neglect; 1 to 10: Immediate danger to self or others or self-neglect; and 0 – inadequate information.

Then give the formulation....

15. Formulation—theoretical framework for understanding patient's presentation
1. Diagnostic: This section clarifies the diagnoses in Axes I and II. It prioritizes the diagnoses that were chosen and provides reasons for the priority. It also provides a link between the primary and the secondary diagnoses.
2. Etiologic: Consider the biological, psychological, and social aspects of illness etiology in the context of the predisposing, precipitating, perpetuating, and protective factors.
3. Therapeutic: This section describes the basic framework of treatment for patients, giving reasons for why these treatment modalities would be most effective in helping the patient.
4. Prognostic: This section describes the overall prognosis for the patient. It takes into account the diagnoses, treatment compliance, psychological stability, social issues, and the patient's motivation level.

Then give the treatments....

16. Treatments

Consider biological, psychological, and social aspects of treatment in the context of the predisposing, precipitating, perpetuating, and protective factors (include full history, collateral sources, physical examination, past treatment records, laboratory tests, etc. Also include medication classes and psychotherapies that will be helpful, vocational rehabilitation, community reintegration, support groups, case management, etc.).

Then give the prognosis....

17. Prognosis

Consider biological, psychological, and social aspects of prognosis in the context of the predisposing, precipitating, perpetuating, and protective factors. Break prognosis down into the short- and long-term risks of worsening of the following issues.

- Worsening of primary illness
- Worsening of comorbid conditions: psychiatric/medical
- Worsening of substance abuse/dependence
- Suicide risk
- Homicide risk
- Medication nonadherence
- Worsening of social issues: education/occupation/relationships

These factors can be further assessed based on the following factors:

- Previous history
- Severity of symptoms/disorders
- Motivation for change
- Previous treatments
- Adherence to treatments

2. INTERVIEW CHECKLIST (30 MINUTES)

Name:
Age:
Sex:
Religion:
Employment Status:
Marital Status:

Inpatient/outpatient:

Presenting Complaints:
1.
2.
3.

Review of Systems

Mood:	Energy:		Sleep:	Appetite/weight:	Interests:
Concentration:	Helpless:		Hopeless:	SI:	HI:
Anxiety:	1. GAD 4. OCD		2. Panic d/o 5. PTSD	3. Agoraphobia	
Psychoses:	A. Delusions: B. Hallucinations:		1. Persecutory 1. AH	2. Grandiose 2. VH	3. Bizarre 3. Others
Substance Abuse:	1. Alcohol		2. Tobacco	3. Others	
Memory Problems:	1. Basic ADLS:	a. Dressing d. Toileting	b. Eating e. Hygiene	c. Ambulation	
	2. I-ADLS:	a. Shopping d. Transportation	b. Housework	c. Accounting	

Somatic Complaints:

Past psychiatric history (PPH):

Past medical history (PMH):

Medications:

Allergies:

Social and Developmental History:

Family History:

Mental Status Examination:

Summary:

DSM-IV-TR Multiaxial Diagnosis:
Axis I:
Axis II:
Axis III:
Axis IV:
Axis V:

Formulation:

	Predisposing	Precipitating	Perpetuating	Protective
1. Diagnostic:				
2. Etiologic:				
A. Biological				
B. Psychological				
C. Social				
3. Therapeutic:				
4. Prognostic:				

Prognosis:	Short-term	long-term
A. Worsening of primary illness		
B. Treatment noncompliance		
C. Substance use		
D. SI/HI		
E. Self-care		
F. Relationship issues		

Treatment Plan:
A. Biological
B. Psychological
C. Social

Note:
Suicidal ideation (SI); Homicidal ideation (HI); Generalized anxiety disorder (GAD); Obsessive compulsive disorder (OCD); Post traumatic stress disorder (PTSD); Auditory hallucinations (AH); Visual hallucinations (VH); Activities of daily living (ADLs)

3. CYTOCHROME P-450 SYSTEM

System	Inhibitors		Inducers
1A2	Cimetidine Ciprofloxacin Diltiazem Erythromycin Fluoroquinolones	Fluvoxamine Grapefruit (juice) Mexiletine Norfloxacin Ritonavir	Modafinil Nicotine Omeprazole Phenobarbital Primidone Rifampin
2D6	Amiodarone Bupropion Celecoxib Chlorpromazine Cimetidine Clomipramine Cocaine Fluoxetine Fluphenazine Fluvoxamine Haloperidol	Metoclopramide Methadone Norfluoxetine Paroxetine Perphenazine Propafenone Ranitidine Ritonavir Sertraline Thioridazine Venlafaxine	Dexamethasone Rifampin
3A4	Amiodarone Cimetidine Ciprofloxacin Clarithromycin Clotrimazole Diltiazem Erythromycin Fluconazole Fluoxetine Fluvoxamine Grapefruit juice Indinavir Itraconazole Ketoconazole Metronidazole	Miconazole Nefazodone Nelfinavir Nevirapine Norfloxacin Norfluoxetine Omeprazole Paroxetine Propoxyphene Quinidine Ranitidine Ritonavir Saquinavir Sertindole Verapamil	Barbiturates Carbamazepine Dexamethasone Modafinil Nevirapine Phenobarbital Phenylbutazone Phenytoin Pioglitazone Primidone Rifabutin Rifampin St John's Wort Sulfinpyrazone

SUGGESTED READINGS

http://www.anaesthetist.com/physiol/basics/metabol/cyp/Findex.htm, last accessed on May 10, 2009.

http://www.atforum.com/SiteRoot/pages/addiction_resources/P450%20Drug%20Interactions.PDF, last accessed on May 10, 2009.

4. COMMON PSYCHOTROPIC MEDICATIONS

Class of Medication/ Name of Medications	Half-life (h)	Dosage/Levels	Major Side Effects/Risks
Anxiolytics			
1. **Benzodiazepines**			
• Alprazolam	6–20	0.25–3 mg/day	Sedation, drowsiness, fatigue, memory disturbance, muscle weakness, and respiratory depression. Sudden withdrawal causes agitation, anxiety, insomnia, seizures, and hallucinations.
• Clonazepam	18–40	0.5–2 mg/day	
• Diazepam	30–100	5–15 mg/day	
• Lorazepam	10–20	1–3 mg/day	
2. **Nonbenzodiazepines**			
• Buspirone	2–11	20–60 mg/day in divided doses	Dizziness, headache, lightheadedness, gastrointestinal (GI) disturbance, nausea, parasthesia, restlessness, and drowsiness.
• Hydroxyzine	7–20	50–200 mg qhs	Anticholinergic toxicity, dry mouth, and urinary retention. Use with caution in elderly.
Antidepressants			
1. **MAOIs**			
• Phenelzine	11 h	15–90 mg/day	Postural hypotension, insomnia, agitation, daytime somnolence, hyperadrenergic crises, weight gain, dry mouth, urinary retention, constipation, nausea, flushing, hepatotoxicity, and edema.
• Tranylcypromine	4.4–8 h	10–90 mg/day	Same as above.
• Selegiline	2 h	10 mg/day in two divided doses	Hypertensive crisis, depression, hallucination, vivid dreams, postural hypotension, rash, urticaria, nausea, headache, and dry mouth.
2. **Mirtazapine**	Females 37 h	15–60 mg/day	Sedation, increased appetite, weight gain, dizziness, dry mouth, sexual dysfunction, headache, and nausea. Rarely neutropenia.
3. **SNRIs**	Males 26 h		
• Duloxetine	12.5 h	30–120 mg/day	Nausea, anxiety, dry mouth, and insomnia. Sedation, sexual dysfunction, and headache. Sweating and dizziness.
• Venlafaxine	5–11 h	75–450 mg/day	Nausea, insomnia, anxiety, nervousness, sedation, sexual dysfunction, headache, tremor, dizziness, constipation, sweating, tachycardia, palpitation, and blood pressure elevation.

4. SSRIs			
• Citalopram	30 h	10–60 mg/day	Nausea, reduced appetite, weight loss, sweating, tremor, flushing, agitation, anxiety, jitteriness, sedation, insomnia, headache, sexual dysfunction, diarrhea, syndrome of inappropriate antidiuretic hormone secretion (SIADH), hyponatremia, galactorrhea, hyperprolactinemia, dry mouth, prolonged bleeding time, bleeding tendencies, bruxism, hair loss, cognitive impairment, serotonin syndrome, and weight gain with long-term treatment.
• Escitalopram	27–32 h	10–30 mg/day	Same as above.
• Fluoxetine	2–4 days-fluoxetine and 7–9 days-metabolite	5–80 mg/day	Same as above.
• Fluvoxamine	15 h	50–300 mg/day	Same as above.
• Paroxetine	24 h	10–50 mg/day	Same as above. Significant weight gain, sedation, constipation, and GI disturbance.
5. TCAs			
• Amitriptyline	12–24 h	50–300 mg/day	Sedation, orthostatic hypotension, anticholinergic effects (dry mouth, constipation, urinary retention, blurred vision, diminished working memory, and dental cavities), cardiac conduction defects, significant weight gain, sexual dysfunction (erectile), cardiotoxicity, seizures, and respiratory arrest in overdose.
• Clomipramine	35 h	50–250 mg/day	Same as above.
• Nortriptyline	60–90 h	25–150 mg/day. Therapeutic plasma level 50–150 ng/mL.	Same as above.
6. Bupropion	20 h	150–450 mg/day	Seizures, agitation, dry mouth, restlessness, diminished appetite, weight loss, headache, constipation, insomnia, anxiety, and GI disturbance. Rarely blood pressure elevation, cognitive dysfunction, and dystonia.
Antipsychotics			
1. Atypicals			
• Aripiprazole	75 h	10–15 mg/day	Agitation and insomnia.
• Clozapine	6–26 h	12.5–25 mg/day starting dose, titrated up to 300–450 mg/day	Agranulocytosis, weight gain, seizures, postural hypotension, sedation, tachycardia, transient hyperthermia eosinophilia, and rebound psychosis.

• Olanzapine	35 h	10–20 mg/day	Sedation, dizziness, and weight gain associated with new-onset diabetes mellitus.
• Risperidone	3–20 h	1–6 mg/day in divided doses	Insomnia, postural hypotension, dizziness, galactorrhea, sexual dysfunction, weight gain, and extra pyramidal symptoms (EPS) at higher doses.
• Quetiapine	6–8 h	300–800 mg/day in divided doses	Initial sedation, weight gain, orthostatic hypotension, insomnia, dry mouth, sedation.
• Ziprasidone	4–5 h	80–160 mg/day	Sedation, dry mouth, and constipation.
2. **Typicals**			
• Chlorpromazine	18–40 h	75–400 mg/day	Urinary retention, weight gain, rash, leucopenia, agranulocytosis, cholestasis, decreased seizure threshold, EPS (tremor, parkinsonism, akathisia, and tardive dyskinesia), neuroleptic malignant syndrome, QTc prolongation, and torsade de pointes.
• Fluphenazine	15–30 h	2.5–10 mg/day	Same as above.
• Haloperidol	12–36 h	0.5–20 mg/day	Same as above.
• Perphenazine	8–20 h	12–64 mg/day	Same as above and closed-angle glaucoma.
• Trifluoperazine	10–20 h	2–40 mg/day	Same as above and hepatotoxicity.
Cognitive Enhancers			
Cholinesterase inhibitors			
• Donepezil	70 h	5–10 mg/day	Nausea, diarrhea, anorexia, insomnia, fatigue, and muscle cramps.
• Galantamine	7 h	8–24 mg/day	Nausea, vomiting, and diarrhea.
• Rivastigmine	1.5 h	1.5–12 mg/day	Nausea, vomiting, and diarrhea.
NMDA antagonist			
• Memantine	60–100 h	20 mg/day	Agitation, urinary incontinence, urinary tract infection, and insomnia.
Hypnotics			
1. **Benzodiazepines**			
• Temazepam	8–20 h	7.5–30 mg qhs	Sedation, drowsiness, memory difficulties, fatigue, and muscle weakness.
• Triazolam	1.5–5.5 h	0.125–0.25 mg qhs	Drowsiness, dizziness, unpleasant taste, and memory difficulties.
2. **Nonbenzodiazepines**			
• Eszopiclone	6 h	Elderly 1–2 qhs <65 years of age 2–3 mg qhs	Drowsiness, GI disturbances, headache, and dizziness.
• Zaleplon	1–2 h	5–20 mg qhs	Same as above.
• Zolpidem	2–3 h	5–10 mg qhs	Somnolence, fatigue, nausea, headache, dizziness, cognitive dysfunction, and angioedema.
3. **Others**			
• Ramelteon	1–2.6 h	8 mg qhs	Fatigue, nausea, headache, and dizziness.

Mood Stabilizers			
• Carbamazepine		200–1,800 mg/day in divided doses. Therapeutic level 4–12 mg/L.	Dizziness, ataxia, clumsiness, sedation, dysarthria, diplopia, GI disturbance, blood dyscrasias, abnormal liver function test, tremor, memory disturbance, confusional state, conduction defect, syndrome of inappropriate antidiuretic hormone secretion (SIADH), rash, lenticular opacities.
• Divalproex sodium	8–12 h	750–1,800 mg/day. Therapeutic level 50–150 μg/mL.	GI disturbance, thrombocytopenia, platelet, dysfunction, sedation, tremor, ataxia, alopecia, weight gain, hepatotoxicity, pancreatitis, rash, and erythema multiforme.
• Lamotrigine	25 h	Usual starting dose is 25 mg/day. Gradually increased up to 100–400 mg/day.	Rash, Stevens-Johnson's syndrome, headache, diplopia, ataxia, blurred vision, and nausea and vomiting.
• Lithium	20 h	Usual starting dose is 300 mg t.i.d. Target plasma level 0.8–1.2 meq/L.	Thirst, polyuria, weight gain, and tremor. GI disturbance, interstitial nephritis, nephrotic syndrome, edema, benign intracranial hypertension, thyroid dysfunction, cardiac arrhythmias, acne, psoriasis, exfoliative dermatitis, alopecia, rash, and relative leukocytosis.
• Topiramate	21 h	200–400 mg in divided/Single evening dose	Sedation, ataxia, somnolence, parasthesia, nystagmus, and cognitive impairment. Nonanion gap metabolic acidosis leading to kidney stones and osteoporosis.
• Gabapentin	5–7 h	900–2,000 mg/day	Nausea, diplopia, glaucoma, hypotension, and cardiac conduction defects. Drowsiness, dizziness, unsteadiness, headache, tremor, edema, diplopia, nausea, and vomiting.
• Oxcarbazepine	2–9 h	600–1,500 mg/day	Drowsiness, dizziness, unsteadiness, headache, tremor, edema, diplopia, nausea, vomiting, hyponatremia, photosensitivity, rash, Stevens-Johnson's syndrome.
Substance Dependence			
1. Alcohol dependence			
• Acamprosate	3 h	1,333 mg/day if wt < 60 kg 1,998 mg/day if wt > 60 kg Given in three divided doses	Nausea, diarrhea and flatulence, insomnia, headache, confusion, sexual dysfunction, and pruritus. Contraindicated in pregnancy, lactation, and liver and kidney dysfunction.

• Disulfiram	60–120 h	250 mg/day taken in the morning	Fatigue, drowsiness, halitosis, body odor, tremor, headache, impotence, dizziness, hepatotoxicity, neuropathy, psychosis, catatonia.
• Naltrexone	4 h	50 mg/day	GI disturbance, abnormal liver function test (LFT), anorexia, insomnia, anxiety, arthralgia, myalgia, and rarely rhabdo myolysis.
2. Nicotine dependence			
• Bupropion	11–14 h	200–450 mg/day	Seizure, agitation, dry mouth, anorexia, insomnia, weight loss, anxiety, constipation, GI disturbance, blood pressure elevation, cognitive dysfunction, and dystonias.
• Varenicline	24 h	1 mg b.i.d.	Nausea, headache, insomnia, dreams, abnormal taste, GI disturbance, and suicidal ideation.
3. Opioid dependence			
• Buprenorphine	37 h	8–16 mg once daily or 32 mg 3 times/week	Dizziness, sedation, constipation, vertigo, nausea, vomiting, and respiratory depression.
• Methadone	25 h	60–100 mg/day	Nausea, vomiting, constipation, bowel obstruction, euphoria, sedation, coma, bradycardia, hypotension, sexual dysfunction, gynecomastia, and hyperprolactinemia.

Suggested Readings

Albers LJ, Hahn RK, Reist C. *Handbook of Psychiatric Drugs*. Laguna Hills: Current Clinical Strategies Publishing, 2008:8–115.

Rosenbaum JF, Arana GW, Hyman SE, et al. *Handbook of Psychiatric Drug Therapy*. 5th Ed. Philadelphia: Lippincott Williams & Wilkins, 2005:5–297.

INDEX

Page numbers followed by a "t" indicate tables.